English 4 Nurses

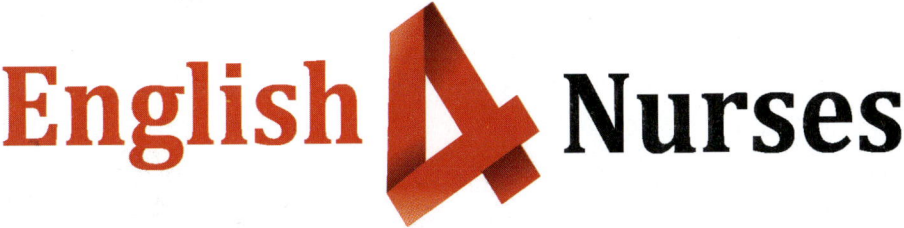

As per the syllabus of Kerala University of Health Sciences for BSc Nursing Students

Dr Liza Sharma MA (Eng), BEd, PhD, MBA
Former Associate Professor
Gian Sagar Group of Institutions
Banur, Rajpura, Punjab

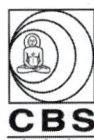

CBS
Dedicated to Education

CBS Publishers & Distributors Pvt Ltd

• New Delhi • Bengaluru • Chennai • Kochi • Kolkata • Lucknow
• Mumbai • Hyderabad • Nagpur • Patna • Pune • Vijayawada

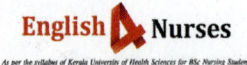

English 4 Nurses

As per the syllabus of Kerala University of Health Sciences for BSc Nursing Students

ISBN: 978-93-90619-33-7

First Edition: 2022

Published by **Satish Kumar Jain** and produced by **Varun Jain** for

CBS Publishers & Distributors Pvt Ltd

4819/XI Prahlad Street, 24 Ansari Road, Daryaganj, New Delhi 110 002, India.
Ph: +91-11-23289259, 23266861, 23266867   Website: www.cbspd.com
Fax: 011-23243014
e-mail: delhi@cbspd.com; cbspubs@airtelmail.in.

Corporate Office: 204 FIE, Industrial Area, Patparganj, Delhi 110 092
 Ph: +91-11-4934 4934   Fax: 4934 4935
e-mail: feedback@cbspd.com; bhupesharora@cbspd.com

Branches

- **Bengaluru:** Seema House 2975, 17th Cross, K.R. Road, Banasankari 2nd Stage, Bengaluru 560 070, Karnataka
  Ph: +91-80-26771678/79   Fax: +91-80-26771680   e-mail: bangalore@cbspd.com
- **Chennai:** 7, Subbaraya Street, Shenoy Nagar, Chennai 600 030, Tamil Nadu
  Ph: +91-44-26680620, 26681266   Fax: +91-44-42032115   e-mail: chennai@cbspd.com
- **Kochi:** 68/1534, 35, 36-Power House Road, Opp. KSEB, Cochin-682018, Kochi, Kerala
  Ph: +91-484-4059061-65   Fax: +91-484-4059065   e-mail: kochi@cbspd.com
- **Kolkata:** 6/B, Ground Floor, Rameswar Shaw Road, Kolkata-700 014, West Bengal
  Ph: +91-33-22891126, 22891127, 22891128   e-mail: kolkata@cbspd.com
- **Lucknow:** Basement, Khushnuma Complex, 7-Meerabai Ma Rg, (Behind Jawahar Bhawan), Lucknow-226001, Uttar Pradesh
  Ph: +0522-4000032   e-mail: tiwari.lucknow@cbspd.com
- **Mumbai:** PWD Shed, Gala No. 25/26, Ramchandra Bhatt Marg, Next to J.J. Hospital Gate No. 2, Opp. Union Bank of India, Noor Baug, Mumbai-400009
  Ph: +91-22-66661880/89   Fax: +91-22-24902342   e-mail: mumbai@cbspd.com

Representatives

- **Hyderabad**   +91-9885175004   • **Patna**   +91-9334159340
- **Pune**   +91-9623451994   • **Vijayawada**   +91-9000660880

Printed at: SDR Printers, Trans Delhi Signature City, Ghaziabad, UP, India

"The English Language is a Work in Progress.
Have Fun With It."

—Jonathan Culver

Dedicated to

My Parents

LATE DR SURJIT SINGH SETHI
&
LATE DR MANOHAR RAJ SETHI

Whose blessings have always been my
source of inspiration which led
to my academic pursuit.

Preface

The stage of transition from senior secondary school to professional and vocational education is a very crucial stage. English has a very vital role to play at this stage. The aim of writing this book is to make it accessible to the students pursuing their degree course in nursing. It will provide ample guidance and practice in grammar, various forms of composition, listening, comprehension and other allied areas. Apparently, initiation and repetition of correct expressions are far more efficacious in forming correct habits than grammatical knowledge. Hence, the emphasis is on the repetition of correct sentence patterns as we learn by doing things and we learn then better by doing correctly.

Maximum exercises have been provided with solutions. Sincere efforts have been made to cover the entire syllabus of BSc Nursing for KUHS and also to develop students' communication skills. This book has been designed in such a way that it can improve language skills of nursing students aspiring to go abroad and also build confidence in speaking or writing English.

No work is entirely free from errors and flaws, so valuable suggestions from our patrons for improvement of this book are invited. I assure you that efforts will continue to be made to further improve this book with every new edition.

Dr Liza Sharma

Acknowledgments

My heartfelt thanks and appreciations are due to all the members of publishing industry and academic institutions for sharing their skills, knowledge and experiences with me. Since I am a teacher, I want to repay it by writing this book and this is because I love this profession as it has given me an opportunity to learn so much.

I would like to extend my sincere gratitude to my father late Dr SS Sethi and my mother late Dr Manohar Sethi, who although are not present with me physically, continuously inspired and motivated me. My mother always showed her confidence in me and was a pillar of strength till her last breath.

Besides, I owe a great deal to my family. I am thankful to my husband, Mr SP Sharma, and sons Parth and Avish for their literary criticism, encouragement, support and constantly putting up with me in this great endeavor.

I want to thank **Mr Satish Kumar Jain** (Chairman) and **Mr Varun Jain** (Managing Director), M/s CBS Publishers and Distributors Pvt Ltd for their immense support and guidance in the publication of this book. One more person who has acted like the backbone, as far as the publication of this book is concerned, is **Mr Bhupesh Aarora** [Sr. Vice President – Health Science Division (Publishing & Marketing)], without whom this book wouldn't have been what it is today.

I would also like to convey my special thanks to the entire team of CBS Publishers and Distributors for their extreme hard work at every stage. I extend my special thanks to Ms Nitasha Arora (Publishing Head & Content Strategist-PGMEE & Nursing), and Dr Anju Dhir (Product Manager cum Commissioning Editor Medical) for their editorial support. I would also extend my thanks to Mr Shivendu Bhushan Pandey (Sr. Manager & Team Lead), Mr Manoj K Yadav (Production Manager), Mr Ashutosh Pathak (Sr. Proofreader cum Team Coordinator) for putting their hard work and efforts to bring out this book on time.

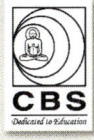

CBS Nursing Knowledge Tree

Extends its Tribute to

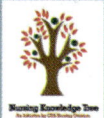

Florence Nightingale

For glorifying the role of women as nurses,
For holding the title of " The Lady with the Lamp,"
For working tirelessly for humanity—
Florence Nightingale will always be
remembered for her
selfless and memorable services to the
human race.

Florence Nightingale
(May 1820 – August 1910)

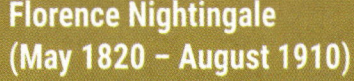

Nursing Knowledge Tree
An Initiative by CBS Nursing Division

"Coming together is a beginning. Keeping together is progress. Working together is success."

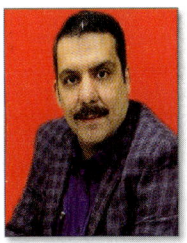

It gives us immense pleasure to share with you that the Nursing Knowledge Tree—An Initiative by CBS Nursing Division, has successfully established itself in the field of nursing as we have been able to stand as a strong contender by sharing approximately 50% of the market share. This growth could not have been possible without your invaluable contribution as our reader, author, reviewer, contributor and recommender, and your outstanding support for the growth of our titles as a whole. You people are the pillars of our series and we are so glad that you all have strengthened our basic foundation.

Nursing Knowledge Tree has been a pioneer and specialist in publishing best quality books for nursing education. Keeping in mind the changing trends in nursing education, we, at Nursing Knowledge Tree, have taken up a mission to bring student-friendly and syllabus-based books written by Subject Experts PAN India.

Our Noteworthy Achievements:

- Our nationally-acclaimed titles
  - *PGIMER NINE Clinical Nursing Procedures*—**Sandhya Ghai**
  - *Target High Staff Nurse Entrance Examination*—**Muthuvenkatachalam S, Ambili M Venugopal**
  - *CBS Nursing Drug Guide*—**Yogesh Gulati/Rakesh Sharma**
  - *Textbook of Nursing Foundations*—**Harindarjeet Goyal**
  - *Essentials of Biochemistry*—**Harbans Lal**
  - *Textbook of Nursing Education*—**Ratna Prakash**
  - *Nursing Research in 21st Century*—**Sukhpal Kaur and Amarjeet Singh**
  - *Essentials of Applied Microbiology*—**D R Arora and Brij Bala Arora**
  - *Textbook of Pediatric Nursing*—**Meharban Singh and Raman Kalia**
- Liaised with the topmost institutes of the country, like **AIIMS, NIMHANS, PGIMER NINE, CMC-Vellore, Manipal University, JIPMER, RAK-Delhi**, etc.
- Published **100+ Quality Nursing Books** and more than **50 New Books** on various subjects for Nursing Undergraduates, Postgraduates and Nursing superspecialty are under process and will be releasing in 2021.
- Increased our social presence by participating in more than **200+ National Conferences, CME's, College Exhibitions & Webinars** in previous years.
- We have come out with **Nursing Next Live**, an EdTech platform, the Next Level of Nursing Education, where we bring learning to people, instead of people going for learning. Through NNL App we are providing various study modules/plans covering All Subjects/ All Topics, Video Lectures, Question Banks, E-notes and a Variety of Tests. Students can choose the plan according to their needs and requirements.
- We are excited to announce that we are coming out with our new initiative—**Nursing Next Live Social**, where nursing faculties can share as well as gain knowledge, with the aim to revolutionize the way the nursing segment connects. It's going to be India's first networking platform for Nursing Segment.

Our Journey towards providing Quality Nursing Education is Incomplete without YOU ! Join Us Now !

We specialize in publishing nursing books of superior quality, going ahead we see us publishing more and more quality content and it will only be possible when intellectuals from across the nation come together. Keeping pace with the advancements, we want to strengthen the nursing sector, which was long neglected, and establish a strong foundation when it comes to quality content for the segment.

We are determined to bring about changes in the Nursing Education system and with your support and contributions, we will do it for sure. We will be delighted if you join hands with us in the form of Author, Contributor or Reviewer and take the vision of quality education for nursing students ahead.

Let's join hands together and share our ideas and knowledge. Be the part of this Revolution. We are looking forward to your cooperation in future as well. Share your CVs at **bhupesharora@nursingnextlive.in** or scan the given QR code and fill the form or you can talk to me directly at +9555353330.

With Best Wishes
Mr Bhupesh Aarora
Sr. Vice President – Health Science Division
(Publishing & Marketing)

Syllabus

ENGLISH (THEORY)

Placement : *First Year*   **Time** (Theory) : *30 hours*

Course description: The Course is designed to enable students to enhance ability to comprehend spoken and written English for effective communication in their professional work.

Unit	Time (hrs)	Learning objectives	Content	Teaching learning activities	Assessment
I	8	• Speak and write grammatically correct English	**Introduction** • Review of Grammar • Building vocabulary • Phonetics • Public speaking	• Exercise on use of Grammar • Practice in Public Speaking	• Objective type test • Fill in the blanks • Paraphrasing
II	4	• Develop ability to read and understand the prescribed text	**Reading** • Read and comprehend prescribed course books	**Exercise on:** • Reading • Summarizing • Comprehension	• Short answers • Essay type test
III	8	• Develop writing skills	**Various forms of composition** • Letter writing • Note taking • Precise writing • Nurses notes • Anecdotal records • Diary writing • Reports on client's health status • Preparation of resume/CV	**Exercise on writing:** • Letter writing • Nurses notes • Precise • Diary • Anecdote • Story writing • Resume/CV • Essay writing • Discussion on written reports/documents	• Prepare letters, diary, resume
IV	6	• Develop skill in spoken English	**Spoken english** • Oral report • Discussion • Debate • Telephonic conversation	**Exercise on:** • Debating • Participating in seminar • Panel, symposium	• Assessment of the various skills

Contd...

Unit	Time (hrs)	Learning objectives	Content	Teaching learning activities	Assessment
V	4	• Develop skill in listening comprehension	**Listening comprehension** • Media, audio, video, speeches, etc.	**Exercise on:** • Listening to audio, video, tapes and identify the key points	• Assessment of the various skills

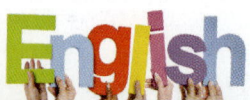

Contents

Unit I	Review of Grammar

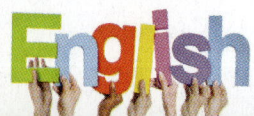

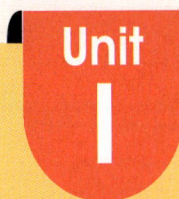

Unit
I

Review of Grammar

Unit Outline

Chapter 1

English: A Global Tool

INTRODUCTION

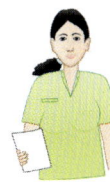

The British Council estimates that the world has about 375 million people who speak English as a first language, another 375 million who speak it regularly as a second language in a country where English has some semi-official status (such as India) and about 750 million more people who speak English as a foreign language.

Communication is a key skill in today's corporate world. In order to attain success one needs to communicate and the base of any communication is a language. The world is growing smaller and it is very rightly said that, today we are living in a 'Global Village'. English plays a central role in this 'globalization' and it has become the language of choice for communication between the various people of the Earth.

English has gained immense importance in today's competitive world. In this growing race one does not wish to be left out and in order to be a part of the race, fluency in this language is imperative.

Although English is not our mother tongue, we are fortunate to be well versed with this language, as it is taught to us right at the school level. This gives us a leading edge and prepares us for an enriched future.

Unfortunately, this advantage over time has been eroded due to improper teaching-learning, the mother-tongue influence, the rise of *'Hinglish'* (Hindi + English) and *Indianisms*. All these are serious barriers to effective communication. They comprise both clarity and personality.

Some common Indianisms are:

- Entry from the backside
- "Myself" as an introduction
- My good name is ......
- Words and phrases to avoid:
  - Basically, actually, having, around about (together)
  - Myself What is your 'good' name?
  - Very very, again again, fastly fastly
  - 'Very much' easy, 'too much' beautiful

- ❏ Tags-also, no? Isn't it?
- ❏ Doing job, backside, my place, marketing (for shopping)
- ❏ Means, what you can say, what you call, same to same
- ❏ *Mutlab, toh, voh, ekdum, jaise*, madam, sir (only when appropriate)
- ❏ Strong **t, d** ending sounds, e.g., good, **didn't**

LEARNING A LANGUAGE

Language as defined by the Oxford dictionary is "the means of human communication, consisting of the use of spoken or written words in a structured way."

Hierarchy of skills is depicted in Figure 1.

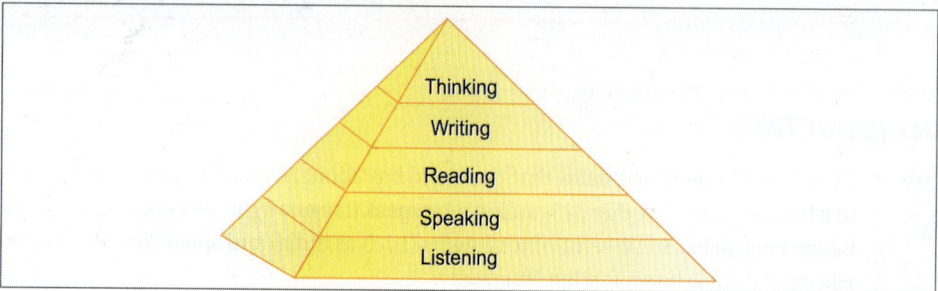

Fig. 1: Hierarchy of skills

To learn a language or to have a command over a language certain steps are followed in both formal and informal methods of learning. If viewed as a pyramid it would be something like this.

Listening

As you can see in the figure given above, the first skill required to learn a language is 'Listening'—a *receptive* skill. We learn to speak our native language effortlessly simply because we are constantly exposed to the language. Our mind learns to process the different sounds we hear (receive) into a form and flow (grammar and fluency) and recall it as and when required without formal tutoring. Maximum learning takes place at this level.

- ❏ Did I first learn to listen or speak?
- ❏ What are the informal sources/methods of learning a language through listening?
- ❏ How can I increase my exposure to listening to correct English sounds?

Speaking

The second level of proficiency in a language is 'Speaking'. It is a *productive* skill. Once a person has a storehouse of sounds and words (vocabulary) in his memory, he can express himself, as he is able to establish meaning and thought flow when speaking. This level takes the longest to master. The other two higher levels are a natural outcome of this level.

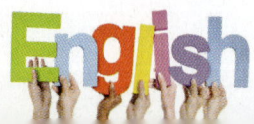

❑ How long was it before I learnt to speak (native language)?

❑ What does the term fluency mean to me?

❑ How long will it take for me to become fluent in English?

❑ What do I need to do for it?

Reading

The third level of skill required for proficiency is 'Reading', which again like listening is a receptive skill. Reading implies the ability to understand the meaning of the written or printed word. This skill enables a person to enhance and expand his knowledge and reinforce the other skills.

❑ When did I develop the ability to read?

❑ Are there different kinds of reading, what are they? (Silent/aloud/cursory/assimilate)

❑ What are the things we read other than books?

❑ Are there any smart ways to read?

Writing

Writing is the fourth level, a higher skill which again is a productive skill. It involves the ability to communicate ideas through the written or printed word. For this skill you need to have an understanding of grammar of the language as there is no face-to-face contact. In absence of gestures and expressions to support or convey meaning, you rely solely on the written/printed word.

❑ What is the difference between writing and handwriting?

❑ What do I need to do to improve my writing ability?

❑ Are spellings important?

❑ Is punctuation needed?

Thinking

A person is considered proficient in a language when he/she can effortlessly think in that language. The reason is, it is the culmination or combination of all the skills and therefore is at the highest level. People who are considered good orators or writers are those who have this skill. At the simplest level, it means one who is fluent in the language.

❑ Why do I need to think in English?

❑ What do I need to do to be able to think in English?

WHAT IS GRAMMAR?

Grammar is the system of a language. People sometimes describe grammar as the 'rules' of a language; but in fact no language has rules. If we use the word 'rules', we suggest that somebody created the rules first and then spoke the language, like a new game. But Languages did not start like that. Languages started by people making sounds which evolved into words, phrases and sentences. No commonly spoken language is fixed. All languages change over time. What we call 'grammar' is simply a reflection of a language at a particular time.

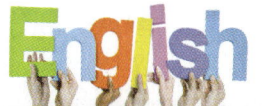

WHAT IS THE STUDY OF GRAMMAR?

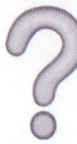

Grammar is a branch of linguistics dealing with the form and structure of words (morphology) and their interrelation in sentences (syntax). The study of grammar reveals how language works.

❏ Do we need to study grammar to learn a language? The short answer is 'no'. Very many people in the world speak their own, native language without having studied its grammar. Children start to speak before they even know the word 'grammar'. But if you are serious about learning a foreign language, the long answer is "yes, grammar can help you to learn a language more quickly and more efficiently." It is important to think of grammar as something that can help you, like a friend. When you understand the grammar (or system) of a language, you can understand many things yourself, without having to ask a teacher or look in a book.

❏ So think of grammar as something good, something positive and something that you can use to find your way—like a signpost or a map.

PARTS OF SPEECH

The fundamental building block of all languages is the word. Words are classified into parts of speech according to the way the words function in a sentence. It is important to realize that a word's part of speech is not inherent in the word itself but in the way the word is used. It is not unusual for a word to belong to more than one part of speech and class depending on how the word is used. For example, the word *round* can be used as a noun, a verb or an adjective:

Noun: Should we get another *round*?

Verb: The horses *round* the last post and head for home.

Adjective: He puts a small, round pebble in his pocket.

So, instead of asking the question, "What part of speech is X?," we should always ask the question, "What part of speech is X in this sentence?"

There are seven functional parts of speech: **nouns, verbs, adjectives, adverbs, pronouns, conjunctions,** and **prepositions**. There is also by some reckoning an eighth part of speech, **interjections**. Interjections are like asides or commentaries that are really not part of the actual grammar of a sentence. For example, 'well' and 'damn' in the following sentences are interjections:

❏ *Well*, I don't know what to tell you.

❏ Damn I locked my keys in the car.

Well, because interjections, by definition, play no grammatical role in a sentence, we will ignore them from this point onward and concentrate on the remaining seven functional parts of speech.

❏ I don't know what to tell you.

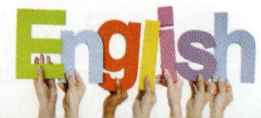

It is important to be able to recognize and identify the different types of words in English, so that you can understand grammar explanations and use the right word form in the right place. Here is a brief explanation of what the parts of speech are:

- **Noun:** A noun is a naming word. It names a person, place, thing, idea, living creature, quality or action. Examples: *cowboy, theatre, box, thought, tree, kindness, arrival.*
- **Verb:** A verb is a word, which describes an action (doing something) or a state (being something). Examples: *walk, talk, think, believe, live, like, want.*
- **Adjective:** An adjective is a word that describes a noun. It tells you something about the noun. Examples: *big, yellow, thin, amazing, beautiful, quick, important.*
- **Adverb:** An adverb is a word, which usually describes a verb. It tells you how something is done. It may also tell you when or where something happened. Examples: *slowly, intelligently, well, yesterday, tomorrow, here, everywhere, etc.*
- **Pronoun:** A pronoun is used instead of a noun, to avoid repeating the noun. Examples: *I, you, he, she, it, we, they, etc.*
- **Conjunction:** A conjunction joins two words, phrases or sentences together. Examples: *but, so, and, because, or, etc.*
- **Preposition:** A preposition usually comes before a noun, pronoun or noun phrase. It joins the noun to some other part of the sentence. Examples: *on, in, by, with, under, through, at, etc.*
- **Interjection:** An interjection is an unusual kind of word, because it often stands alone. Interjections are words, which express emotion or surprise, and they are usually followed by exclamation marks. Examples: *Ouch!, Hello!, Hurray!, Oh no!, Ha! etc.*
- **Article:** An article is used to introduce a noun. Examples: *the, a, an.*

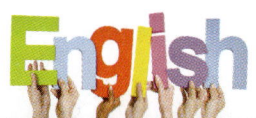

NOTES

Chapter 2

Nouns

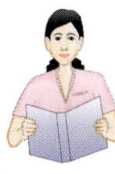

The word *noun* comes from a Latin word that means 'name'. Accordingly, nouns are often defined by their naming ability. A noun is a word used to name a person, a place, a thing, or an idea.

There are two types of nouns: Proper nouns and common nouns. Proper nouns are the names of specific individuals or entities. Proper nouns are normally capitalized. While common nouns are the names of generic categories.

Here are some examples of proper and common nouns:

Proper Noun: Abraham Lincoln, Barack Obama, Agra, Red Fort.

Common Noun: President, cat, chair and table.

Nouns are of five different kinds:

1. Proper Nouns
2. Common Nouns
3. Collective Nouns
4. Material Nouns
5. Abstract Nouns

Proper Nouns

A proper noun is the name given to a particular person, place or thing to single it out from others of its kind, as:

- ❑ Ram, James, Ahmad, Peter, Surjit, Ajoy.   ... Persons
- ❑ Kolkata, London, India, Asia, Park Street.   ... Places
- ❑ Geeta, Quran, Diwali, Friday, Ganga.   ... Things

Remember that a proper noun will always begin with a capital letter.

Common Nouns

A common noun is the common name given to person, place or a thing of the same kind, as:

- ❑ Boy, man, lady, child, postman.   ... Persons
- ❑ Village, park, town, street, ground.   ... Places
- ❑ Book, river, chair, shirt, sound.   ... Things

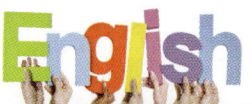

Collective Nouns

A collective noun is the name given to a collection of similar common nouns, like groups of persons, animals or things which are treated as one complete 'whole', as:

- ❏ Class, mob, team, army, gang. ... of persons
- ❏ Flock, herd, pack, litter, brood. ... of animals
- ❏ Gross, heap, pile, cluster, collection. ... of things

Material Nouns

A material noun is the name given to a material substance, as:

- ❏ Stone, paper, glass, gold, iron, cement, etc.

Abstract Nouns

An abstract noun is the name given to some feeling, action, quality, state, art or subject, etc. as:

- ❏ Happiness, sorrow, surprise, fear. ...Feelings
- ❏ Deed, treatment, motion, race. ...Actions
- ❏ Justice, mercy, politeness, rudeness. ...Qualities

Defining a noun as a 'name' seems quite natural for proper nouns. However, the definition of *noun* as a 'name' does not work well for common nouns. It is not that common nouns are not names; of course they are. The problem is that the concept of 'name' is so broad that it is easy to extend 'name' to parts of speech that are not nouns. For example, jump is the 'name of an action' and blue is the 'name of a color, but in the following sentences, *'jump,'* is a verb and blue is an adjective:

- ❏ The children tried to jump over the ditch.
- ❏ The new dishes are *blue in color*.

Another way to identify common nouns is by taking advantage of a unique property of 'how they are used'. Only common nouns are commonly and routinely modified by adjectives. Thus, if a word can be readily modified by an adjective, then that word must be a common noun. A particularly convenient adjective to use as a test word is 'the'.

Gender

We know that according to sex ,things fall into two chief classes—**males** or **females**. The word for sex in Grammar is **gender**. So, there are two chief genders:

1. *Masculine Gender* *(male sex)*
2. *Feminine Gender* *(female sex)*

1. *Masculine Gender*

Nouns denoting males are Masculine Gender; as—

Boy husband he-goat tiger ram

2. *Feminine Gender*

Nouns denoting females are Feminine Gender; as—

Girl wife she-goat tigress ewe

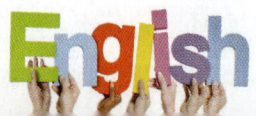

3. Common Gender

Sometimes we name a noun, but its sex or gender remains unexplained though its meaning is clear.

For example:

1. The **child** is sleeping.
2. My **cousin** is reaching here today.

In these sentences, nouns—*child, cousin*—are clear as far as their meanings are concerned, but their gender is not clear at all. A **child** can be a boy or a girl. Similarly, the **cousin** can be a man or woman. Such nouns are **common** to both the sexes.

Nouns denoting either sex are of Common Gender; as—

1. *parent*—father or mother
2. *friend*—male or female
3. *enemy*—male or female
4. *bird*—male or female
5. *baby*—male or female
6. *person*—man or woman
7. *pupil*—boy or girl
8. *Servant*—man or maid
9. *orphan*—boy or girl
10. *neighbour*—man or woman
11. *teacher*—man or woman
12. *spouse*—husband or wife
13. *monarch*—king or queen
14. *minister*—man or woman

4. Neuter Gender

Lifeless things have no sex, i.e., they are neither males nor females.
In other words, they belong to **neither sex** or **Neuter Gender**.

Nouns denoting neither sex are of Neuter Gender; as—

Chair   pencil   house   arrow   book

Note 1: In English the gender is purely a matter of sex—

a.   **Girl**   : She is girl.   (Feminine)
    Actress : She is an actress.   (Feminine)
    Boy   : He is a boy.   (Masculine)
    Man   : He is a man.   (Masculine)

Note 2. Collective nouns naming collections of living things too are of neuter gender; as—

Crowd   class   team   army

Note 3. Lifeless things are sometimes described as persons, i.e., they are personified. So, they must be some gender in that case. Remember the following facts about personified inanimate (lifeless) things:

a.   A personified noun begins with a capital letter.

b.   Personified nouns remarkable for strength, toughness and superiority are of **Masculine Gender; as—**

The sun	Summer	Winter	Death
Storm	Time	War	Wind
Thunder	Ocean	Fear	Majesty

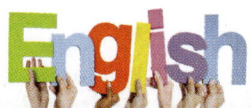

1. The sun sheds his light on all planets alike.
2. The Atlantic Ocean is notorious for its storms.
3. The war is a bad thing and even worse are its results

c. Personified Nouns remarkable for *beauty, grace, gentleness, fertility* and inferiority are of **Feminine Gender; as—**

The Moon	The Earth	Hope	Nature
Spring	Justice	Mercy	Peace
odesty	Liberty	Charity	Autumn
Fame	Truth	Ship	Beauty

1. The Moon has no light of her own.
2. The Earth is different from other planets as she is livable.
3. During Spring, Nature is at her best.

Change of Gender

Feminine of Masculines can be made in three different ways; as—

1. **Using a new word:**

Masculine	Feminine	Masculine	Feminine
bachelor	maid	horse	mare
boar	sow	husband	wife
boy	girl	king	queen
brother	sister	lord	lady
buck	doe	man	woman
bull	cow	monk	nun
bullock	heifer	nephew	niece
cock	hen	papa	mamma
colt	filly	ram	ewe
dog	bitch	sir	madam
drake	duck	son	daughter
drone	bee	stag	hind
father	mother	swain	nymph
gander	goose	uncle	aunt
gentleman	lady	wizard	witch

2. **Adding a word:**

Masculine	Feminine	Masculine	Feminine
brother-in-law	sister-in-law	god-son	god-daughter
buck-rabbit	doe-rabbit	grand-father	grand-mother
cock-sparrow	hen-sparrow	great-uncle	great-aunt
he-goat	she-goat	land-lord	land-lady

Contd...

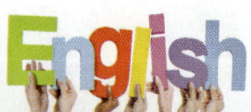

Masculine	Feminine	Masculine	Feminine
jack-ass	she-ass	pea-cock	pea-hen
man-servant	maid-servant	washer-man	washer-woman

3. Adding—ess:

Masculine	Feminine	Masculine	Feminine
author	authoress	mayor	mayoress
giant	giantess	poet	poetess
god	goddess	priest	priestess
heir	heiress	prince	princess
host	hostess	prophet	prophetess
lion	lioness	shepherd	shepherdess

There are different rules for changing Singular Nouns into Plural forms:

a. Adding *s* to the singular form:

Singular	Plural	Singular	Plural
act	acts	hut	huts
boy	boys	idea	ideas
cat	cats	jeep	jeeps
door	doors	kite	kites
egg	eggs	lamp	lamps
fowl	fowls	male	males
gate	gates	nib	nibs
hammer	hammers	pupil	pupils
hand	hands	question	questions
house	houses	window	windows

b. Adding *es* to singular ending in s, ss, sh, ch, x, z:

Singular	Plural	Singular	Plural
bus	buses	princess	princesses
ass	asses	tax	taxes
bush	bushes	box	boxes
bunch	bunches	quiz	quizzes

Note: If the ending 'ch' of a singular Noun sounds as 'k', its plural is formed by adding 's' only; as—

Monarch – monarchs   stomach – stomachs

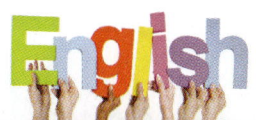

c. **Adding s to Singulars ending in 'y' after a vowel:**

Singular	Plural	Singular	Plural
day	days	storey	storeys
ray	rays	monkey	monkeys
key	keys	donkey	donkeys
boy	boys	guy	guys

d. **Changing the 'y' of Singular nouns, ending in 'y' after a consonant, into 'ies':**

Singular	Plural	Singular	Plural
baby	babies	army	armies
duty	duties	lady	ladies
fairy	fairies	story	stories
family	families	victory	victories
dictionary	dictionaries	ally	allies

e. **Adding es to Singular Nouns ending in *o* after a consonant:**

Singular	Plural	Singular	Plural
buffalo	buffaloes	mango	mangoes
cargo	cargoes	motto	mottoes
echo	echoes	negro	negroes
flamingo	flamingoes	potato	potatoes
hero	heroes	volcano	volcanoes
mosquito	mosquitoes	zero	zeroes

f. **Adding s to Singular ending in *oo, eo, io, yo* and some words ending to:**

Singular	Plural	Singular	Plural
bamboo	bamboos	halo	halos
cuckoo	cuckoos	piano	pianos
embryo	embryos	studio	studios
folio	folios	dynamo	dynamos
curio	curios	photo	photos
manifesto	manifestos	rhino	rhinos

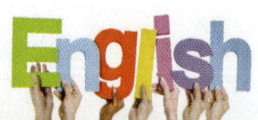

g. Changing *f* and *fe* into ves:

Singular	Plural	Singular	Plural
calf	calves	myself	ourselves
elf	elves	shelf	shelves
half	halves	thief	thieves
knife	knives	wife	wives
leaf	leaves	wolf	wolves
Exception:			
belief	beliefs	cliff	cliffs
chief	chiefs	reef	reefs
dwarf	dwarfs	roof	roofs
grief	griefs	relief	reliefs
gulf	gulfs	turf	turfs
handkerchief	handkerchiefs	sheriff	sheriffs
mischief	mischiefs	safe	safes
proof	proofs	fief	fiefs
Double Plurals of Singulars ending in 'f':			
hoof	hoofs	staff	staffs
	Hooves		staves
Scarf	scarfs	wharf	wharfs
	Scarves		wharves

h. Miscellaneous:

Singular	Plural	Singular	Plural
child	children	man	men
foot	feet	mouse	mice
dormouse	dormice	tooth	teeth
goose	geese	ox	oxen
louse	lice	woman	women

i. Adding an apostrophes ('s):

Singular	Plural	Singular	Plural
5	5's	B.A.	B.A's
p	p's	P.O.W	P.O.W's

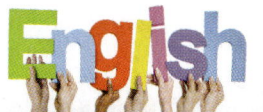

j. Adding 's' to the main word of a compound-noun:

Singular	Plural
coat-of-mail	coats-of-mail
commander-in-chief	commanders-in-chief
court-martial	courts-martial
daughter-in-law	daughters-in-law
foot-man	foot-men
governor-general	governors-general
hanger-on	hangers-on
looker-on	lookers-on

Some Nouns are always used in a Plural sense:

1. *cattle*—The cattle are grazing.
2. *goods*—The goods are lying on the floor.
3. *people*—People of India are peace-loving.
4. *swine*—Whose swine are these?
5. *vermin*—The vermin do much harm to crops.
6. *ashes*—His ashes were immersed in the Ganga.
7. *assets*—His assets are very small.
8. *thanks*—My thanks for this help are due to you, sir.
9. *tidings*—What are the latest tidings, man?
10. *contents*—The contents of this book are at page 3.
11. *wages*—The wages for daily labour are very low.
12. *bellows*—The bellows are used to fan the furnace-fire.
13. *arms*—Arms are kept in an armoury.
14. *scissors*—Scissors are an important tool of a barber.
15. *pants*—These pants do not fit on you nicely.
16. *trousers*—Your trousers are a bit tight. Aren't they?
17. *riches*—Riches have wings; they do not stick to one place.
18. *alms*—Alms were given to the poor on festivals.
19. *odds*—The odds against me were very heavy.
20. *repairs*—The repairs of the building are yet to be carried out.
21. *vacations*—The vacations are over.

k. Some Nouns are Plural in appearance but are used in a Singular sense:

1. *athletics*—Athletics is so dear to me.
2. *innings*—The first innings is over.
3. *mathematics*—Mathematics is my favorite subject.
4. *news*—This news is just untrue.
5. *politics*—Politics is very dirty these days.
6. *physics*—Physics is an important branch of science.
7. *summons*—This summons was never served on me.
8. *gallows*—The murderer was brought to the gallows which was fixed up for him.

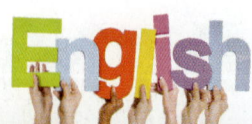

l. **These Nouns always take a Singular verb:**

1. *abuse*—He gave me much abuse.
2. *advice*—All his advice was useless.
3. *furniture*—This furniture is very fine.
4. *alphabet*—The English alphabet has 26 letters in all.
5. *information*—This information is all wrong.
6. *poetry*—Poetry is one of the five fine arts.
7. *scenery*—The scenery on the stage was very imposing.

m. **Some Nouns have two forms in Plural—either of them with a separate meaning.**

Singular	Plural	Meanings
1. brother	1. *brother*	sons of the same mother
	2. *brethren*	members of the same society
2. cloth	1. *cloths*	pieces of unsewn cloth
	2. *clothes*	sewn clothes
3. die	1. *dies*	moulds or dies
	2. *dice*	small cubes used in games
4. index	1. *indexes*	tables of content
	2. *indices*	exponents in algebra
5. staff	1. *staves*	sticks
	2. *staffs*	worker in a firm, etc.

n. **Some Nouns have Plurals which have two meanings each:**

Singular	Plural	Meanings
1. *customs*	*customs*	1. practices
		2. tax
2. *letter*	*letters*	1. characters of the alphabet
		2. letters sent through post
3. *effect*	*effects*	1. influences
		2. goods
4. *manner*	*manners*	1. ways
		2. behavior
5. *part*	*parts*	1. portions
		2. ability
6. *spectacle*	*spectacles*	1. sights
		2. glasses worn on eyes
7. *quarter*	*quarters*	1. fourth parts
		2. dewellings

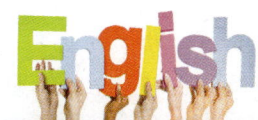

Errors in the use of Nouns

A noun is the name of a person or place or a thing as:
Kapil, Agra, college, match, honesty, class, gold, India, bench, the Ganges, etc.

Incorrect Sentences	*Correct Sentences*
❑ The sceneries of Shimla are charming.	❑ The scenery of Shimla is charming.
	Or
	❑ The scenes of Shimla are charming.
❑ He gave me many advices.	❑ He gave me many pieces of advice.
	Or
	❑ He gave me much advice.
❑ Alya loves the poetries of Keats.	❑ Alya loves the poetry (or poems) of Keats.
❑ She gave us no informations.	❑ She gave us no information.
❑ Amit has many works to do.	❑ Amit has much work to do.
❑ I have sold my old furnitures.	❑ I have sold my old furniture.
❑ She has packed her luggages.	❑ She has packed her luggage.
❑ You did many mischiefs yesterday.	❑ You did many acts of mischief yesterday.
	Or
	❑ You did much mischief yesterday.
❑ Mohan gave the beggar two breads.	❑ Mohan gave the beggar two loaves (or pieces) of breads.
❑ Radha has no issues.	❑ Radha has no issue.
❑ India is importing new machineries.	❑ India is importing new machinery.
❑ We shall spend our summer vacations at Shimla.	❑ We shall spend our summer vacation at Shimla.
❑ You must help the poors and the blinds.	❑ You must help the poor and the blind.
❑ The naughty boy does not avoid bad companies.	❑ The naughty boy does not avoid bad company.
❑ Good children do not move in bad companies.	❑ Good children do not move in bad company.
❑ His hairs are grey.	❑ His hair is grey.

(*Note:* When 'hair' is taken as a single thread, the word 'hairs' should be used in the plural form, e.g., There are four grey hairs in his beard).

Certain nouns, such as scenery, furniture, hair, advice, stationery, machinery, luggage, information, expenditure, abuse, business, damage, poetry, issue, vacation, etc. are used in the singular form and carry the singular verb.

❑ I have purchased a new scissors.	❑ I have purchased a new pair of scissors.
❑ Punam does not like vegetable.	❑ Punam does not like vegetables.

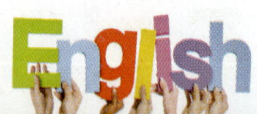

Some nouns, like thanks, contents, trousers, circumstances, alms, ashes, scissors, spectacles, vegetables, annals, remains, tongs, proceeds, meals, orders, sorts, means, riches, wages, etc. are used in the plural.

- In this circumstance, he cannot help me.
- His thank is due to me.
- These are happy news.
- Politics are a dirty game.
- English are my favorite subject.

- In these circumstances, he cannot help me.
- His thanks are due to me.
- This is a happy news.
- Politics is a dirty game.
- English is my favorite subject.

Some nouns as politics, news, Economics, English are plural in form but singular in content.

- There are twenty fishes in this tank.
- I saw a flock of sheeps.
- He killed some deers.
- She gave ten rupees to the beggar.
- The farmer has four horse.

- There are twenty fish in this tank.
- I saw a flock of sheep.
- He killed some deer.
- She gave ten rupees to the beggar.
- The farmer has four horses.

Some nouns, like fish, sheep, deer, piece, yoke, etc. have the plural.

- She bought two dozens oranges.
- I bought this for eight hundreds rupees.
- He lent me a hundred rupees note.
- They had a four hours talk.

- She bought two dozen oranges.
- I bought this for eight hundred rupees.
- He lent me a hundred rupee note.
- They had a four-hour talk.

Some nouns as dozen, score, hundred, thousand, pound, etc. (signifying exact numbers or measure) are used in the singular when they come after numerical.

- The cattles are grazing.
- Gentry of the town was present at the function.
- All the peoples laughed at her dialogue.
- The officer deserve credit for this.

- The cattle are grazing.
- Gentry of the town were present at the function.
- All the people laughed at her dialogue.
- The officer deserves credit for this.

Gentry, folk, cattle, people, poultry, public, peasantry, officer, vermin, alphabet are some of the collective nouns. They are singular in form but plural in meaning. They require a plural verb.

- My house is built of bricks and stones.
- The Taj is built of white marbles.

- My house is built of brick and stone.
- The Taj is built of white marble.

When material nouns are used to denote a mass of matter, they are used as singular.

- I shall dine at my aunt's house today.
- I shall dine at my aunt's house today.

The word house, church, school, shop, are often omitted after a possessive case.

- It is a boy's hostel.
- I shall wait for you in the fresher's party.

- It is a boys' hostel.
- I shall wait for you in the freshers' party.

In case of plural form ending in 's' indicate the possessive case by adding an apostrophe 's'. But when the plural noun does not end in 's', indicate the possessive by adding 's'.

- His shirt's color is red.
- His pen's ink is green.

- The color of his shirt is red.
- The ink of his pen is green.

As a rule 's' is used for indicating persons, living beings and personified objects.

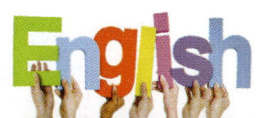

More Common Errors in the Use of Nouns and Noun Phrases

Incorrect Sentences	Correct Sentences
❏ There was no place on the bench for you.	❏ There was no room on the bench for you.
❏ He is my cousin brother.	❏ He is my cousin.
❏ We saw a theatre.	❏ We saw a play.
❏ Please put your sign here.	❏ Please put your signatures here.
❏ They like the play of tennis.	❏ They like the game of tennis.
❏ Good night mam, I have come to consult you.	❏ Good evening mam, I have come to consult you.
❏ A hundred miles are a long distance.	❏ A hundred miles is a long distance.
❏ There were many males in the compartment.	❏ There were many men in the compartment.
❏ Renu stays in the boarding.	❏ Renu stays in the boarding house.
❏ Meenu failed by ten numbers.	❏ Meenu failed by ten marks.
❏ He has no issues.	❏ He has no issue.
❏ Her hairs are black.	❏ Her hair is black.
❏ Politics are a dirty game.	❏ Politics is a dirty game.
❏ They gave you many advices.	❏ They gave you much advice.
❏ Ramu has packed my luggages.	❏ Ramu has packed my luggage.
❏ She sent us many informations.	❏ She sent us much information.
❏ I am reading the poetries of Keats.	❏ I am reading the poetry of Keats.
	Or
	❏ I am reading the poems of Keats.
❏ The sceneries of Kashmir are very charming.	❏ The scenery of Kashmir is very charming.
❏ The boys did many mischiefs.	❏ The boys did many acts of mischief.
❏ She found two long hair in her food.	❏ She found two long hairs in her food.
❏ The summons were served by a bailiff.	❏ The summon was served by a bailiff.
❏ In the first inning our team scored eighty runs.	❏ In the first innings our team scored eighty runs.
❏ Your trouser is new.	❏ Your trousers are new.
❏ The poultry is Sohan's.	❏ The poultry are Sohan's.
❏ He bought three dozens eggs.	❏ He bought three dozen eggs.
❏ He ran a 1500 meters race.	❏ He ran a 1500 meter race.
❏ The village folk is simple minded.	❏ The village folks are simple minded.
❏ The cattles are grazing in the field.	❏ The cattle are grazing in the field.
❏ The leaders of two countries had a two hours meeting.	❏ The leaders of two countries had a two hour meeting.
❏ A five-men delegation waited on the Minister.	❏ A five-man delegation waited on the Minister.
❏ He hopes to secure the job by these means.	❏ He hopes to secure the job by this means.
❏ The price of this table is five hundreds rupees.	❏ The price of this table is five hundred rupees.
❏ Thousand of people attended the meeting.	❏ Thousands of people attended the meeting.
❏ A five years old child won the first prize.	❏ A five-year-old child won the first prize.

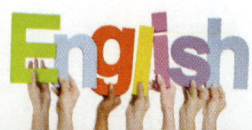

- The people of this town is educated.
- My circumstance is not favorable.
- He gave me ten thousands rupees.
- You have broken your spectacle.
- Mathematics are a difficult subject.
- The wages of sin are death.
- These news are not true.
- His means is limited.
- He stays in the boarding.
- This shirt's color is nice.
- One of my friend is going abroad.
- Do not find faults with others.
- The girl's hostel has been closed.
- His family members are not here.
- This house is built of bricks and stones.
- The weather of Shimla is good for health.
- He is a member of young Mens Club.
- You have carried away someone's else's book.
- Ram's and Shyam's shop is in the main market.
- This room's roof leaks in the rainy season.
- Ram and Shyam's shops are in the main market.

- The people of this town are educated.
- My circumstances are not favorable.
- He gave me ten thousand rupees.
- You have broken your spectacles.
- Mathematics is a difficult subject.
- The wages of sin is death.
- This news is not true.
- His means are limited.
- He stays in the boarding-house.
- The color of this shirt is nice.
- One of my friends is going abroad.
- Do not find fault with others.
- The girls hostel has been closed.
- The members of his family are not here.
- This house is built up of brick and stone.
- The climate of Shimla is good for health.
- He is member of Young Men's Club.
- You have carried away someone else's book.
- Ram and Shyam's shop is in the main market.
- The roof of this room leaks in the rainy season.
- Ram's and Shyam's shops are in the main market.

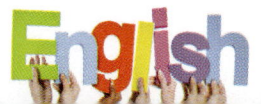

NOTES

Chapter 3

Pronouns

A pronoun is a word that is used in place of a noun to avoid its repetition.

- ❐ Remember that the word 'noun' has a wide meaning here. It applies to all the five kinds of nouns as well as noun equivalents.

Kinds of Pronouns

Pronouns are of seven chief kinds:
1. Personal Pronouns
2. Demonstrative Pronouns
3. Indefinite Pronouns
4. Distributive Pronouns
5. Interrogative Pronouns
6. Relative Pronouns
7. Reflexive Pronouns

Personal Pronouns

A personal pronoun is a pronoun used for any of the three persons, as:
1. The person who is speaking: I, we, me, us, mine, ours, etc.
2. The person spoken to: you, yours, etc.
3. The person or thing spoken of and other than the above two persons: he, she, it, hers, its, his, etc.

Pronouns of First Person		**Pronouns of Second Person**	
(Masculine and Feminine)		(Masculine and Feminine)	
Singular	I, me, mine	Singular	You, yours
Plural	We, us, ours	Plural	You, yours

Pronouns of Third Person
(Masculine, Feminine and Neuter Genders)

Singular	Masculine		Feminine	Neuter
	He, him, his		She, her, hers	It, it, its
Plural	They, them, theirs (All genders)			

Note 1: Most of the personal pronouns have two possessive forms each, as:

I → my, mine   We → our, ours
You → your, yours   She → her, hers
They → their, theirs

Out of the two possessive forms of each pronouns, one has been given in italics. This form is never used as a pronoun but as an adjective before nouns; as:

◻ This is *my* book.
◻ Those are *our* bags.
◻ Here is *your* pen.
◻ There is *her* ribbon.
◻ Where are *their* bats?

These adjectives are called possessive adjectives.
The other possessive forms of each pronoun is used as a possessive pronoun, as:

◻ This book is mine.
◻ Those bags are ours.
◻ That pen is yours.
◻ This ribbon is hers.
◻ These hats are theirs.

Note 2: 'He' and 'it' have one possessive form each, as:

He → his   it → its

These single forms are used both as possessive adjectives and possessive pronouns, as:

◻ This is his book.   (Possessive Adjective)
◻ This book is his.   (Possessive Pronouns)

Demonstrative Pronouns

A demonstrative pronoun is a pronoun that points to a noun going before it and is used in place of it.

Chief demonstrative pronouns are: this, that, these, those, one, such, etc:

◻ This book is better than that.
◻ That pen is superior to this.
◻ Tobacco and wine are not good things. These are harmful to health.
◻ Streets of Delhi are broader than those of Kolkata.
◻ Your shirt is white but mine is a red one.
◻ I never thought such.

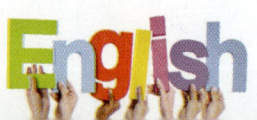

Indefinite Pronouns

An indefinite pronoun is a pronoun that refers to a person or thing generally and indefinitely and not in a particular way.

Chief indefinite pronouns are: one, none, they, all, some, someone, somebody, nobody, other, etc:

- One must take care of one's health.
- None of my lost books was found.
- They say (people say) that truth is evergreen.
- All are brothers and sisters.
- Some are born great but some achieve greatness.
- Someone (somebody) has broken the windowpane.
- Nobody (no one) can do such a mean act.
- Always help others as far as you can.

Distributive Pronouns

A distributive pronoun is a pronoun that refers to nouns, one at a time.

Chief distributive pronouns are: each, either, neither, etc:

- Each of them is to blame.
- The soldiers had each a gun.

Interrogative Pronouns

An interrogative pronoun is a pronoun that is used to ask a question.

There are five chief interrogative pronouns: what, who, which, whose, whom, as:

- *Who* is there at the door?
- *What* do you want of me?
- *Which* is the best boy of these all?
- *Whose* is the beautiful painting?
- *Whom* are you looking for?

Note: You must note what each of the three interrogative pronouns: what, who, which – imply when used in regard to persons. Remember that:

a. 'Who' enquires the name or family connection, as:
   - Who is he?
   - What is his name?
   - Who is Mohan?
   - Whose son is Mohan?
                    Or
   - Which family is Mohan from?

b. 'What' enquires profession or social status, as:
   - What is he?

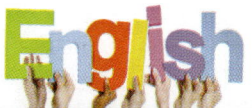

- What is he by occupation?

Or

- What is his social status?

c. 'Which' enquires identity or choice, as:

- Which is he?
- Which of the present persons is he?

Relative Pronouns

A relative pronoun is a pronoun that refers to a noun going before it and also joins two sentences together.

Chief relative pronouns are: who, what, which, whom, whose, that, but, as, etc:

☐ He is the boy who stole my purse.

☐ This is what I want.

☐ That is the book which I am looking for.

☐ This is the house that my uncle has built.

☐ Where is the girl whom you have helped?

☐ Call in the child whose bag has been lost.

☐ This is not the same book as that of mine.

☐ Such men who are honest are loved by all.

☐ There is no man who does not wish to be happy.

Note:

a. Sometimes the relative pronoun is omitted also, as:

- We must suffer the punishment for the deeds (that) we do.
- This is the house (which) I bought last year.

b. The relative pronoun is of the same number and person as the noun or pronoun for which it stands, as:

- It is I who am to blame.
- It is Mohan who is to blame.

c. The relative pronoun must be placed as near its noun or pronoun as possible; as:

- The boy who broke my slate is my friend's brother.   (Correct)
- I live in a house in Delhi which is made of bricks.   (Incorrect)

It should be:

I live in Delhi in a house which is made of bricks.   (Correct)

Or

In Delhi, I live in a house which is made of bricks.

d. Some compound relative pronouns are also used in English. They are: whoever, whatever, whichever etc.

- Whoever saves the princess, shall be her husband.
- You can choose whichever book you like.
- Whatever I do, I do whole-heartedly.

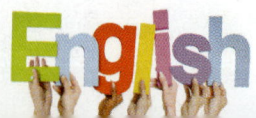

Reflexive Pronouns

A reflexive pronoun is a compound personal pronoun used to reflect the subject of an action or to make a pronoun more emphatic.

Reflexive pronouns are formed by adding self or own to some personal pronoun and adjectives, as:

1. My + self = Myself
2. Your + self = Yourself
3. Him + self = Himself
4. Her + self = Herself
5. It + self = Itself
6. Our + selves = Ourselves
7. Your + selves = Yourselves
8. Them + selves = Themselves

Reflexive pronouns must have an antecedent in the same sentence. A common mistake is to use a reflexive pronoun as a way of avoiding the choice between a subject and object pronoun, for example:

❏ Snow-white smiled at the dwarves and myself   (Incorrect)

In this sentence, the writer is not sure whether to use 'I' or 'me'. The writer thought to duck the choice by using the reflexive myself. This is a mistake because there is no antecedent for 'myself'. If the writer had stuck with I and me, the writer would have had a fifty-fifty chance of being right. But the reflexive without an antecedent is wrong (100 percent of the time).

Here is the reflexive 'myself' used correctly with an antecedent:

❏ I smiled at myself.   (Correct)

The antecedent of myself is the subject pronoun.

Indefinite pronouns: A large number of pronouns are referred to unspecified persons, things, or groups.

Some common indefinite pronouns are all, another, both:

Here is an example of a sentence with two indefinite pronouns:

❏ Many are called, but few are chosen.

It is easy to confuse indefinite pronouns with the same words used as adjectives. Remember: Indefinite pronouns stand alone and adjectives modify nouns. Here is an example that illustrates the difference:

Indefinite pronoun: Popeye would like some. (The pronoun 'some' stands alone.)

Modifying adjective: Popeye would like some spinach. (The adjective 'some' modifies spinach.)

Errors in the use of Pronouns

A pronoun is a word used in place of a noun as: I, we, you, your, he, him, she, her, it, etc.

❏ Myself can do it.	❏ I can do it myself.
❏ Let he and I do it.	❏ Let him and me do it.
❏ It was me who did it.	❏ It was I who did it.
❏ I and you will help the poor.	❏ You and I will help the poor.
❏ This action of her's was not liked by us.	❏ This action of hers was not liked by us.
❏ We enjoyed much at the hill-station.	❏ We enjoyed ourselves much at the hill-station.

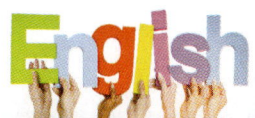

- Everybody were in their best clothes.
- Everybody was in his best clothes.
- Neither of these two boys are going to pass.
- Neither of these two boys is going to pass.
- Each of the guests must bring their invitation card.
- Each of the guests must bring his invitation card.
- I think Ram or Shyam have lost their books.
- I think Ram or Shyam has lost his books.
- One of the boys has lost one's books.
- One of the boys has lost his books.
- One must keep up his dignity.
- One must keep up one's dignity.
- Whom do you want to invite?
- Who do you want to invite?
- The boy who they praised has failed.
- The boy whom they praised has failed.
- I and my friend were invited to the party.
- My friend and I were invited to the party.
- I, you and he should attend the meeting.
- You, he and I should attend the meeting.
- You, he and I broke the rules of this game.
- I, he and you broke the rules of this game.
- Each of the students have done their homework.
- Each of the student has done his homework.
- She is one of those girls who never waste her time.
- She is one of those girls who never waste their time.
- Whom do you think will be appointed?
- Who do you think will be appointed?
- Let Lata and I try.
- Let Lata and me try.
- Do you like him accompanying us?
- Do you like his accompanying us?
- Let we all solve this problem.
- Let us all solve this problem.
- I availed of the opportunity.
- I availed myself of the opportunity.
- Your need is greater than that of mine.
- Your need is greater than mine.
- They who are honest need fear no one.
- Those who are honest need fear no one.
- The climate of Shimla is better than Delhi.
- The climate of Shimla is better than that of Delhi.
- If I were him, I would not behave that way.
- If I was he, I would not behave that way.
- I and you are classmates.
- You and I are classmates.
- He and you must go out for a gymn.
- You and he must go out for a gymn.
- I, he and you are playing a match.
- You, he and I are playing a match.
- You and we must work together.
- We and you must work together.
- They and you can go now.
- You and they can go now

While referring to persons, it is customary to place pronouns like this-IInd person, IIIrd Person, Ist Person (II, III, I). But in case of plural pronouns, 'we' comes before 'you' and 'you' before 'they'.

- Each of the girls must bring their own books.
- Each of the girls must bring her own book.
- Every girl was in their best dress.
- Every girl was in her best dress.

Each, every, everyone, everybody, anyone, either, neither, none are followed by the verbs and pronouns in the singular.

- None are allowed to miss their class.
- None is allowed to miss her class.
- The two brothers love one another.
- The two brothers love each other.
- Parth, Shiva and Bablu help each other.
- Parth, Shiva and Bablu help one another.

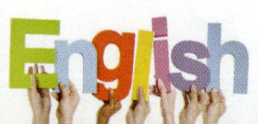

'Each other' is used for two persons or things, 'one another' for more than two persons or things.

- Distribute these mangoes among two boys.
- Distribute these mangoes between the two boys.
- Distribute sweets between four girls.
- Distribute sweets among four girls.

'Between' is used for two persons or things 'among' for more than two persons or things.

- Who did you beat yesterday?
- Whom did you beat yesterday?
- Whom do you think will win the prize?
- Who do you think will win the prize?

'Who' denotes subject and 'whom' stands for object.

- One must do his duty.
- One must do one's duty.
- It is one of the best books that has been written by Arvind.
- It is one of the best books written that have been written by Arvind.
- He is one of those persons who never shirks work.
- He is one of those persons who never shirk work.

A relative pronoun always agrees with its antecedent in gender, number person.

- Let you and I play here.
- Let you and me play here.
- Between you and I she is a lazy girl.
- Between you and me she is a lazy girl.
- These toys are for he and I.
- These toys are for him and me.

When a pronoun appears as object of a verb or of a preposition, it should be used in the objective case.

- Any of these two umbrellas will serve my purpose.
- Either of these two umbrellas will serve my purpose.
- You can take either of the four books.
- You can take any of the four books.
- None of these two boys are sincere.
- Neither of these two boys is sincere.
- Neither of my ten friends have helped me.
- None of my ten friends has helped me.

Either and neither should be used for two persons or things; anyone and none for more than two persons or things. The verb in each case will be singular.

- This is the chair whose leg is broken.
- This is the chair the leg of which is broken.

Pronouns like who, whose, whom are used for persons while 'which' is used for animals and things. But 'which' is also used for animate objects when there is a mention of two such objects.

- Whom do you think is the best artist?
- Who do you think is the best artist?
- Whom you think is your sister between Sarla & Gita?
- Which is your sister between Sarla & Gita?
- You must avail of this chance.
- You must avail yourself of this chance.
- Radha absented from the class.
- Radha absented herself from the class.
- I amused by reading a book.
- I amused myself by reading a book.

The reflexive pronoun is used after such verbs as enjoy, avail, absent, amuse, resign, apply, over-sleep, revenge, distinguish, over reach, exert, etc.

- I kept myself away from the class.
- I kept away from the class.
- She qualified herself for this post.
- She qualified for this post.

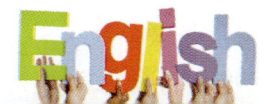

No reflexive pronoun is used after such verbs as keep, qualify, hide, rest, break, enlist, bath, dash, open, spread, turn, steal, stop, repent, gather, burst, feed, etc.

Incorrect Sentences	*Correct Sentences*
❐ It was her who stole your purse.	❐ It was she who stole your purse.
❐ It is me.	❐ It is I.
❐ If I were him, I would not disobey my teacher.	❐ If I were he, I would not disobey my teacher.

The complement of the verb 'to be', when it is expressed by a Pronoun, should be in the nominative form.

❐ You are clever than me.	❐ You are cleverer than I.
❐ She is wiser than him.	❐ She is wiser than he.
❐ He and myself went to Patiala	❐ He and I went to Patiala.
❐ Her brother and herself are fond of cakes	❐ Her brother and she are fond of cakes.
❐ I am yours faithful servant.	❐ I am your faithful servant.
❐ I take your leave now.	❐ I take leave of you now.
❐ She cannot bear my separation.	❐ She cannot bear separation from me.
❐ At my sight she started screaming.	❐ At the sight of mine, she started screaming.

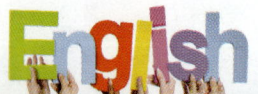

Chapter 4

Verbs

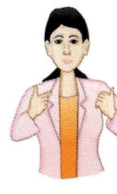

The traditional definition of verb is 'a word used to express action or describe a state of being.' As the definition implies, there are two different types of verbs: action verbs and linking verbs that describe the subjects. Here are some examples of each type:

Action Verbs:
- Donald laughed.
- Jane wrote a novel.

Linking Verbs:
- Donald is funny.
- The novel became a best-seller.
- The soup smelled wonderful.

The defining characteristic of all verbs is that verbs (and only verbs) have tenses: present, past and future. Unless a word can be used in the present, past and future tense, it is not a verb no exceptions. Verbs come in two flavours: regular and irregular. Regular verbs form their past tenses in an absolutely regular way by adding -'ed' (sometimes just -'d' the verb already ends in an 'e'). Irregular verbs form their past tense in some other irregular ways, often by 'changing the vowel of the verb.' Here are two examples, one with the regular verb 'remember' and the other with their regular verb 'forget':

Present: Wilbur always remembers his mother's birthday.
Past: Wilbur remembered his mother's birthday this year.
Future: Wilbur will remember his mother's birthday next year.

The helping verb 'will', which we use to form the future tense, is a convenient test word for identifying verbs.

Kinds of Verbs

Verbs have two main kinds:
1. Principal or main verbs.
2. Helping or auxiliary verbs.

Auxiliary Verbs

An auxiliary verb is the verb that helps a principal verb to form its tense, mood or voice, etc. as:

- ❏ I can play hockey very well.
- ❏ Did you beat his brother?
- ❏ One must obey one's parents.

In these sentences, the verbs, like 'can, did, must', help their principal verbs 'play, beat, obey' to form tenses and moods, etc. So, they are helping or auxiliary verbs.

Common examples of auxiliary verbs used in English are as follows:

1. Be	2. Have	3. Do	4. Can
5. May	6. Must	7. Need	8. Used
9. Will	10. Shall	11. Ought	12. Dare

Principal Verbs

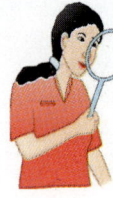

A principal verb is the verb that can express an action or a fact all by itself without the help of any other verb, as:

- ❏ The postman brought me a letter.
- ❏ Parents love their children.
- ❏ The teacher taught us a new lesson.

Kinds of Principal Verbs

Principal verbs have four chief kinds:

- ❏ Transitive verbs
- ❏ Intransitive verbs
- ❏ Defective verbs
- ❏ Incomplete verbs

Transitive Verbs

A transitive verb is the verb that denotes an action which does not stop with the subject but passes on to some object, as:

- ❏ The player kicked the ball.
- ❏ Tom whitewashed the fence.
- ❏ The fox gulped the cheese.
- ❏ The driver applied the brakes.
- ❏ The farmer reaped the harvest.

Intransitive Verbs

An intransitive verb is the verb that denotes an action which stops with the subject and does not pass on to any object, as:

- ❏ The child is sleeping.
- ❏ The onlookers were laughing.
- ❏ Our school opens at 9 a.m. and closes at 4 p.m.
- ❏ She smiled at my words.
- ❏ There are five errors in your essay.

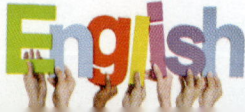

Defective Verbs

There are verbs (both transitive and intransitive) that suffer from a serious defect. They cannot be used in all tenses and moods as most of the verbs can be. That is why these verbs are called defective verbs.

A defective verb is the verb that cannot be used in all tenses and moods, etc, as:

'Will' can be used in only two tenses – present (will) and past (would). We cannot use it in future tense.

Common Defective Verbs are:

Shall	May	Can	Ought
Must	Need	Dare	Will

Incomplete Verbs

There are verbs (both transitive and intransitive) that fail to make complete sense even after taking an object. They require some more word or words to make complete sense. That is why they are called incomplete verbs.

An incomplete verb is the verb that needs some word or words to complete its predicate, as:

- ❑ They *elected* him king. (Transitive)
- ❑ The dog *became* mad. (Intransitive)
- ❑ The medicine *tasted* bitter. (Intransitive)
- ❑ The judge *found* him guilty. (Transitive)

All the four kinds of principal verbs shall be studied in detail in separate chapters.

Conjugation of Verbs

To conjugate a verb means to provide its three forms which are used in various tenses. These three forms of verb are:

1. Present
2. Past
3. Past Participle

Conjugation of Verbs

There are four principal forms which English verbs take in order to indicate tense.

1. The base form: This is the form which the verb takes to indicate the Simple Present Tense:
   - I play hockey every day.
   - We go for a walk in the morning.
2. The base form of the verb takes an -s or -es after it when the subject or the verb is in the third person singular:
   - He plays hockey every day.
   - Raju goes for a walk in the morning.
3. The Simple Past form:
   - The gardener watered the plants.
   - It rained heavily yesterday.

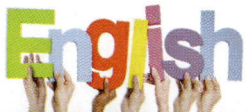

4. The Past Principle form: This is the form which the verb takes after the auxiliary has/have, had and will/shall have to express the present perfect, the past perfect and the future perfect tense respectively:
   - I have taken my lunch.
   - The patient had died before the doctor reached.
   - I shall have finished this work by 5 o'clock.
5. The Present Participle (ing) form: This is the form which the verb takes after the auxiliary be (in its various forms) to express a continuous action:
   - Anil is flying a kite.
   - The old man was sitting under a tree.
6. Besides these fur forms, verbs also take the form to+verb. This form is called the infinitive form. It does not express any tense, but is used to convey various meanings.
   - I forgot to post the letter.
   - His aim is to become a doctor.
   - Mangoes are good to eat.

Regular and Irregular Verbs

In the case of most verbs in English the past tense and past participle forms are got by adding -d or -ed to the base form. These verbs are called Regular Verbs.

Examples:

Base	Past	Past Participle
Call	Called	Called
Play	Played	Played
Hope	Hoped	Hoped
Try	Tried	Tried

In the case of the other verbs in English, the past tense and past participle forms are got, not by adding -d or -ed, but in various other ways. These verbs are known as Irregular Verbs.

Examples:

Base	Past	Past Participle
Break	Broke	Broken
Eat	Ate	Eaten
Meet	Met	Met
Shut	Shut	Shut

Study carefully the four principal forms of the following irregular verbs:

Present	Past	Past Participle	Present Participle
Arise	Arose	Arisen	Arising
Awake	Awoke	Awoken	Awaking

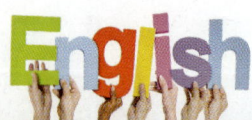

Be (am, is/are)	Was/Were	Been	Being
Bear	Bore	Born, Borne	Bearing
Beat	Beat	Beaten	Beating
Become	Became	Become	Becoming
Begin	Began	Begun	Beginning
Bend	Bent	Bent	Bending
Bid (command)	Bade	Bidden	Bidding
Bid (make a bid)	Bid	Bid	Bidding
Bind	Bound	Bound	Binding
Bite	Bit	Bitten	Biting
Bleed	Bled	Bled	Bleeding
Blow	Blew	Blown	Blowing
Break	Broke	Broken	Breaking
Bring	Brought	Brought	Bringing
Build	Built	Built	Building
Burn	Burnt	Burnt	Burning
	Burned	Burned	
Burst	Burst	Burst	Bursting
Buy	Bought	Bought	Buying
Catch	Caught	Caught	Catching
Choose	Chose	Chosen	Choosing
Come	Came	Come	Coming
Cost	Cost	Cost	Costing
Creep	Crept	Crept	Creeping
Cut	Cut	Cut	Cutting
Deal	Dealt	Dealt	Dealing
Dig	Dug	Dug	Digging
Do	Did	Done	Doing
Draw	Drew	Drawn	Drawing
Dream	Dreamt	Dreamt	Dreaming
	Dreamed	Dreamed	Dreaming
Drink	Drank	Drank	Drinking
Drive	Drove	Driven	Driving
Dwell	Dwelt	Dwelt	Dwelling
Eat	Ate	Eaten	Eating
Fall	Fell	Fallen	Falling
Feed	Fed	Fed	Feeding

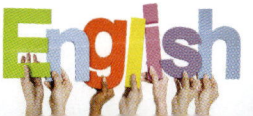

Feel	Felt	Felt	Feeling
Fight	Fought	Fought	Fighting
Find	Found	Found	Finding
Fling	Flung	Flung	Flinging
Fly	Flew	Flown	Flying
Forbid	Forbade	Forbidden	Forbidding
Forget	Forgot	Forgotten	Forgetting
Freeze	Froze	Frozen	Freezing
Get	Got	Got	Gotton
Give	Gave	Given	Giving
Go	Went	Gone	Going
Grow	Grew	Grown	Growing
Hang	Hung	Hung	Hanging
	Hanged	Hanged	
Have	Had	Had	Having
Hear	Heard	Heard	Hearing
Hide	Hid	Hidden, Hid	Hiding
Hit	Hit	Hit	Hitting
Hold	Held	Held	Holding
Hurt	Hurt	Hurt	Hurting
Keep	Kept	Kept	Keeping
Kneel	Knelt	Knelt	Kneeling
Know	Knew	Known	Knowing
Lay	Laid	Laid	Laying
Lead	Led	Led	Leading
Leap	Leapt	Leapt	Leaping
Learn	Learnt	Learnt	Learning
	Learned	Learned	
Lend	Lent	Lent	Lending
Let	Let	Let	Letting
Lie	Lay	Lain	Lying
Light	Lit	Lit	Lighting
	Lighted	Lighted	
Lose	Lost	Lost	Losing
Make	Made	Made	Making
Mean	Meant	Meant	Meaning

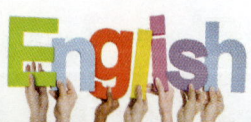

Meet	Met	Met	Meeting
Pay	Paid	Paid	Paying
Put	Put	Put	Putting
Read	Read	Read	Reading
Ride	Rode	Ridden	Riding
Ring	Rang	Rung	Ringing
Rise	Rose	Risen	Rising
Run	Ran	Run	Running
Say	Said	Said	Saying
See	Saw	Seen	Seeing
Seek	Sought	Sought	Seeking
Sell	Sold	Sold	Selling
Send	Sent	Sent	Sending
Set	Set	Set	Setting
Shake	Shook	Shaken	Shaking
Shed	Shed	Shed	Shedding
Shine	Shone	Shone	Shinning
Shoot	Shot	Shot	Shooting
Show	Showed	Shown	Showing
Shrink	Shrank	Shrunk	Shrinking
Shut	Shut	Shut	Shutting
Sing	Sang	Sung	Singing
Sink	Sank	Sunk	Sinking
Sit	Sat	Sat	Sitting
Sleep	Slept	Slept	Sleeping
Smell	Smelt	Smelt	Smelling
Sow	Sowed	Sown	Sowing
Speak	Spoke	Spoken	Speaking
Spell	Spelt	Spelt	Spelling
	Spelled	Spelled	
Spend	Spent	Spent	Spending
Spin	Span	Spun	Spinning
	Spun		
Spit	Spat	Spat	Spitting
Split	Split	Split	Splitting

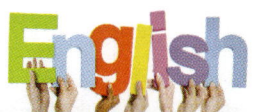

Spoil	Spoilt	Spoilt	Spoiling
	Spoiled	Spoiled	
Spread	Spread	Spread	Spreading
Spring	Sprang	Sprung	Springing
Stand	Stood	Stood	Standing
Steal	Stole	Stolen	Stealing
Stick	Stuck	Stuck	Sticking
Strike	Struck	Stricken	Striking
Strive	Strove	Striven	Striving
Swear	Swore	Sworn	Swearing
Sweep	Swept	Swept	Sweeping
Swim	Swam	Swum	Swimming
Take	Took	Taken	Taking
Teach	Taught	Taught	Teaching
Tear	Tore	Torn	Tearing
Tell	Told	Told	Telling
Think	Thought	Thought	Thinking
Throw	Threw	Thrown	Throwing
Understand	Understood	Understood	Understanding
Wake	Woke	Woke	
		Waked	Waking
	Waked	Woken	
Wear	Wore	Worn	Wearing
Weave	Wove	Woven	Weaving
Weep	Wept	Wept	Weeping
Win	Won	Won	Winning
Wind	Wound	Wound	Winding
Wring	Wrung	Wrung	Wringing
Write	Wrote	Written	Writing

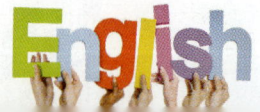

Correct Usage

Study the use of the following verbs:

1. Born, borne

    When bear means to bring forth, the past participle is born; but when it means to carry; the past participle is borne.
    - He was born with a silver spoon in his mouth.
    - The wounded were borne to the hospital.

2. Fell, felled

    Fell is the past tense of the verb fall. Felled is the past tense of the verb fell which means to cause to fall.
    - His father fell ill yesterday.
    - The woodcutter felled a tree.

3. Found, founded

    Found is the past tense or the past participle of the verb find. Founded is the past tense or the past participle of the verb found, which means to lay the foundation of or to set up.
    - I found a ring on the way.
    - My father founded this dispensary.

4. Hanged, Hung

    When hang means to put a person to death by hanging, its past tense or past participle is hanged. But when it is used to other senses, the past or past participle is hung.
    - Saddam Hussein, the ousted President of Iraq, was hanged on 30th December 2006.
    - We hung the pictures on the wall.

5. Lie, Lay

    To lie has two different sets of forms, when it means to say untrue things, the three forms are lie, lied, lied. When it means to rest, the three forms are lie, lay, lain.

    To lay means to put or place something down or to produce eggs. Its three forms are lay, laid, laid.

    (a) He Lied to me.

      I am going to lie here and rest.

      He lay awake the whole night. The patient had lain down to rest.

    (b) Please lay the table.

      I laid the facts before my father.

      The hen has laid an egg.

6. Rise, Raise

    Rise means to get up or to come up; raise means to lift up.
    - I rise at 6 o'clock every day.
    - The Sun rises in the east.
    - Please raise your right hand.

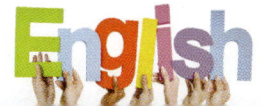

Errors in the use of Verbs

A verb is a word that tells us something about a person, place or thing as: see, read, laugh, write, enjoy, sing, build, weep, etc.

Incorrect Sentences	*Correct Sentences*
❏ Every boy and girl were present.	❏ Every boy and girl was present.
❏ Everyone of them are going.	❏ Everyone of them is going.

Each, every, neither, either, nobody, anyone, anybody, none, are followed by verbs in the singular.

❏ Either you or your sister have done it.	❏ Either you or your sister has done it.
❏ Neither you or nor I are guilty.	❏ Neither you nor I am guilty.
❏ Sita or Tanu are at fault.	❏ Sita or Tanu is at fault.

Two or more singular. Nouns or pronouns connected by the conjunctions 'either' 'or', 'neither' 'nor' require a singular verb. If the subjects differ in number or in person, the verb, agrees with the number or person which stands nearest to it.

Incorrect Sentences	*Correct Sentences*
❏ Slow and steady win the race.	❏ Slow and steady wins the race.
❏ Law and order are to be maintained at all costs.	❏ Law and order is to be maintained at all costs.
❏ Noodle and rice are my favorite food.	❏ Noodle and rice is my favorite food.

When two different nouns combine to form one idea or are treated as a unity, the verb is singular.

❏ Hundred rupees are a big sum.	❏ Hundred rupees is a big sum.
❏ Ten miles are not a long distance.	❏ Ten miles is not a long distance.
❏ Fifty Thousand rupees are not a small sum.	❏ Fifty thousand rupees is not a small sum.

When a plural noun is considered collectively, the verb is singular.

❏ The 'Tale of Two Cities' are an interesting novel.	❏ The 'Tale of Two Cities' is an interesting novel.
❏ 'The United States' have a big navy.	❏ 'The United States' has a big navy.

When a plural noun is a proper name for some collective unit or some single object or denotes some specific quality or amount, the verb is in the singular.

❏ The teacher together with her students were there.	❏ The teacher together with her students was there.
❏ Shalu along with her sisters were present.	❏ Shalu along with her sisters was present there.

Two nouns or pronouns connected by and not, with, in addition to, like, besides, together, as well as, not only but also, are followed by a verb in the singular when the former of the two nouns or pronouns is in the singular.

❏ I have seen him yesterday.	❏ I saw him yesterday.
❏ He has passed the examination last year.	❏ He passed the examination last year.

When two actions or events take place in the past, the action or event taking place first is shown in the Past Perfect Tense, the other one in the Past Indefinite Tense.

❏ I shall help you if you will speak the truth.	❏ I shall help you if you speak the truth.
❏ She will repent if she will waste her time.	❏ She will repent if she wastes her time.

English

Don't use two future tenses together The sentence beginning with 'when' or 'if' should be in the Present Indefinite Tense.

- Many a girls were playing.
- Many a boys have left the class.

- Many girls were playing.
- Many boys have left the class.

'Many a' should be followed by a singular noun and a singular verb.

- I knew that she will disobey me.
- You told us that honesty was the best policy.

- I knew that she would disobey.
- You told us that honesty is the best policy.

If the Principal Clause is in the Past Tense the Sub ordinate Clause must be in the Past Tense unless it has a universal truth or a historical truth or a habitual truth.

- This is one of the best books that has been published.
- He is one of the greatest leaders who has served his country.

- This is one of the best books that have been published.
- He as one of the greatest leaders who have served their country.

The plural antecedents of the relative pronoun should have plural verb.

- I do not know where is he going.
- Can you tell when will she come back?

- I do not know where he is going.
- Can you tell when she will come back?

If there are two clauses in a sentence, the Subordinate Clause should not be in the question form.

- You behave as if you are a princess.
- I wish I was a child again.

- You behave as if you were a princess.
- I wish I were a child again.

Expressions like 'as if' 'as though', or expression of a wish should be followed by a Past tense and in the plural form but if the Principal clause is in the Indefinite tense, it should be followed by Past Perfect Tense.

- Walking on the road, he met an old man.
- Entering the office, I heard the telephone ring.

- While (or when) he was walking on the road, he met on old man.
- As I was entering the office, I heard the telephone ring.

The participle should not be left without proper agreement. It must be attached with a noun or a pronoun to which it refers.

- The difficulty of getting houses in big cities are great.
- Your choice of friends are not good.

- The difficulty of getting houses in big cities is great.
- Your choice of friends is not good.

When the subject is in the singular form, it must have a singular verb.

- The poet and the novelist is dead.
- The white and black cow are grazing.

- The poet and the novelist are dead (two persons)
- The white and black cow is grazing. (one)

When two or more persons refer to one person or thing, the verb is singular. But when the article is repeated before every person, the verb should be in the plural form.

Incorrect Sentences

- I have never and will never disobey you.
- She has never and will never tell a lie.

Correct Sentences

- I have never disobeyed and will never disobey you.
- She has never told and will never tell a lie.

Use 3rd form of the verb after have and has.
- ❐ Our only guide were the stars.
- ❐ The stars was our only guide.
- ❐ Our only guide was the stars.
- ❐ The stars were our only guide.

A verb should agree with its subject and not with the complements.
- ❐ A large number of students was present today.
- ❐ The rest of the students was on leave.
- ❐ A large number of students were present today.
- ❐ The rest of the students were on leave.

Some nouns, like number, plenty, rest, variety, army, etc. are plural in meaning though they are singular in form; so the verb is in plural.
- ❐ Not riches but education ensure success.
- ❐ Not wealth but health count in life.
- ❐ Not riches but education ensures success.
- ❐ Not wealth but health counts in life.

When collective nouns, like committee, crowd, army, fleet is thought of as a whole, acting together as one unit, it is used in the singular sense.
- ❐ The ministry is divided on the language issue.
- ❐ The ministry are divided on the language issue.

When a collective noun is not acting as a unit, it takes a plural verb.
- ❐ My brother prevented me to go to the bazaar.
- ❐ She insisted to marry an actor.
- ❐ My brother prevented me from going to the bazaar.
- ❐ She insisted on marrying an actor.

Verbs, like succeed, insist, persist, prevent, check, desist, avoid, restrain, addict, hinder, bent, prohibit etc. are followed by a gerund. (i.e., a verbal noun).
- ❐ You had better not to go there.
- ❐ None can dare to touch me.
- ❐ You had better not go there.
- ❐ None can dare touch me.

No infinitive (i.e., 'to') is used after the phrase-Had better, had rather and after some verbs, like dare, need, make, let.
- ❐ My brothers as well as I am playing.
- ❐ She as well as her friends are reading.
- ❐ My brothers as well as I are playing.
- ❐ She as well as her friends is reading.

When two subjects, not of the same person, are joined by as well as, the verb agrees with the first subject.
- ❐ You did not do so, nor he did.
- ❐ No sooner he reached the station than the train steamed off.
- ❐ You did not do so, nor did he.
- ❐ No sooner did he reach the station than the train steamed off.

The Verb comes before its subject when it is introduced by neither, nor or hardly or no sooner.
- ❐ She did not see you for six months.
- ❐ I am working in this office for 2000.
- ❐ She has not seen you for six months.
- ❐ I have been work in this office since 2000.

Use Perfect Continuous Tense where time is given.

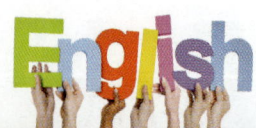

Chapter 5

Adverbs

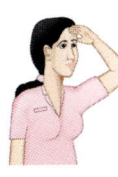

Adverbs are words that modify verbs, adjectives or other adverbs. By far the most common use of adverbs is to modify verbs, so we will deal with them first.

Adverbs that Modify verbs

Here are some examples of adverbs (in italics) that modify verbs (in bold):

- ❑ They **parked** the truck *yesterday*.
- ❑ They **loaded** the truck *there*.
- ❑ They **drove** truck *carefully*.
- ❑ They **use** the truck *frequently*.

Adverbs that modify verbs have several characteristics that make them (relatively) easy to identify. They answer adverb questions and they are movable.

An adverb is a word that modifies a verb, an adjective or another adverb; as:

- ❑ The shepherd shouted loudly.   (modifying a verb)
- ❑ He is very mischievous boy.   (modifying an adjective)
- ❑ She walks very gracefully.   (modifying an adverb)

An adverb may modify a phrase also, as:

- ❑ At noon the sun is right above us.
- ❑ Everything is just out of order.
- ❑ She was walking close behind me.
- ❑ You are always in a hurry.

An adverb may modify an entire sentence too, as:

- ❑ Finally *Nurjahan agreed to marry Jahangir*.
- ❑ Unluckily, *we were caught in a storm*.
- ❑ Probably, *he is not at fault*.
- ❑ Apparently, *the sun looks moving*.

I. Kinds of Adverbs

Adverbs have four chief kinds:
1.   Simple Adverbs
2.   Interrogative Adverbs
3.   Relative Adverbs
4.   Adverbs of Affirmation or Negation

Simple Adverbs

Observe the following sentences:
- She **walks** gracefully.
- I get up **early**.
- Come **here**, Mohan.

Each sentence has a word in bold type. It modifies the verb in a simple way. It does not ask any question nor does it act as a connective. So, it is a simple adverb.

A simple adverb is an adverb that modifies a verb etc. in a simple way.

Interrogative Adverbs

Observe the following sentences:
- **When** did you pass your class 10th examination?
- **How** are you?
- **Where** do you hail from?
- **Why** did you beat him?

Each sentence has a word in bold type. It is an adverb but it has been used to ask a question. So, it is an interrogative adverb.

An interrogative adverb is an adverb that modifies a verb and at the same time asks a question.

Relative Adverbs

Observe the following sentences:
- This is **where I** spent my childhood.
- I know **why you** have beaten him.
- She knows **when** he will come back.
- Tell me **how I** can solve this sum.

Each sentence has a word in bold type. It is an adverb but it has been used as a connective. So, it is a relative adverb.

A relative adverb is an adverb that modifies a verb and at the same time acts as a connective.
Note: You must have noted that interrogative and relative adverbs are the same words. But they differ in their uses and functions.

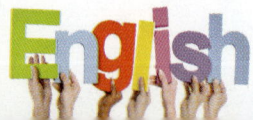

Adverbs of Affirmation and Negation

Observe the following sentences:

1. Do you have a race daily? Yes, I do.
2. Did she marry your brother? No, she didn't.
3. Are you happy here? Certainly, I am.
4. He hates you, I think. You are perhaps right.
5. Will you help me? By all means, I will.
6. Is he a cheat? Of course, he is.

An adverb of affirmation is an adverb that affirms a statement or fact.

An adverb of negation is an adverb that negates a statement or fact.

II. Comparison of Adverbs

Some Adverbs, like Adjectives have the Degree of Comparison. Such Adverbs are generally compared like Adjectives.

(i) If the Adverb is of one syllable, we form the comparative by adding -er and the superlative by adding -est to the positive; as:

Positive	Comparative	Superlative	Positive	Comparative	Superlative
Fast	faster	fastest	Hard	harder	hardest
Long	longer	longest	Soon	sooner	soonest
Late	later	latest	Near	nearer	nearest

(ii) Adverb ending in *ly* form the comparative by adding *more* and the superlative by adding *most*; as:

Positive	Comparative	Superlative
Swiftly	more swiftly	most swiftly
Skillfully	more skillfully	most skillfully
WIsely	more wisely	most wisely
Beautifully	more beautifully	most beautifully
Exception		
Early	earlier	earliest

Note that only Adverbs of *Manner, Degree* and *Time* can be compared. Adverbs, like *now, then, where, there, once* cannot be compared.

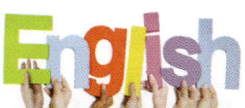

(iii) Some Adverbs form their comparative and superlative degrees irregularly, thus:

Ill, bad	worse	worst
Well	better	best
Much	more	most
Little	less	least
Nigh, near	nearer	nearest
Far	farther	farthest
Forth	further	furthest
Late	later	last

III. Formation of Adverbs

Adverbs are formed:

(i) By adding 'ly'; as:

Gently, happily, honestly, wisely, highly, etc.

Weekly, yearly, daily, fortnightly, quarterly, etc.

(ii) By adding prepositions; as:

ahead, asleep, abroad, today, tomorrow, etc.

afresh, alone, beyond, below, besides, etc.

hereby, hitherto, wherein, herewith, etc.

thenceforth, henceforth, etc.

(iii) By combining a noun and an adjective; as:

Midnight, meantime, otherwise

IV. Position of Adverbs

Order of Adverbs is very elastic in English and many shades of emphasis, etc. can be expressed by a change of position, e.g.,

I want only you.

Only I want you.

In the first sentence there is a choice (between you and others) and I choose you. But the second sentence means that nobody else except I (want you)

1. An Adverb is placed before an Adjective or another Adverb it modifies.

You are *quite* wrong.

She sings very *sweetly*.

Do not speak *so fast*.

Exception: Adverb *enough* is always placed after the word it modifies.

He spoke loud *enough* to be heard.

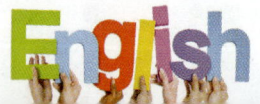

2. After an Intransitive verb:

They fought *bravely.*

She spoke *fluently.*

Exception: Adverbs of time such as always, ever, often, seldom, never, etc., are placed before the verb they modify.

She *seldom* writes to me.

He *often* comes to meet me.

He *always* speaks the truth.

Nothing wrong *ever* happened to him.

But these Adverbs are placed after the verb 'to be':

He is *never* angry.

3. When a verb is Transitive, the adverb follows an object.

He faced his *losses bravely.*

He does his work *carefully.*

4. An Adverb is placed between the auxiliary and the principal verb.

I shall *certainly* help you.

5. The world *'only'* should be placed immediately before the word it modifies.

He lent me *only* five rupees.

He worked for *only* two hours.

V. Use of Some Adverbs

1. **Very, much:**

Very as an Adverb qualifies *adverbs, certain adjectives* in the positive degree and *present* and *some* past participles.

You look *very* bright today.

We have had a *very* trying time.

I was *very* pleased to hear from you.

Hindi can be *very* easily learnt.

Much qualifies a *verb,* a *past participle* or a *comparative* or *superlative* adjective.

I *much* prefer this book to that.

I am *much* annoyed with you.

The man is *much* better today.

She is *much* the prettiest girl of the family.

Note that *'very tired,' 'very pleased'* are exceptions.

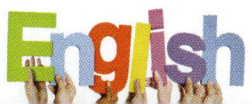

2.   **Too very:**

'**Too**' implies 'more than enough' and, therefore, should never be used in place of '*very*'. It is wrong to say, 'I am *too* tired'. I am *very* tired' is the correct way of putting it.

'**Too**' has a negative sense, and is equal to "so...that......not". When it is used in this sense, it is followed by an infinitive or by a phrase beginning with '*for*'.

He is *too* proud to beg.

My heart is *too* full for words.

It should be used when we are sure of a negative meaning otherwise the sentence will give just the opposite meaning, e.g.,

I am *too* glad to see you.

Here the use of '*too*' is wrong. It should have been "I am very glad to see you".

'*Too*' is also used in the sense of '*also*'; as:

he was fined and punished *too*.

3.   **Enough:**

Enough implies that the proper limit has been reached and it is used after the word it modifies.

He was clever *enough* to see through the trick.

He was kind *enough* to comply to my request.

It is used in front of a noun and after an adjective or adverb.

I have *enough* money; I can pay the bill.

It was cold *enough* to freeze our fingers.

4.   **Since, ago, before:**

Since and *ago* mean a period of time, dating back from now. They are preceded by a verb in the Past Indefinite Tense and a noun or phrase expressing period of time.

I came here a week *ago (since)*.

He passed his Senior Secondary Examination six months ago *(since)*.

Before means formerly.

I had never seen much a sight *before*.

Before is used in the Indirect speech and not 'ago'.

I said, "I sold my book a year *ago*".

I said that I had sold my book a year *before*.

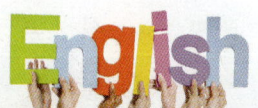

Errors in the use of Adverbs

An Adverb is a word that modifies a verb, an adjective or another adverb as: always, enough, seldom, much, sometimes, extremely, etc.

- ❏ He stood behind just me.
- ❏ He stood just behind me.
- ❏ We sat in the shade almost.
- ❏ We sat almost in the shade.
- ❏ A snake creeps very silent.
- ❏ A snake creeps very silently.
- ❏ He is an almost drunkard.
- ❏ He is almost a drunkard.
- ❏ More men have, more they desire.
- ❏ The more men have, the more they desire.
- ❏ That box is very heavy to lift.
- ❏ The box is too heavy to lift.
- ❏ He seized my hand quite roughly.
- ❏ He seized my hand rather roughly.
- ❏ He well lived and happily died.
- ❏ He lived well and died happily.
- ❏ He stayed seldom with me for long.
- ❏ He seldom stayed with me for long.
- ❏ He came often here to see me.
- ❏ He often came here to see me.
- ❏ I like only a mango when it is ripe.
- ❏ I like a mango only when it is ripe.
- ❏ He merely did this because he was ordered to.
- ❏ He did this merely because he was ordered to.
- ❏ I forbade you not to enter the room.
- ❏ I forbade you to enter the room.
- ❏ The air is very hotter today than yesterday.
- ❏ The air is much hotter today than yesterday.
- ❏ We not have seen him since Monday last.
- ❏ We have not seen him since last Monday.
- ❏ This news is much shocking.
- ❏ This news is very shocking.
- ❏ I cannot walk no further today.
- ❏ I cannot walk further today.
- ❏ He bore cheerfully his losses.
- ❏ He bore his losses cheerfully.
- ❏ 1 quite have forgotten you.
- ❏ I have quite forgotten you.
- ❏ He almost dying.
- ❏ He is almost dying.
- ❏ I am little tired.
- ❏ I am a little tired.
- ❏ 1 built this house long before.
- ❏ I built this house long ago.
- ❏ He seldom or ever comes late,
- ❏ He seldom or never comes late.
- ❏ He is very old to work hard,
- ❏ He is too old to work hard.
- ❏ Yes, 1 did not find him at home.
- ❏ No, I did not find him at home.
- ❏ The air today is enough cold for me.
- ❏ The air today is cold enough for me.
- ❏ The roof of this house is too strong.
- ❏ The roof of this house is very strong.
- ❏ I expected little that he would die so soon.
- ❏ I little expected that he would die so soon.
- ❏ This cold wind is quite dangerous for the child.
- ❏ This cold wind is very dangerous for the child.
- ❏ Two hours have passed since he had fallen asleep.
- ❏ Two hours have passed since he fell asleep
- ❏ It is too cold today.
- ❏ It is very cold today.
- ❏ You are too busy.
- ❏ You are very busy.

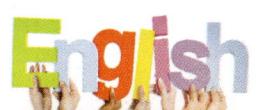

'Too' should not be used in the sense of 'very' or 'much'. 'too' means some kind of excess or more than enough.

- He is enough rich to help you.
- I am enough tired to go farther.

- He is rich enough to help you.
- I am tired enough to go farther.

The adverb 'enough' is generally used after the word it modifies.

- I visit his house often.
- Driver smokes Seldom.

- I often visit his house.
- Driver seldom smokes.

The adverbs of time, seldom, often, sometimes frequently, never, ever, always etc., are generally used before the verbs they modify.

- It is nothing else than pride.
- You can call him anything else than a fool.
  'Else' should be followed by 'but' and not by 'than'.
- She is wonderful beautiful.
- You are regular irregular.

- It is nothing else but pride.
- You can call him anything but a fool.

- She is wonderfully beautiful.
- You are regularly irregular.

'Wonderful' and 'regular' are adjectives. Use the correct adverbs here.

- He was compelled to at once leave the place.
- She tried to hurriedly reach there.

- He was compelled to leave the place at once.
- She tried to reach there hurriedly.

An adverb should not be used before an infinitive.

- Satish will tomorrow call on you.
- I last night visited the circus.

- Satish will call on you tomorrow.
- I visited the circus last night.

Adverb or adverbial phrases of definite time, like yesterday, tomorrow, last night, today, four months ago are usually placed at the end of the sentences.

- It is very hot to go out.
- Rihan is very poor to help you.
- You are too proud.

- It is too hot to go out.
- Rihan is too poor to help you.
- You are very proud.

"Too' means enough' while 'very' is used simply to make the adjective or adverb stronger.

- I only spend ten rupees.
- I only worked two sums.

- I spent only ten rupees.
- I worked only two sums.

'Only' should be placed immediately before the word it qualifies.

- He does carefully his work.
- You have almost reached, at your goal.
- I fluently spoke.

- He does his work carefully.
- You have almost reached your goal.
- I spoke fluently.

With a 'transitive verb' as adverb generally comes after the object. But when the verb is intransitive, the adverb or adverbial phrase is placed after the verb.

- I fortunately passed the test.
- We reached our goal at length.

- Fortunately I passed the test.
- At length we reached our goal.

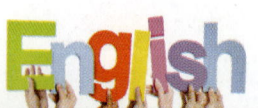

An adverb should be placed at the beginning of a sentence when it is intended to qualify not any word in particular, but the sentence as a whole.

- ❑ You are speaking much fluently.
- ❑ Mohini is very wiser than Manisha
- ❑ You are speaking very fluently.
- ❑ Mohini is much wiser than Manisha.

'Very' modifies adjectives or adverbs in a positive degree and 'much' in the comparative degree.

- ❑ I shall come back just now.
- ❑ My friend has met me presently.
- ❑ I shall come back presently.
- ❑ My friend has met just now.

'Presently' should be used for near future while 'just now' refers to present or past time.

- ❑ She is so nice.
- ❑ Reena is very proud as Sheena.
- ❑ I work quicker than he.
- ❑ You should know to respect others!
- ❑ She is very nice.
- ❑ Reena is as proud as Sheena.
- ❑ I work more quickly than him.
- ❑ You should know how to respect others.

Adjectives should not be used as adverbs.

- ❑ We seldom or ever tell a lie.
- ❑ We seldom or never tell a lie.

Use seldom or never.

- ❑ Firstly you should be obedient and secondly dutiful.
- ❑ First you should be obedient and secondly, dutiful.

'First' is an adverb. Therefore, in an enumeration, use first, secondly, thirdly, etc.

- ❑ She never remembers having sent me a letter.
- ❑ I never saw him today.
- ❑ She does not remember having sent me a letter.
- ❑ I did not see him today.

Here 'never' incorrectly used for 'not'. Never means 'not ever'.

- ❑ Are you an obedient girl? Yes, you are not an obedient girl.
- ❑ Are you at obedient girl? Yes, you are an obedient girl. (or No, you are not an obedient girl.

If the answer to a question is, the verb following must be in the affirmative. But if the answer is no, the verb following must be in the negative.

- ❑ Your father is very miser.
- ❑ The widow feels sadly.
- ❑ Radha speaks very hasty.
- ❑ She hurriedly reached there.
- ❑ Please carry carefully my bag.
- ❑ Firstly you should be regular and secondly hard-working.
- ❑ The bag is too much heavy for me.
- ❑ My grandfather peacefully died.
- ❑ He exactly came in time.
- ❑ You must come at 6 p.m. sharply.
- ❑ Your father is very miserly.
- ❑ The widow feels sad.
- ❑ Radha speaks very hastily.
- ❑ She reached there hurriedly.
- ❑ Please carry my bag carefully.
- ❑ First you should be regular and secondly, hardworking
- ❑ The bag is much too heavy for me.
- ❑ My grandfather died peacefully.
- ❑ He came exactly in time.
- ❑ You must come at 6 p.m. sharp.

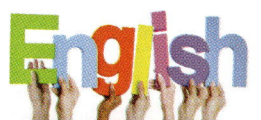

NOTES

Chapter 6

Adjective

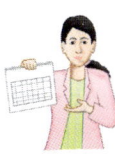

An adjective is a word that is used to add something to the meaning of a noun or a pronoun. Observe the following sentences:

- She is proud of her *charming* looks.
- The *fourth* boy in this row is Atul.
- Give me *some* money as a loan.
- *This* boy is very rude and naughty.
- *My* watch is superior to yours.

In these sentences:

- The word 'charming' describes the quality of the noun that is looks.
- The word 'fourth' describes the number of the noun that is boy.
- The word 'some' describes the quantity of the noun that is money.
- The word 'this' demonstrates the noun that is boy.
- The word 'my' describes the possession of the noun that is watch.

All these words, 'charming, fourth, some, this, my', describe or qualify their respective nouns that follow them. These nouns have been printed in italics. So, these words are adjectives. Each of them describes its noun in a different way by giving its number, quantity, quality, possession or by demonstrating it. Accordingly, adjectives are of different kinds too, as are as follows:

Adjectives play two distinct roles: noun modifiers and predicate adjectives. As noun modifiers, adjectives always precede the nouns they modify. Predicate adjectives, they follow linking (descriptive) verbs and describe the subject. Here are some examples of both types:

Adjectives as noun modifiers (adjectives in italic, nouns in bold)

- An *awful* **noise**
- That *dreadful* old **man**
- Five *golden* **rings**
- The *special, deep*-**dish**, *Chicago-style* **pizza**.

Adjectives as predicate adjectives (adjectives in italics)

- The play was *terrific.*
- Harry sounded *excited.*

I. Kinds of Adjectives

Adjectives have five different kinds:
1. Adjectives of Quality
2. Adjectives of Quantity
3. Adjectives of Number
4. Demonstrative Adjectives
5. Possessive Adjectives

Adjectives of Quality

An adjective of quality is the adjective that denotes the quality or kind of its noun or pronoun, as:
- Rama sang a sweet song.
- Horatius was a brave soldier.
- The clever jackal pleased the lion.
- Indian wives are mostly faithful.
- Where is my white shirt?

Adjectives of Quantity

An adjective of quantity is the adjective that denotes the quantity of its noun or pronoun, as:
- I bought some tea.
- He is a little proud of his position.
- You have no right to say so.

Adjectives of Number

An adjective of number is the adjective that denotes the number or order (serial) of its noun or pronoun, as:
- A hand has four fingers and one thumb.
- A few boys are there in the room.

Demonstrative Adjectives

A demonstrative adjective is the adjective that points out or demonstrates its noun or pronoun, as:
- This painting is very fine.
- That girl is very modest.
- These pets are mine, not hers.

Possessive Adjectives

We will read in the chapter on pronouns that each personal pronoun has two possessive forms. One of these forms is used as a possessive adjective. These adjectives are:

I → My	We → Our	She → Her	You → Your
He → His	It → Its	They → Their	Ram → Ram's

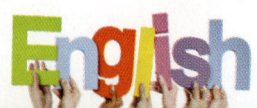

- My friend is an industrious boy.
- Our flag is called the tricolor:
- Her charms are the talk of the town.

II. Comparison of Adjectives

Adjectives have *three* Degrees of Comparison
  I. Positive Degree
  II. Comparative Degree
  III. Superlative Degree

Look at the following sentences:

Rani is *clever.*
      Rani is *cleverer* than her sister.
      Rani is the *cleverest* of all her sisters.

In the first sentence, the word 'clever' is the simple form of the Adjective. It is called the *Positive Degree.* In the second sentence, Rani possesses the quality of being clever in a greater degree than her sister. 'Clever' in this sentence is, therefore, an adjective of the *Comparative Degree.* In the third sentence, however, Rani possesses the quality of being clever in the greatest degree of all. It is, therefore, in the *Superlative Degree.*

      Thus, we see that when we compare two persons or things. We use the *Comparative Degree* and when we compare more than two objects or persons, we use the *Superlative Degree.*

Note that an adjective in the comparative Degree is followed by than and an adjective in the superlative Degree is preceded by 'the' and is followed by a preposition 'of' or 'in'; as:

I am cleverer *than* he (is).

He is the cleverest *of* all the boys in the class.

kolkata is the biggest town in India.

III. Formation of Degrees of Comparison

Comparatives and Superlatives are formed according to the following rules:

(i) By adding -*er* and -*est* to the positive; as:

Positive	Comparative	Superlative
Great	greater	greatest
Long	longer	longest
Short	shorter	shortest
Small	smaller	smallest
Thick	thicker	thickest
Deep	deeper	deepest

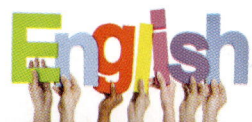

If the positive ends in 'e', only 'r' and 'st' are added respectively; as:

Positive	Comparative	Superlative
Large	larger	largest
Brave	braver	bravest
Wise	wiser	wisest
True	truer	truest

(ii) If the positive ends in 'y' preceded by a consonant then 'y' is changed into 'i' before adding 'er' and 'est'; as:

Easy	easier	easiest
Happy	happier	happiest
Dry	drier	driest

If, however, the final 'y' in the positive is preceded by a vowel, only 'er' or 'est' are added; as:

Gay	gayer	gayest
Grey	greyer	greyest

(iii) If the positive ends in a consonant preceded by a short vowel, the final consonant is double; as:

Hot	hotter	hottest
Fat	fatter	fattest
Thin	thinner	thinnest
Wet	wetter	wettest

(iv) Adjectives of more than two syllables and many adjectives of two syllables form the comparative by adding *more* and *most*; as:

Beautiful	more beautiful	most beautiful

(v) Some Adjectives are compared in an irregular way; as:

Good, well	better	best
Bad, ill	worse	worst
Little	less, lesser	least
Many, much	more	most
Late	latter, later	latest, last
Fore	former	foremost, first
Far	farther, further	farthest, furthest
Old	older, elder	oldest, eldest
Near	nearer	nearest, next
In	inner	innermost, inmost
Out	outer, utter	outermost, uttermost
Up	upper	uppermost, upmost

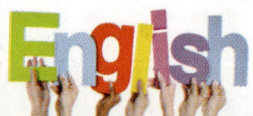

(vi) Some Adjectives expressing qualities as *excellent, ideal, perfect, unique, supreme,* cannot be compared; as:

> It is an *ideal* house to live in.
>
> He is a *perfect* rogue.
>
> It was an *excellent* piece of work.

(vii) Certain Comparative Adjectives ending in 'ior' have no positive or superlative; as:

> He is *inferior* to me in intelligence.
>
> He is *junior* to me in service.
>
> This event is *prior* to that.

Note that these Adjectives are followed by 'to' instead of 'than'.

IV. Correct use of Some Adjectives

1. Some, any:

Some is used in *Affirmative* sentences to express quantity or degree; *any* is used in Negative and *Interrogative* sentences to express quantity or degree; as:

> I shall buy *some* good books.
>
> I shall not buy *any* books.
>
> Has he written *any* book?

But *some* is used correctly in questions which are really commands or requests; as:

> Will you please lend me *some* money?
>
> Can you spare me *some* time on Monday?

2. Each, every:

Each is used in speaking two or more things; *every* is used only in speaking of more than two; as:

> *Each* boy was given a prize.
>
> Four boys sat on *each* bench.
>
> *Each* one of these stools is broken.
>
> It rained *every* day during Christmas.

3. Little, a little. the little:

Little means 'not much' (hardly any). It has, therefore, a negative meaning.

> There is *little* hope of his recovery. (i.e., he is not likely to recover).
>
> He showed *little* concern for him.
>
> He has *little* influence over him.

A little means 'some, though not much'. It is used in the positive sense; as:

> A *little* tact would have saved the situation.
>
> A *little* knowledge is a dangerous thing.
>
> The *little* means 'not much, but all that there is'; as
>
> He must make the best use of the *little* money he has.
>
> He has spent the *little* money he had.
>
> Tell me the *little* you know about him.

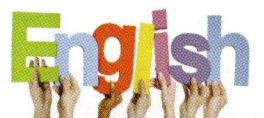

4. **Few, a few, the few:** These are Adjective of Quality.

    Few is used in a negative sense and means 'not many' (hardly way);

    > *Few* men are free from faults.

    > *Few* persons are so hopeless as drunkards.

    A *few* means 'some'. It is used in a positive sense and is the opposite to 'none'; as:

    > A *few* days' rest will help you recover.

    > He spoke a *few* words.

    The *few* means, 'not many, but all there are; as:

    > He has forgotten the *few* friends he had in his youth.

    > I have read *the few* books I have.

5. **Much, many:**

    Much denotes quantity while many denotes number; as:

    > My cow gives *much* milk.

    > We did not have *much* rain this summer.

    > *Much* can be said in his favor.

    > *Many* people came to meet him at his departure abroad.

    > *Many* happy returns of the day.

    Note. The modern tendency is to use *much* and *many* in negative sentences only. While 'a lot of, plenty of, a number of,' are used in affirmative sentences; as:

    > My cow gives *plenty of* milk.

    > A *number of* people came to meet him at his departure abroad.

    Note that 'many a' is followed by a singular noun and takes a singular verb; as:

    > *Many a* man visits the Taj every year.

6. **Few, less:**

    Few refers to number, while *less* refers to size or quantity; as:

    > The *less* said the better.

    > No *fewer* that five hundred people witnessed the show.

7. **Either, neither:**

    Either means one of the two or both; as:

    > *Either* book will do.

    > There were trees on *either* side of the road.

    Neither is a negative of *either* and means 'neither the one nor the other'.

    > I took *neither* side.

    > *Neither* of the two answer she gave was correct.

8. **All, whole:**

    All denotes numbers as well as quantity while 'whole' denotes quantity; as:

    > *All* men mourned his loss.

    > She was so hungry that she ate the 'whole' loaf.

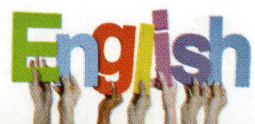

9. **Older, oldest; elder, eldest:**

Older and *oldest* refer to age and are used for both persons and things while *elder* and *eldest* apply to persons only and convey the idea of seniority or of the first born in a family. *Elder* is not followed by than.

    She is *older* than her brother.

    This is the *older* of the two trees.

    This is the *oldest* buildings in the town.

    He is my *elder* brother.

    Ram is the *eldest* of us all brothers.

    My elder brother is *older* than I.

10. **Further, farther:**

Farther refers to a greater distance between two points while *further* refers to something more in advance or something additional. *Farther* is, therefore, used where distance is referred to; as:

    Delhi is *farther* from Chennai than Nagpur is.

    Speak *further.*

11. **Later, latest; latter, last:**

Latter and *latest* imply time whereas *latter* and *last* imply position. *Latter* is used when there are only two things to be compared and *last*, when there are more than two.

Latter and *last* express order of time; as:

    I was *late* for school, but Sohan came *later* still and Ahmed was the *last* to come.

    This is the *last* chapter of this book.

    This is the *latest* edition of this book.

    Robin and Robert are brothers but the *latter* is more clever than the former.

12. **Another, any other, other:**

'*Another*' (with singular nouns) and '*other*' (with plural nouns) are used in affirmative statements; whereas '*any other*' is used in negative ones; as:

    We saw *another* man yesterday

    We did not see *any other* man yesterday.

13. **Each other, one another:**

Each other is used which two persons or things are meant while *one another* is used for more than two persons or things; as:

    The two brothers love *each other.*

    Little children love *one another.*

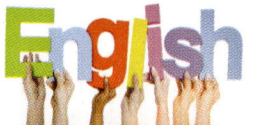

Errors in the use of Adjectives

An adjective is a word used to modify or qualify a noun or a pronoun as black, small, happy, proud, thin, etc.

Incorrect Sentences	*Correct Sentences*
❑ He is a worst student.	❑ He is a very bad student.
❑ He wrote a best book.	❑ He wrote a very good book.
❑ He is the cleverer than the two.	❑ He is the cleverer of the two.
❑ He is my most greatest friend.	❑ He is my greatest friend.
❑ This pen is much more cheaper than that.	❑ This pen is much cheaper than that.
❑ This boy is no less cleverer than that.	❑ This boy is no less clever than that.
❑ He is the abler of the three sons.	❑ He is the ablest of the three sons.
❑ O the dearest one, when shall we see you again?	❑ O dearest one, when shall we see you again?
❑ The doctor called to see him each other day.	❑ The doctor called to see him every other day.
❑ They all loved each other.	❑ They all loved one another.
❑ The two men struck one another.	❑ The two men struck each other.
❑ He is cleverer than any boy in the class.	❑ He is cleverer than any other boy in the class.
❑ I am very fond of these kind of flowers.	❑ I am very fond of this kind of flowers.
❑ Don't mix with those sort of people.	❑ Don't mix with that sort of people.
❑ He stood at the extremest edge of the rock.	❑ He stood at the extreme edge of the rock.
❑ Which was the best of the two?	❑ Which was the better of the two?
❑ Which was the most famous Rome or Athens?	❑ Which was more famous, Rome or Athens?
❑ He had the shortest memory than any other person.	❑ He had a shortest memory than any other person.
❑ There were trees on every side of the road.	❑ There were trees on each side of the road.
❑ I am senior by him in service.	❑ I am senior to him in service.
❑ My pen is superior than yours.	❑ My pen is superior to yours.
❑ Knowledge is more preferable than riches.	❑ Knowledge is preferable to riches.
❑ He was the laziest of all other workmen.	❑ He was the laziest of all workmen.
❑ He is as clever as any boy in the class.	❑ He is as clever as any other boy in the class.
❑ He has read the two first chapters of the book.	❑ He has read the first two chapters of the book.
❑ The population of Kolkata is greater than Delhi.	❑ The population of Kolkata is greater than that of Delhi.
❑ This is the last news.	❑ This is the latest news.
❑ He is our mutual friend.	❑ He is our common friend.
❑ He failed in the verbal test.	❑ He failed in the oral test.
❑ He is my older brother.	❑ He is my elder brother.
❑ I sent him an oral message.	❑ I sent him a verbal message.
❑ He is elder than his sister.	❑ He is older than his sister.
❑ He is house is nearest to mine.	❑ His house is next to mine.

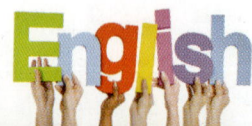

- He is the eldest of my sons.
- My oldest son died at the age of twelve.
- I prefer English than Hindi.
- She is senior than I by two years.

- He is the oldest of my sons.
- My eldest son died at the age of twelve.
- I prefer English to Hindi.
- She is senior to me by two years.

Use 'to' after prefer, senior, junior, preferable, superior and inferior, superior, Don't use 'more' before these words.

- You are wise than I.
- She is beautiful than her sister.

- You are wiser than me.
- She is more beautiful than her sister.

Use the comparative degree when there is a comparison between two persons or two things.

- He is more taller than I.
- I am more cleverer than you.

- He is taller than me.
- I am cleverer than you.

Double comparatives should be avoided.

- Manu is taller in his four brothers.
- She is more intelligent of all her class-mates.

- Manu is the tallest of his four brothers.
- She is the most intelligent of all her classmates.

Superlative Degree should be used when there is a comparison among more than two persons or things.

- Renuka is the most happiest girl.
- You are the most smartest girl.

- Renuka is the happiest girl.
- You are the smartest girl.

Double Superlatives should be avoided.

- Robin is better than any player in the team.
- Salman is more famous than any actor of Hindi films.

- Robin is better than any other player in the team.
- Salman is more famous than any other actor in Hindi films.

In a comparative degree use than any 'other'.

- You are the richest of all other friends.
- She is the most charming of all other girls.

- You are the richest of all the friends.
- She is the most charming of all the girls.

In a superlative degree, don't use 'other' or 'any other'. Definite article 'the' should be used before the superlative degree.

- Madhu is comparatively weaker in English.

- Madhu is comparatively weak in English.

Don't use comparative degree with 'comparatively'.

- She is cleverer than industrious.

- She is more clever than industrious.

When two qualities in the same person are compared we use 'more' before the positive degree.

- You are the most ideal teacher.
- Your performance is the most excellent.

- You are an ideal teacher.
- Your performance is excellent.

Certain adjectives, like ideal, unique, impossible. extreme, perfect, excellent; complete, entire, chief etc. do not admit of any comparison.

- She is my oldest daughter.
- You are the eldest player in the team.

- She is my eldest daughter.
- You are the oldest player in the team.

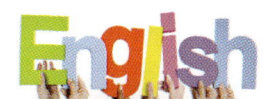

Older or oldest is used when comparative age is in question. Elder or eldest is used when comparative age of the members of the same family is in question. Moreover, 'older' and 'oldest' may be used both for persons and things but 'elder' and 'eldest' are used only for persons.

- Few girls are present in the class.
- A poor man has a few friends.

- A few girls were present in the class.
- A poor man has few friends.

'Few' is negative and means practically none. 'A few' is positive and means 'some'. 'The few' conveys negative as well positive idea. It means some but all.

- Little knowledge is a dangerous thing.
- I have spent little money I had.

- A little knowledge is a dangerous thing.
- I have spent the little money I had.

'Little' is negative and means 'not much'. A little means 'some'. 'The little' implies both negative and positive meanings, i.e., not much and all the money.

- No less than forty students were present.
- She needs no fewer than five kilos of rice.

- No fewer than forty students were present.
- She needs not less than five kilos of rice.

'Fewer' denotes number and 'less' refers to quantity.

- I have much friends.
- You have many works to do.
- Rashi bought as many as five kilos of wheat.
- Kareena needs as much as sixty rupees.

- I have many friends.
- You have much work to do.
- Rashi bought as much as five kilos of wheat.
- Kareena needs as many as sixty rupees.

'Many' and 'as many as' refer to number while 'much' and 'as much as' denote quantity.

- Reena came latter than Meena.
- Of these two friends the later is more intelligent.
- What is the last news?
- The latest chapter of this book is very interesting.

- Reena came later than Meena.
- Of these two friends, the latter is more intelligent.
- What is the latest news?
- The last chapter of this book is very interesting.

'Later' and 'latest' are used to show time. 'Latter' and 'last' are used to show position.

- Vanshika is the ablest and intelligent of all the girls.
- Mango is the best and sweet fruit.

- Vanshika is the ablest and the most intelligent of all the girls.
- Mango is the best and the sweetest fruit.

When adjectives are used for the same subject and one of them is superlative, the other one must also be superlative.

- I shall not buy some chocolates.
- The teacher gave him any books.

- I shall not buy any chocolate.
- The teacher gave him some books.

'Any' is used in the negative sentence while 'some' is used in a positive one. Both can be used in the Interrogative also.

- He knows both girls.
- Ritesh lost both legs.
- I shall attend both meetings.

- He knows both the girls.
- Ritesh lost both of his legs.
- I shall attend both the meetings.

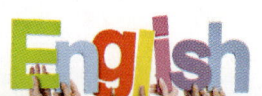

Use 'article 'the' after 'both' when it is used as an adjective. It is placed before the noun or possessive pronoun.

- ❑ Mumbai is further from Delhi than Chennai.
- ❑ Bombay is farther from Mumbai than Chennai.
- ❑ The PM made no farther remarks.
- ❑ The P.M. made no further remarks.

'Farther', refers to distance while 'further', means more or additional.

- ❑ Smeera is rather richer than her friend.
- ❑ Smeera is richer than her friend.
- ❑ I am rather happier than you.
- ❑ I am happier than you.

'Rather' has force of comparative. Avoid the use of double comparatives.

- ❑ The climate of Srinagar is cooler than Shimla.
- ❑ The climate of Srinagar is cooler than that of Shimla.
- ❑ My notes are superior to you.
- ❑ My notes are superior to those of you (or yours).

Comparison is always made between things of the same kind.

- ❑ The whole India loved Nehru and Gandhi.
- ❑ The whole of India loved Nehru and Gandhi.
- ❑ His all friends were insincere.
- ❑ All his friends were insincere.

When 'whole' is used as and adjective it is preceeded by 'the' and followed by 'of'. All' is placed before the noun or possessive noun?

- ❑ She is two years smaller than me.
- ❑ She is two years younger than me.
- ❑ You are two inches younger than him.
- ❑ You are two inches smaller than him.

'Young' or 'old' show age while, 'big' or 'small' show size.

- ❑ Sugar tastes sweetly.
- ❑ Sugar tastes sweet.
- ❑ Quinine tastes bitterly.
- ❑ Quinine tastes bitter.

Use an adjective (not an adverb) after such verbs as look, feel, taste, smell, etc.

- ❑ I do not like these kind of books.
- ❑ I do not like this kind of books.
- ❑ These sort of pictures are not liked by me.
- ❑ These sorts of pictures are not liked by me.

'Kind' and 'sort' should be used in the singular.

- ❑ Rich should help poor.
- ❑ The rich should help the poor.
- ❑ Only brave deserve the fair.
- ❑ Only the brave deserve the fair.

If we place 'the' before an adjective, it becomes a plural noun.

- ❑ Karan and Manu are brothers, the first is wiser than the second.
- ❑ Karan and Manu are brothers, the former is wiser than the latter.
- ❑ The best team won the final match.
- ❑ The better team won the final match.
- ❑ Car, scooter or bicycle, either will do.
- ❑ Car, scooter or bicycle, any will do.
- ❑ He behaved friendly when I met him.
- ❑ He behaved in a friendly manner when I met him.
- ❑ Television is terrible harmful for eyes.
- ❑ Television is terribly harmful for the eyes.
- ❑ I have strong headache.
- ❑ I have severe headache.
- ❑ He is my fast enemy.
- ❑ He is my sworn enemy.
- ❑ He has money enough to support you.
- ❑ He has enough money to support you.
- ❑ This room is too much small for me.
- ❑ This room is much too small for me.
- ❑ She is suffering from severe cold.
- ❑ She is suffering from bad cold.

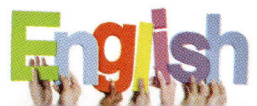

NOTES

Chapter 7

Conjunctions

CONJUNCTIONS

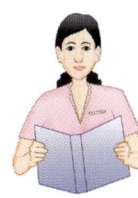

Conjunctions are words used to join words, phrases and groups of words. There are two fundamentally different types of conjunctions: coordinating conjunctions and subordinating conjunctions.

Conjunctions are mainly of two types:
1.   Coordinate conjunctions
2.   Subordinate conjunctions

Let's discuss them one by one in detail:

Coordinate Conjunctions

Observe the following sentences:
- ❑ He is old *yet* he can run fast
- ❑ Two *and* two make four
- ❑ Obey me *or* be off.

Each sentence has a conjunction printed in bold letters. It joins two sentences of equal rank. If we take away the conjunction, two independent sentences are there, Neither of them depends on the other. So, each of these conjunctions is a **coordinate conjunction**.

A coordinate conjunction is the conjunction that joins together words, phrases or sentences of equal rank.

Coordinating conjunctions are words like: and, but, and, or which join words or group of words of equal status. Subordinating conjunctions join group of words of unequal status. Now, we will deal only with coordinating conjunctions.

Here are some examples using coordinating conjunctions to join single words (The joined words are underlined):
- ❑ Tarzan loves coconuts <u>and</u> bananas.
- ❑ Jane wanted coconuts <u>or</u> bananas.
- ❑ Tarzan's parents were poor <u>but</u> honest.

Here are examples using the remaining coordinating conjunctions to join group of words (The joined group of words are underlined):

- Jane <u>and</u> Tarzan are in love, <u>yet</u> they still can't agree on their china pattern.
- It was my turn to cook, <u>so</u> we had something simple.
- We turned back, <u>for</u> it was getting dark.
- I didn't want to leave <u>nor</u> did anybody else.

Kinds of Coordinate Conjunctions

Coordinate conjunctions are of four kinds:
- Cumulative Conjunctions
- Alternative Conjunctions
- Adversative Conjunctions
- Illative Conjunctions

Cumulative Conjunctions

Observe the following sentences:
- Jack came in and John went out.
- He plays football as well as hockey.
- He is rich and generous too.
- The robbers gagged the traveller also they beat him up.

Each sentence has a conjunction which joins one statement to another with a sense of addition or commutation. So, it is a cumulative conjunction.

Alternative Conjunctions

Observe the following sentences:
- Walk fast **or** you will miss the train
- She must work hard **else** she will fail.
- Pay my money **otherwise** I shall thrash you.
- Either he is really mad **or** he just pretends to be mad.

Each conjunction joins two statements expressing an alternative so, it is an alternative conjunction.

Adversative Conjunctions

Observe the following sentences:
- He is brilliant **but** the brother is dull.
- He is poor **yet** he is honest.
- I am strong **still** I do not boast.
- She is charming **however** she is not proud.
- The goods are blessed **while** the bad have to suffer.
- Do anything **only** don't bother me.

Each conjunction joins two statements expressing a contrast or opposition So, it is an adversative conjunction

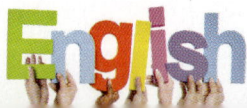

Illative Conjunctions

Observe the following sentences:
- ❐ It is time to take tea so let us go home.
- ❐ He was at fault therefore he was scolded.
- ❐ You must take rest for you are unwell.
- ❐ The triangles are congruent hence they are equal.

Each conjunction joins two statements expressing an inference or illation so, it is an illative conjunction.

Subordinate Conjunctions

Subordinate Conjunctions express a number of things.

Subordinate conjunctions express time, place, manner, condition, comparison, cause or reason, purpose, effect and contrast.

1. **Time** : *when, while, as soon as, before, till, until, no sooner.... than.*
   I don't know *when* he will come.
   Wait *till* you are called.
   He played *while* I worked.

2. **Place** : *where, wherever, whether,* etc.
   I shall accompany you *wherever* you go.
   He does not know *where* he comes from.

3. **Manner** : *as, so far as, as if,* etc.
   He is a good man so *far as* his nature is concerned.
   You should behave *as* you have been told.
   He eats *as if* he were an animal.

4. **Condition** : *if, unless, provided, whatever.*
   You can be punished *if* you don't finish your homework.
   I shall not get to his house *unless* he comes to me first.
   We can show good result *provided* that we cooperate with our teachers.

5. **Comparison** : *so.......as, as.........as, than,* etc.
   Eat green vegetables *as* much *as* you can.
   Suneeta is taller *than* her brother.
   Bombay is not *so* big *as* Calcutta.

6. **Reason or cause** : *because, since,* etc.
   I like him *because* he helped me.
   Since he stood first in the class, he must be a good student.

7. **Purpose** : *in order, so that, lest,* etc.
   He reads a lot *so that* he may top the class.
   Walk carefully *lest* you should stumble.

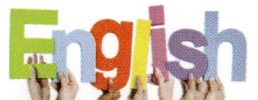

8. **Effect** : *so......that, that,* etc.

He ran so fast *that* he got the first place.

That you may get good marks, a tutor has been engaged for you.

9. **Contrast or concession** : *though, although, however,* etc.

Though he works hard yet he does not get good marks.

Although he is poor, he is honest.

He will never succeed, *however* hard he tries.

USAGE OF CONJUNCTIONS

Since

❑ *Since* is a conjunction of time and implies 'from which time'. It is preceded by a verb in the Present Perfect or Perfect Tense and is followed by a verb in the Past Indefinite Tense.
  - It is long *since* I heard from you.
  - It is now two weeks *since* the schools broke up for the holidays.
  - *Since* is also used to show reason; as,
  - *Since* you did not turn up in time, you have lost the chance.

❑ **Unless, until, lest:**

Unless and *lest* show condition; *until* means time before; *Unless* means 'if not'; *lest* means 'so that......not'.
  - He worked hard *lest* he should fail.
  - He cannot read *unless* he wears spectacles.
  - He remained a minor *until* he was seventeen years old.

Note that *lest* is followed by *should*. We do not use 'not' after *unless* or *until*.

❑ *As long as* (or *so long as*) refers to time during which an action or event takes place; e.g.,
  - *As long as* the world lasts, such happenings will take place.
  - *So long as* the bombardment continues, we must keep indoors.

❑ *While* is both a Subordinate and a Coordinate Conjunction. As a Subordinate Conjunction, it denotes 'time'.
  - Make hay *while* the sun shines.

As a Coordinate Conjunction, *while* denotes a contrast; as:

He is clever *while* his brother is a duffer.

❑ *However* is also used as a Subordinate as well as a Coordinate Conjunction. As a Subordinate Conjunction, it precedes some Adjective or Adverb.
  - *However* hard he may work, he cannot succeed.
  - As a Coordinate Conjunction, it stands along and is not placed in the beginning of a clause.

❑ He did not work hard; *however* he Passed.

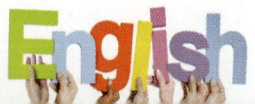

Errors in the use of Conjunctions

A conjunction is a part of speech that connects words; clauses or sentences, or shows relations between sentences as: and, but, as-as, either, or, as well as, unless, etc.

Incorrect Sentences	*Correct Sentences*
❑ Though she is poor but she is honest.	❑ Though she is poor yet she is honest.
❑ I like such boys who are industrious.	❑ I like such boys as are industrious.
❑ Work hard lest you may not fail.	❑ Work hard lest you should fail.
❑ No sooner the sun rose; the mist disappeared.	❑ No sooner did the sun rise; than the mist disappeared.
❑ Hardly had we reached the ground, than the match started.	❑ Hardly had we reached the ground, when the match started.

Unless is already negative. It means 'If not'.

❑ Unless you do not speak the truth, I shall not forgive you.	❑ Unless you speak the truth, I shall not forgive you.

'Until' is already negative; so don't use 'do not' with it.

❑ Wait here until I do not return.	❑ Wait here until I return.
❑ The choice is between glorious death and shameful life.	❑ The choice is between glorious death and shameful life.

Function of 'or' is to express alternative or choice but 'and' denotes addition.

❑ College life is charming and school life is dull.	❑ College life is charming but school life is dull.
❑ You are very rich but you help the poor.	❑ You are very rich and you help the poor.

'And' joins two words or clauses of the same nature while 'but' is to join two antithetical clauses.

❑ Lions are both found in Asia and Africa.	❑ Lions are found both in Asia and Africa.
❑ Both as well as Sonu and Monu are lazy.	❑ Both Sonu and Monu are lazy.

'Both' should be followed by and not by 'as well as', moreover, it should be used immediately before the words to which it refers.

❑ Both Parveen and Vishal are not clothe merchants.	❑ Neither Parveen nor Vishal is a clothe merchant.

'Both' is used in the positive sense. In the negative sense we should use 'neither-nor'.

❑ Neither did she attend the class nor he.	❑ Neither did she attend the class nor did he.
❑ Neither did Manik finish the work nor his brother finished it.	❑ Neither did Manik finish the work nor did his brother finish it.

If neither is followed by an auxiliary verb, nor should also be followed by the same auxiliary verb.

❑ My pen is as good if not better than yours.	❑ My pen is as good as yours if not better than yours.

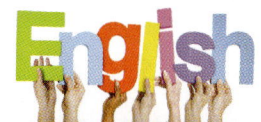

Use of as:

- She is as noble or even nobler than he.
- She is as noble as for even nobler than he.

Don't use 'because' and 'therefore' in the same sentence.

- Because she is dull, therefore she cannot pass.
- She is dull, therefore, cannot pass.

'Supposing' and 'If' and 'when' and then' should not be used together.

- Supposing if you miss the bus where will you go.
- Supposing (or if) you miss the bus where will you go.

- When you abuse me then I shall punish you.
- When you abuse me, I shall punish you.

- Do not be indifferent about your health.
- Do not be indifferent to your health.

- We should pray God daily.
- We should pray to God daily.

- The soldier saluted to the officer.
- The soldier saluted the officer.

- She is very anxious for the health of her children.
- She is very anxious about the health of her children.

- He failed as he lacks in common sense.
- He failed as he lacks common sense.

- They are leaving to America tomorrow.
- They are leaving for America tomorrow.

- She always ride on a car.
- She always rides in a car.

- The cat pounced at the mouse.
- The cat pounced on (or upon) the mouse.

- My child is precious for me.
- My child is precious to me.

- The publisher ran out a thousand copies of his book.
- The publisher ran off a thousand copies of his book.

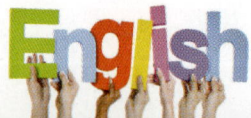

Chapter 8

Interjection

The word Interjection means 'sudden interference.'

Sometimes a speaker interjects words almost in a shouting tone. They startle the hearer as they express a sudden feeling of the mind—joy, grief, surprise, approval, rebuke, hatred or attention etc.

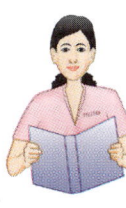

Observe the following sentences:

1. **Hello**! how r u?   *(attention)*
2. **Hurrah**! we have won the match.   *(joy)*
3. **Alas**! I am ruined.   *(grief)*
4. **Ha**! what a charming scenery.   *(surprise)*
5. **Bravo**! a nice hit.   *(approval)*
6. **Lo**! there comes daddy.   *(attention)*
7. **Hush**! The baby is asleep.   *(attention)*
8. **Fie**! how unworthy of you?   *(rebuke)*
9. **Pooh**! how dirty you are?   *(hatred)*

Each word in bold letters expresses sudden feeling of the mind. These feelings are generally exclaimed so, they are called exclamations or interjections.

An Interjection is a word that expresses a 'sudden' feeling of the mind.

Each exclamation is followed by a mark of exclamation (!).

Exclamations include interjected blessings, wishes and prayers also.

NOTES

Chapter 9

Determiners

INTRODUCTION

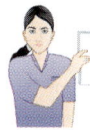

Determiners are the words that are used before a noun to determine or fix its meaning. Determiner is a kind of adjective. The only difference between an adjective and a determiner is that:

An adjective qualifies (adds something to) a noun as, the blue sky, tall girls, red rose, difficult question, sweet mangoes, etc.

A determiner limits the noun that follows it as, a book, an inkpot, the Ramayana, some boys, any book, a few difficulties, a little rest.

About fifty expressions (one or more words) in English are traditionally included among the adjectives, whose major grammatical function is to signal that a noun is followed, are called noun determiners by modern grammarians.

The following are the determiners:

- ❑ **Articles:** A, an, the
- ❑ **Adjectives of number:** Any, some, much, little, a good deal of, a great deal of, number.
- ❑ **Adjectives of quantity:** Any, some, each, every, either, neither, (a) few, both (the), many, more, most, a, all, a lot of, one, two, three, etc. another, other, several, enough.
- ❑ **Demonstrative adjectives:** This, that, these, those.
- ❑ **Interrogative adjectives:** What, which, whose, whichever, whatever.
- ❑ **Possessive adjectives:** My, your, his, her, its, our, their.

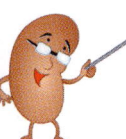

Read these sentences:

- ❑ *My country* is India.
- ❑ *This story* is interesting.
- ❑ *Which boy* is your brother?
- ❑ I want *some salt*.
- ❑ There aren't *many trees* here.

The words *my, this, which, some* and *many* are followed by the nouns *country, story, boy, salt,* and *trees.*

- ❏ *'My'* is a possessive adjective.
- ❏ *'This'* is a demonstrative adjective.
- ❏ *'Which'* is an interrogative adjective.
- ❏ *'Some'* is an adjective of quantity.
- ❏ *'Many'* is an adjective of number.

Such adjectives are called determiners. They are followed by a noun.

Note: A determiner may consist of just one word or a group of words.

Here is a list of different kinds of adjectives used as determiners:

ADJECTIVES OF NUMBER

any	some	each	every
either	neither	both(the)	(a)few
many	more	most	many a
all	a lot of	lots of	one, two, etc.
another	other	several	enough

ADJECTIVES OF QUANTITY

any	some	much	(a)little
no	a great deal	a lot	lots of

INTERROGATIVE ADJECTIVES

what	which	whose
whichever	whatever	

POSSESSIVE ADJECTIVES

my	your	his	her
its	our	their	
these	those		

The indefinite articles (a, an) are used before a singular countable noun. Countable nouns are names of things which can be counted.

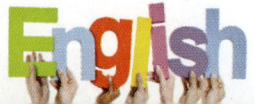

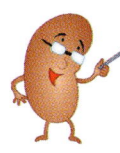

Read these phrases:

A book, a pen, a man, a hat, a fan, a table.

❏ 'a' is used before nouns beginning with a consonant sound.

An apple, an uncle, an egg, an animal

1. 'an' is used before nouns beginning with a vowel (a, e, i, o, u) sound.
2. The initial sound, not the spelling is important.
   a. The following words begin with vowel letters but not with vowel sounds.
      They, therefore, take 'a' before them. For example, a university, a one-rupee note, a European, a unit.
   b. The following words begin with consonant letters but with vowel sounds:
      They, therefore, take 'an' before them. For example, an hour, an heir, an M.P. , an S.P.
3. If a countable noun is preceded by an adjective, 'a/an' is used before the adjective according to its initial sound.
   • He is an honest man.
   • It is a useful book.

The definite article 'the' can be used with both countable nouns (singular as well as plural) and uncountable nouns. Its main purpose is to specify a person, place or thing. For example, there is a duster on my desk, get me the duster.

Do not use 'the' before:

1. Abstract nouns, plural nouns, proper nouns, names of materials, meals, colors when used in general sense.
2. The names of games.
3. Expressions, like, 'all day', 'all night', 'by train', 'by air'.
   a. 'Some' is generally used in affirmative sentences with uncountable and plural countable nouns:
      ▪ I have some good ideas on the subject.
      'Some' can be used in questions when we expect 'yes' answer.
      ▪ Would you like some coffee?
   b. 'Any' is generally used in questions when you ask whether something exists or not. It is also used in negative sentences to say that something does not exist.
      ▪ Are there any jobs that women can't do?
      'Any' is also used in affirmative sentences before plural nouns and uncountable nouns when you refer to a quantity of something which may or may not exist.
      ▪ You can stop at any time you like.
   c. Little and much refer to amount or quantity. 'Little' is used to emphasize that there is only a small amount of something.
      'Much' emphasizes a large amount. Both are used with uncountable nouns.
      ▪ We have made little program.
      ▪ Do you watch much television?

'A little' refers to a small amount of something without any emphasis
      ▪ I am having a little trouble these days.

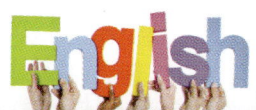

d. 'Few' and 'many' refer to number. These are used before plural countable nouns. 'Few' emphasizes a small number.
    - Few students were present today.

    'A few' refers to a small number without any emphasis.
    - They stayed in London for a few days.

e. 'More', 'less' and 'fewer' are comparative determiners.

    'More' is used before plural and uncountable nouns to refer to a quantity or amount of something which is greater than another quantity or amount.
    - He does more work than do.

    'Less' is used to refer to an amount of something that is smaller than another amount. It is usually used before uncountable nouns.
    - He finds less time for his hobbies.

    'Fewer' is used to refer to a group of things that is smaller than another group before plural nouns.
    - There are fewer trees here.

f. 'All' is a plural verb when followed by countable plural nouns. It includes every person or thing of a particular kind.
    - 'All' is a singular verb when it is followed by an uncountable noun.

g. 'Both' is used to talk about two persons or things of the same kind. It is used to emphasize that the two persons or things are involved, rather than one. It is often followed by 'and'.
    - He held mangoes in both hands.

h. 'Either' is used when one or the other of two people or things are involved. 'Neither' is used when none of the two persons or things is involved
    - I can agree in neither of the cases.

    'Either' can mean both of the two things especially when used with 'end' or 'side'
    - They stood on either side of the bed.

i. 'Each' and 'every' refer to all the members of a group of persons or things.

    When we think about the members as individuals, we use 'each' and when we make a general statement about all of them we use 'every'.
    - Each seat was covered with a white cover.
    - Every child would have milk every day.

j. 'One': When we talk or write about a group of people or things or want to say something about a particular member of the group, we use 'one'.

    It is used instead of 'a' or 'an' and is more emphatic.
    - One should do one's duty.

k. 'Another' is used with singular countable nouns to talk about an additional person or thing of the same type as has already been mentioned.

    He opened another shop last month.

    'Other' is used with plural nouns or sometimes with uncountable nouns.
    - Other people must have thought like this.

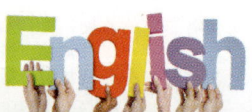

l. 'Enough' is used before uncountable nouns or plural nouns to say that there is as much of something as is needed, or as many things as are needed.

- It had enough room to store all the information.

m. 'Most' indicates nearly all of a group or amount.

- Most people recover but the disease is fatal.

n. 'Several' usually indicates an imprecise number that is not very large, but is more than two.

- Had seen her several times before.

Errors in the use of Articles

A, An, The

A, an = Indefinite Articles

The = Definite Article

'A' is used before a noun that expresses something which is individual but not selected or distinguished from other things of the same kind.

'An' is used before a noun beginning with a vowel or before a word beginning with a silent 'h' or before a consonant which sounds like a vowel.

'The' is used before the names of rivers, seas, buildings, nationality or community, superlative degree of adjectives, names of a class or group of people, group of islands, directions, heavenly bodies, etc.

No article is used:

a. before proper, material or abstract nouns

b. before the names of days and months

c. before the names of arts and subjects

d. before the names of regular meals

e. before the names of sports, diseases, seasons and festivals

f. before certain titles and names which indicate relationship

g. before a noun used in its widest sense

h. before plural nouns, used to denote a class is general sense

i. before the names of the things single in kind

j. before collective nouns used in a general sense

Incorrect Sentences	*Correct Sentences*
❑ This is a news to me.	❑ This is news to me.
❑ He is a M.A., M.Ed.	❑ He is an M.A., M.Ed.
❑ She is a honest lady.	❑ She is an honest lady.
❑ Ganga has overflowed its banks.	❑ The Ganga has overflowed its banks.
❑ The game came to end.	❑ The game came to an end.
❑ He is a honourable man.	❑ He is an honourable man.
❑ She returned after a hour.	❑ She returned after an hour.
❑ It is quarter past three now.	❑ It is a quarter past three now.
❑ The English is spoken by English	❑ English is spoken by the English.
❑ The stitch in time saves nine.	❑ A stitch in time saves nine.

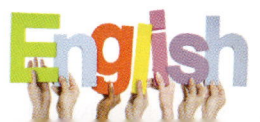

- ❑ Let us go and bathe in river.
- ❑ More one has, more one wants.
- ❑ You are a man who can do it.
- ❑ We shall start after the breakfast.
- ❑ He has settled in United States.
- ❑ Speak a truth and do not tell the lie.
- ❑ Girls of this class are very intelligent.
- ❑ The boys leave the school at four o'clock.
- ❑ There is nothing on the earth so pure as the sea-air.
- ❑ Elizabeth, the Queen of England, ruled very wisely.

- ❑ Let us go and bathe in the river.
- ❑ The more one has, the more one wants.
- ❑ You are the man who can do it.
- ❑ We shall start after breakfast.
- ❑ He has settled in the United States.
- ❑ Speak the truth and do not tell a lie.
- ❑ The girls of this class are very intelligent.
- ❑ The boys leave school at four O'clock.
- ❑ There is nothing on earth so pure as sea-air.

- ❑ Elizabeth, Queen of England, ruled very wisely.

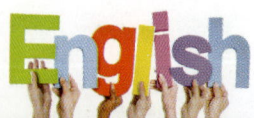

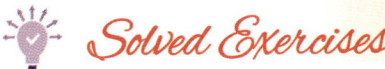

Solved Exercises

I. **Fill in the blanks with suitable determiners:**

1. There aren't _____ good restaurants in this town.
2. We need _____ wood for the fire.
3. Don't worry about lunch. I've bought _____ sandwiches.
4. Shall we have _____ fish? This restaurant is famous for it.
5. You need _____ scissors to cut the paper.
6. Could you bring me _____ glass, please?
7. Have you got _____ brothers and sisters?
8. If you need _____ paper, there is a box on the shelf.
9. I think you owe me _____ money.
10. Would you like _____ rice with your chicken?

II. **Fill in the blanks with suitable determiners:**

1. We'd like to stay longer, but we don't have _____ time.
2. My shirt is dry now. Have you got _____ iron?
3. Could you give me _____ information please?
4. Jack bought _____ glass to repair the broken windows.
5. Can you buy me _____ paper? There's an article I want to read.
6. There are _____ people in the garden.
7. How _____ pages do you have to read?
8. How _____ homework have you got?
9. Are there _____ students in your class?
10. Could you give him _____ information?

III. **Fill in the blanks with suitable determiners:**

1. I'll try to call you tonight, but I don't have _____ time.
2. How _____ times do you brush your teeth every day?
3. Shall I make some more tea? I didn't make _____ .
4. Kitty only ate a sandwich because she didn't have _____ money.
5. There weren't _____ seats so some of us had to stand up.
6. Have you got _____ work, or do you want to come to the cinema?
7. We invited lots of people to our party, but not _____ turned up.
8. You'll have to share, because there aren't _____ books.

IV. **Fill in the blanks with suitable determiners:**

1. How _____ does this cost?
2. Jame has got too _____ luggage.

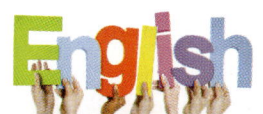

3. Sorry we haven't got _____ cakes left, not a single one.

4. If you haven't got _____ money I can lend you some.

5. There are too _____ people in this room, it's crowded.

6. How _____ books have you got at home?

7. Are there _____ cinemas in this town?

8. There isn't _____ hot water.

V. **Fill in the blanks with suitable determiners:**

1. Do you have _____ minutes? I'd like to ask you _____ questions. I need _____ more information.

2. Devender's previous employer promoted her because she makes _____ mistakes in her work.

3. Unfortunately, he has _____ friends.

4. We're planning to spend _____ days with my relatives and then _____ days with my husband's relatives.

5. I was hungry, so I ate _____ nuts.

6. Because the family is very poor, the children have _____ toys. Both parents have to work, so they have _____ time to spend with their children.

7. Into each life, _____ rain must fall.

8. Hitasha likes sweet tea. She usually adds _____ honey to her tea. Sometimes she adds _____ milk too.

ANSWERS

I. Any, some, some, some, some, a, any, some, some, some.

II. Enough, an, some, some, a, many, many, much, many, enough.

III. Much, many, much, much, many, much, many, many.

IV. Much, much, any, any/enough, many, many, any, any.

V. A few-a few-a little, few, few, a few -a few, a few, few-little, a little, a little-a little.

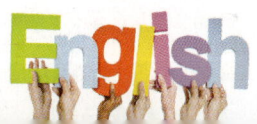

Practice Exercises

I. **The following exercise has been solved to help you understand the use of determiners:**

1. He has <u>center</u> chance of winning the match.
2. <u>The</u> apple is on <u>the</u> table.
3. <u>An</u> apple <u>a</u> day, keeps <u>the</u> doctor away.
4. There were tall trees on <u>either</u> side of the road.
5. We have <u>enough</u> food for ten people.
6. They know <u>their</u> duty.
7. May I have <u>some</u> milk?
8. The teacher did not give him <u>any</u> book.
9. Please give me <u>some</u> water.
10. He sold <u>the few</u> books he had.

II. **Fill in the blanks with a, an or the:**

1. _____ gold is _____ precious metal.
2. Bicycle is made of _____ steel and _____ Rubber.
3. _____ umbrella protects us from _____ rain.
4. _____ wheat and _____ cotton are grown in Punjab.
5. I like jam on _____ piece of _____ bread.
6. I met _____ European on my way to _____ college.
7. This is _____ house made of _____ stone.
8. We can never forget _____ kindness which reached us.
9. They put all _____ money earned into _____ box.
10. She lay unconscious for _____ hour and _____ half.

III. **Fill in the blanks with some, any, much or many:**

1. Would you lend me _____ books?
2. How _____ rice do you need?
3. Can I have _____ coffee?
4. He made _____ mistake in his letter.
5. The beggar hasn't _____ money.
6. How_____milk do you drink every day?
7. How_____stories does this book contain?
8. The ration shop did not have _____ sugar, so I came without it.
9. How _____ boys are present in the class?
10. I haven't _____ time.

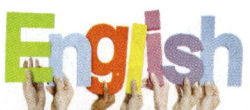

IV. Fill in the blanks with suitable determiners:

1. _____ people were killed in the accident.
2. Bring _____vegetables from the market.
3. _____ honest man is___work of God.
4. Anita resembles_____sister.
5. The camel is _____ship of _____desert.
6. Don't you have _____relatives in Chandigarh?
7. How _____mangoes are there in the box?
8. I would like _____more tea.
9. ____apple contains _____ sugar.
10. How _____sugar is there in _____container?

V. Fill in the blanks with the determiners:

1. You must take care _____ health.
2. I always mind my _____ handwriting.
3. _____ Tripti nor her sister came here.
4. _____ boy has come.
5. I don't want _____ tea now.
6. I'm afraid _____ people don't like you at all.
7. We have _____ funds to raise a memorial.
8. He is so poor that he has _____ money.
9. She doesn't have _____ sense.
10. _____ intentions are quite clear.
11. Do you want _____ food?
12. _____ way did you follow?

VI. Fill in the blanks with the determiners:

1. He has _____ milk now, because the cat drank away _____ milk he had.
2. A cow has _____ legs.
3. I have got _____ pens. So I can lend you _____ pens.
4. _____ people have arrived. Let's begin the show.
5. Nature has given us _____ eyes.
6. He has two sons _____ the sons are educated.
7. _____ house has four rooms.
8. _____ learning is a dangerous thing.
9. _____ man loves freedom.
10. _____ hope is lost.
11. He is a man of _____ words.
12. I have visited _____ senior secondary schools located in this backward tehsil.
13. He is a complete duffer. He has _____ sense.

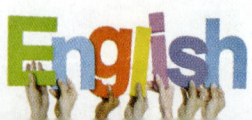

VII.   Fill in the blanks with 'a' or 'an':

1. _____ bad tooth may cause pain.
2. This is _____ chair.
3. I have _____ orange.
4. What _____ exciting match!
5. What _____ happy girl!
6. Is it _____ egg?
7. _____ apple _____ day keeps the doctor away.
8. He is _____ coward.
9. His brother is _____ university student.
10. His uncle is _____ M.P.
11. He considers himself to be _____ Shakespeare.
12. Kurukshetra is _____ historical town in Haryana.
13. _____ hundred rupees will not do.
14. How much _____ dozen are you selling the oranges?
15. Two of _____ trade seldom agree.
16. He made _____ journey round the world.
17. He gave me _____ toy.
18. Do not make _____ noise.
19. _____ honest man never tells a lie.
20. I gave him _____ one-rupee note.

VIII.   Fill in the blanks with 'a' or 'an' where necessary. In case nothing applies, fill it with 'X':

1. _____ horse is _____ animal.
2. _____ cow gives us _____ milk.
3. He drank _____ cup of _____ tea.
4. _____ chair is made of _____ wood.
5. _____ cat eats _____ meal.
6. He filled _____ pen with _____ ink.
7. _____ cake is made from _____ flour and _____ milk.
8. _____ butter and _____ cheese are made from _____ milk.
9. This ring is made of _____ gold.
10. Do you like _____ coffee?
11. He is fond of _____ music.
12. _____ cow feeds on _____ grass.
13. _____ paper is _____ useful thing.
14. There is _____ dirt on this plate.
15. We need _____ air to live.
16. This is _____ class of forty students.
17. He can write _____ poetry. Can you write _____ poem?
18. Add _____ ice to _____ water.

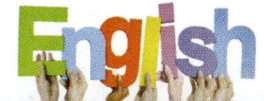

19. He is _____ artist.
20. He doesn't take _____ sugar.

IX. **Fill in the blanks with suitable determiners. In some cases more than one determiner is possible:**

1. Shall I bring you _____ cup of coffee?
2. Have you got _____ books? "Yes, I have one or two."
3. You should mind _____ work.
4. _____ houses belong to me.
5. _____ people don't like to talk to strangers.
6. This is a simple question. I have _____ doubt about it.
7. He is _____ expert in _____ subject. He has read _____ books on it.
8. I'm afraid you don't know that nobody likes _____ bad manners.
9. I can never forget _____ days. I was very happy at that time.
10. He can build _____ house. He has _____ funds.
11. _____ shop is the nearest?
12. He has _____ house. His brother has two.
13. _____ men are born great.
14. I rang him but there was _____ reply
15. There are trees on _____ side of the road.

X. **Fill in the blanks with suitable determiners:**

1. Cancer is _____ dreaded disease which kills thousands of people all over _____ world. Medical researchers have not been able to find _____ cause and so have not been able to find _____ effective cure for it. Experiments are, however going to find out _____ cause and _____ cure. _____ conquest of _____ disease will be great victory for medical science.

2. In city, there lived small girl of about five. _____ little girl had mother and no one else. They lived together, but _____ life of _____ hardships _____ mother was _____ charwoman. Income was meager. But _____ girl was fed, dressed and had shoes on _____ feet. And _____ mother bought different goodies from hospital sometimes candy, sometimes apples.

3. A man had _____ goose that laid _____ golden egg _____ day. _____ day___wife tempted him, saying, "We shall take out all____golden eggs at once. So___man killed goose. But they didn't find golden eggs inside it. Their all____hopes of getting rich quickly were dashed to___ground.

4. My gloomy thoughts probably stem from _____ accident. I had ___years ago. I was crossing _____ street with _____ wife after__ lovely meal together, and____ next minute ___car had hit me and knocked me into___ wife. She was thrown into the ___lane and struck by ___car coming from opposite direction.

5. ___next day, soon after they had set out they found themselves in___ lovely part of country.___ road ran through ___dried up river and on__ side of that rose cliffs, rugged,

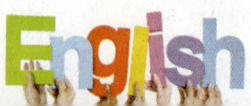

rocky cliffs, which seemed to cut them off from___ sight and sound of ___other human beings. It was ___hot day. ___was still, and__ sun, shining down on them, seemed to set them on fire. Nor were there____ trees to give___ shade. So they walked on.

6. I was one of ___ happiest souls on earth. ___ sweeping of ___room was ___ college examination. I have passed ___ examinations since then, but I have always felt that this was___ best one I ever passed.

7. In former times when ___ window pane in ___house got broken you would call___ glazier to put in___ new one, or if ___ lights fused electrician would be sent for to put them right. Nowadays people are___ own glaziers and electricians.

8. ___ things are more restful at ___ beginning of ___holiday than ___ long journey in ___ swift train, during which traveller in corner seat facing engine and controlling ___window does not read, nor even think, but watches ___ country unroll itself, mile after mile, ___ moving panorama.

9. If I had ___ son I would take him from school at ___ age of fourteen, not ___ moment later, and put him for two years in ___ commercial house.

10. ___ man's dog stands by him in prosperity and in poverty, in health and sickness. He will sleep on ___ cold ground, where ___wintry winds blow and ___snow drives fiercely, if only he may be by___ master's side. He will kiss ___ hand that has ___ food to offer, he will lick ___wounds and sores that come in encounter with ___ roughness of ___world.

THE USE OF DETERMINERS

XI. Fill in the blanks with suitable determiners:

1. It is very difficult to get _____ good job.
2. We wait for _____ postman every day.
3. There isn't _____ paper for me to write on.
4. Is there _____ food for me? I'm very hungry.
5. Some boys have come to college without _____ knowledge of English.
6. How _____ milk will be needed for breakfast?
7. Her father was _____ eminent artist.
8. _____ boys who called on the Prime Minister have gone back.
9. Please give me _____ rice.
10. I have already spent _____ few rupees I had.
11. The Ganges is _____ holy river.
12. I shall not buy _____ mangoes.
13. How _____ trees are there in your garden?
14. French is _____ easy language.
15. I have bought _____ umbrella.
16. I have read _____ book I bought last week.
17. He is _____ honourable man.
18. Will you please lend me _____ money?

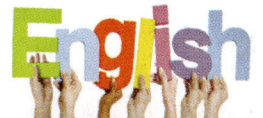

19. He is _____ one-eyed person.
20. She hasn't _____ blue sarees.
21. These are _____ students who have broken the chair.
22. The teacher asked _____ easy question.
23. He is _____ able man.
24. Ramesh is _____ best of all.
25. Please give me _____ one-rupee note.
26. How _____ stories does this book contain?
27. His father is _____ university professor.
28. I brought _____ ice-cream for the children.
29. There is _____ milk in the jug; drink it up.
30. I have lost _____ pen you gave me.
31. Can you give me _____ food to eat? I am very hungry.
32. I am sorry. There isn't _____ food left.
33. Have you found _____ pen you lost yesterday?
34. He applied for _____ post of a lecturer.

Answers

II. The-a, the-the, An-the, The-the, the-a, a-the, a-the, the, the-the, an-a.

III. Some, much, some, some, any, much, many, any, many, any.

IV. Many, some, An ,the, her, a-the, any, many, some, An-little, much-the.

V. Of your, dirty, Neither, The, any, some, much, little, any, Her, some, Which.

VI. Little-the, four, many-some, Many, two, both, The, A little, Every, All, his, some, little.

VII. A, a, an, an, a, an, an-a, a, a, an, a, a, A, a, a, a, a, a, An, a.

VIII. X-an, The-X, a-X, A-X, A-X, X-an, A-X-X, X-X-X, X, X, X, A-X, X-a, X, X, a, X-a, X-X, an, X.

IX. A, some, your, The, Some, no, an-this-many, your, those, a-lot of, which, one, Some, no, the

X 1. A, the, a, any, a, a, The, the.

2. The, the, the, The, a, the, her, the.

3. A, one, a, one, his, the, the, the, the.

4. An, few, the, my, a, the, a, my, the , a.

5. The, the, The, the, the, the, the, a, it, the, any, them.

6. The, The, the, a, my, the.

7. The, the, a, the, the, their.

8. The, the, the, the, a, the, the, the.

9. A, the, a, the.

10. The, the, the, the, the, the, the, the, the, the.

XI. A, a, any, some, any, much, an, The, some, the, the, any, many, an, an, the, an, some, a, any, the, an, an, the, a, many, a, some, a, the, some, any, the, the.

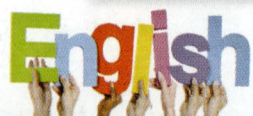

Chapter 10

Modals

INTRODUCTION

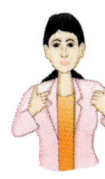

Modal verbs are auxiliary verbs that are used with other main verbs. Modal verbs are: can, could, will, would, may, might, shall, should and must.

Note these important rules:

❑ Two modal verbs cannot be put together.

- Modal verbs are followed by the infinitive without to
- Modal verbs do not have third person
- Modal verbs do not form tenses with '-ing', '-ed', etc.
- Modal verbs use inversion in questions (like the verb 'be'), not do/does.
- Modal verbs show the speaker's attitude or feelings about a situation, e.g., how probable or necessary it is and are also used in offering and requesting. The same modal verb can be used in different ways with different meanings, depending on the situation.

English has many modal verbs. Each modal verb can be used in several different contexts:

Ability

❑ I can speak two languages.
❑ I can't read French because it's too difficult.
❑ I couldn't study it when I was at school.

Permission

❑ You can have more biscuits if you want.
❑ You may take as much as you like.
❑ Could I have another slice of cake?

Request

❑ Can/could you give me a ride home later?
❑ Would you email Ganesh for me please?
❑ Will you lock up the office tomorrow?

Offers

- ❐ Can I help you with those?
- ❐ May I take one of those for you?
- ❐ Shall I carry some of your books?

Suggestions and Advice

- ❐ You should/ought to go to the doctor
- ❐ You could try the new medicine.

Obligation

- ❐ You must arrive on time for work.
- ❐ You must not be late for work.

MODAL VERB FORMATIONS

Modal verbs share certain characteristics. They don't change form to match the subject, and they are always followed by a main verb in its base form. The model verbs are changed to interrogative and negative forms without using 'do'.

Subject	Modal verb	Base form	Rest of sentence
I/you/he/she.	Can	Play	The piano quite well
It/we/they.	The modal verb stays the same for any subject	The main verb stays in its base form	

Negatives are formed by adding 'not' between the modal verb and main verb.
- ❐ You should run a marathon.
- ❐ You should not run a marathon.

Questions are usually formed by swapping the subject and the modal verb.
- ❐ They should visit the castle.
- ❐ Should they visit the castle?

'Ought to' and 'have to 'are exceptions because they use 'to' before the base form. 'Ought to' is a more formal way of saying, 'should' and 'have to' means 'must'. They both act like normal verbs.
- ❐ You ought/have to learn how to drive.

'Can' is a modal verb that describes what someone is able to do. It is used in different forms to describe past and present abilities.

'Can/Cannot/Can't'.

'Can' goes between the subject and the main verb. The verb after 'can' goes in its base form.
- ❐ I can ride a bicycle.

    'Can' is always the same. It doesn't change with the subject.
- ❐ He can play the guitar.

    ⤷ Base form of verb

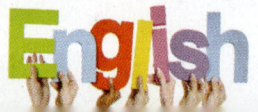

The negative form of 'can' is "cannot" or "can't".

I $\begin{cases} \text{cannot} \\ \text{can't} \end{cases}$ sing pop songs.

the more common short form of cannot

How to form

Subject	Can/cannot/can't	Base form	Object
I/you/he/she	can		
It/we/they	cannot	ride	a bicycle
	can't		

"Could" for past abilities

"Could" is the past form of 'can' and is used to talk about an ability in the past.

"When" plus a time setting can be used to say when someone had the ability.

I can't climb trees now, but I could when I was younger.

Describes a present ability   Describes a past ability.

'Can' in the future.

It is not grammatically possible to talk about the future using 'can'. "Will be able to" is used instead.

At the moment, I can play the instrument quite well.

If I work harder, I will be able to play at concerts.

'Will can' is incorrect.

The negative is formed with 'not able to' or 'unable to'. Unfortunately, I can't read music very well.

If I don't learn, $\begin{cases} \text{I won't be able} \\ \text{will be unable} \end{cases}$ to join the orchestra.

'Will be unable to' can also be used, but it's less common.

Asking Permission and Making Requests

'Can' is the most common modal verb used to ask permission or to make a request.

❑ Can I have some chocolates?

      Yes, you can.

'Could' replaces 'can' for more formal situations, such as in business or to talk to strangers.

❑ Excuse me, could I sit here, please?

   (Please is used in polite requests.)

❑ I'm sorry, but that seat is taken.

   Negative answers can be more polite by adding

❑ 'I'm sorry' or 'I'm afraid'

   'May' can also be used in formal situations.

❑ May I make an appointment?

   Of course.

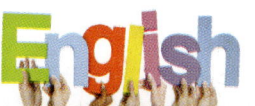

Making Offers

'Can' and 'may' can also be used to offer to do something for someone.

- ❏ Can I help you carry those?
- ❏ May I take your coat?

May is only used for formal situations.

Shall for Offers and Suggestions

'Shall' is used to find out if someone thinks a certain suggestion is a good idea.

- ❏ That bag looks heavy. Shall I carry it for you?

'Should' is used for advice. Should is used when the speaker wants to make a strong suggestion.

- ❏ It's very cold. You should wear a cap.

'Should' comes before advice.

How to Form

Subject	Should	Main verb	Rest of sentence
You	should	wear	a cap

Should is a modal verb.   Base form of main verb (wear)

'Ought to' for advice.

'Ought to' is a more formal and less common way to say 'should'. It is not usually used in the negative or question forms.

- ❏ You should wear a scarf.

You ought to wear a scarf

Obligation

We use 'must' or 'have' to explain that something is necessary.

I must finish my homework before 9.00.

I have to talk to Johnny at 9.30.

'Have to' is not a modal verb, and has all the forms of have.

- ❏ Anil has to leave now.
- ❏ Why does she have to go?
- ❏ You don't have to do it.

There are differences between 'must' and 'have to' in some situations. In formal speech and writing we can use either 'must' or 'have to'.

We use 'have to' when the situation makes something necessary, for example because of official rules, at our school, we have to wear a uniform. Every player in a team has to have a number.

We use 'must' when the speaker personally feels that something is important.

- ❏ You really must stop working so hard and try to relax.
- ❏ You must be here by 9.00, or the bus will leave without you.

Note, that we do not use 'to' after 'must'. There is no future form of 'must'. The future of 'have to' is formed with the auxiliary verb 'will'.

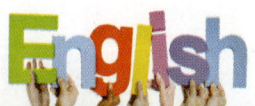

- In some countries, people must recycle, it's the law.
- In the future, I think everyone will have to recycle waste.
  '(Will must' is incorrect)
  'Must not' does not have a future form. 'Don't have to' can be used in the future by changing 'don't' to 'will not' or 'won't'.
- One day, I hope I will not have to work so hard.
  There is no past form of 'must'. The past tense of 'have to' is used instead.
- For most jobs, you must use a computer. In the past, you didn't have to use a computer.

USES OF MODALS

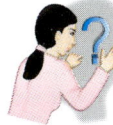

Will is used:

1. To express pure future with second and third person (you, he, she, it, they).
   - You will die of hunger.
   - The chief minister will lay the foundation stone.
2. To express willingness, intention, promise, determination with the first person (I, we)
   - I will write to you again (promise).
   - I will help you (willingness/intention).
   - He will fight to the finish (determination).
3. To express a characteristic habit, assumption, invitation or request and insistence.
   - A dog will usually obey his master (habit).
   - He will be there by now (assumption).
   - Will you come with me (request)?
   (Will is never used with the first person in the interrogative).

Shall is used:

1. To express pure future with the first person (I, we).
   We shall learn this lesson tomorrow.
   - I shall help you.
2. To ask for advice, suggestion, request, etc. with the first person (I, We) in the interrogative.
   - Shall I bring a cup of tea for you (Request)?
   - Shall I open the window (Advice)?
   - Shall we meet tomorrow (Suggestion)?
3. To express command, threat, warning, promise, determination, etc. with the second and third persons (you, he, she, they etc.)
   - You shall do it (Command).
   - He shall be punished if he repeats his mistake (warning).
   - She shall have a reward (Promise).
   - They shall define their honour (Determination).

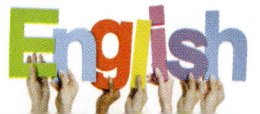

Would (past form of will) is used:

1. To express a habit
   - He would rise early in the morning and go for a walk.
   - He would sit for hours reading the newspaper.
2. To express a polite request.
3. To express a wish, preference.
   - I wish you would come with us.
   - Would that (I wish) he were here.
4. To express an imaginary condition.
   - I would do it, if I were allowed.
   - I would buy a car if I win a lottery.

Should (past form of shall) is used:

1. To express duty/obligation or advisability or desirability
   - We should obey our parents (Duty).
   - You should not be late (Obligation/Desirability).
   - You should go for a walk (Advisability).
   - If he should see me there, he will be angry (Probable condition).
2. To express logical inference, supposition, assumption, possibility/probability
   - They should be at home now (Possibility).
3. To express purpose after lest (In expression of fear)
   - Work hard lest you should fail.
   - They hired a taxi lest they should miss the train.

May is used:

1. To express possibility
   - Ravi may come today.
   - It may rain today.
2. To express permission
   - You may go now.
   - May I come in, Sir?
3. To express wish, faith or hope
   - May you succeed!
   - May God bless you!
4. To express a purpose
   - He is working hard so that he may win a scholarship.

Might (past form of may) is used:

1. To express less possibility
   - He might come today.
   - It might rain tonight.

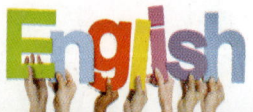

2. To express permission
   - Might I start the discussion?
3. To express guess
   - That might be the postman.

Can is used:

1. To express permission
   - You can borrow my car.
   - Can I smoke here?
2. To express possibility
   - This can be true.
3. To express ability or capacity
   - I can lift this box.
   - He can keep awake the whole night.

Could is used:

1. To express ability/capacity in the past
   - He could swim very well in his youth.
   - I could give him an answer if he had asked me.
2. To express a polite request
   - Could I borrow your book?
   - Could you wait for sometime?
3. To express possibility under certain conditions:
   - If we had money, we could buy a car.
   - It could not be true.

Must is used:

1. To express obligation or duty
   - You must do as you are told.
   - Soldiers must obey the orders of their officers.
2. To express necessity or compulsions.
   - I must go now.
   - The letter must be written today.
3. To express emphatic advice or determination.
   - You must see a doctor at once.
   - We must not leave before we finish the work.
4. To express assumption conclusion/inference, certainty/strong probability.
   - He must be thirty-five.
   - He must have reached by now.
     (Must is not used in the negative or interrogative in this sense, instead, can is used.)
   - Can he be thirty-five?

> ### Remember
>
> - 'Can' never indicates past time.
> - In the sense of ability the past and the future tense forms are: was/were able to and shall/will be able to
>   - He was not able to cross the river (past)
>   - I hope you shall be able to solve this problem (future)

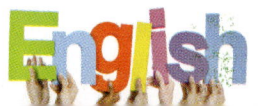

Need is used:

Chiefly to show absence of necessity or compulsion in the negative and interrogative. The negative is formed by need not and the interrogative by inversion.

- ❑ He need not go to the station soon.
- ❑ You need not pay the bill.

It does not take 's' in the third person singular present tense. It's past is 'had' to in the affirmative.

- ❑ Need not have in the negative and need have in the interrogative.
- ❑ Need I have to see my doctor?

Ought is used:

1. To express the subjects obligation or duty
   - We ought to love our neighbours.
   - We ought not to deceive anyone.
2. To give advice
   - You ought to practice for more than two hours.
   - It is less forceful than must.

     Dare means to have courage. It is generally used in the negative and interrogative. The negative is formed by dare not and the interrogative by inversion. It does not take 's' in the third person singular present tense.
   - I dare not go to my father.
   - How dare you talk this?

     Both dare and need can be used as main verbs. Then they take 'S' in the third person singular present tense.

     Used is used To express past habit.
   - I used to go for a walk every morning (I don't go now).
   - I used to play cricket in my young age.
3. To express the existence of something in the past. There used to be a garden in this place long ago.

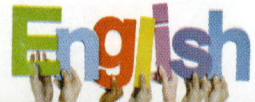

Errors in the use of Auxiliaries

Incorrect Sentences	Correct Sentences

❏ Shall you help me?

❏ Will I go to the garden?

❏ I will be obliged to you.

❏ If she will come to me, I shall help her.

❏ He worked hard lest he may not fail.

❏ I will be drowned and nobody shall save me.

❏ I shall stand by my brother under all circumstances.

❏ You will be turned out of the class if you won't stop talking.

❏ He dare to stand alone.

❏ He dared not to face his father.

❏ He needs not to do any Work.

❏ I dared Mohan fight a duel.

❏ He will know me if he saw me.

❏ He can do this if he tried.

❏ You ought love your parents.

❏ Had you worked hard, you will have passed.

❏ He died that others may live.

❏ I made him to put out the lamp.

❏ He does not need be helped.

❏ He ought have worked hard.

❏ Will you help me?

❏ Shall I go to the garden?

❏ I shall be obliged to you.

❏ If she comes to me, I shall help her.

❏ He worked hard lest he should fail.

❏ I shall be drowned and nobody will save me.

❏ I will stand by my brother under all circumstances.

❏ You shall be turned out of the class if you don't stop talking.

❏ He dares to stand alone.

❏ He dared not face his father.

❏ He need not do any work.

❏ I dared Mohan to fight a duel.

❏ He would know me if he saw me.

❏ He could do this if he tried.

❏ You ought to love your parents.

❏ Had you worked hard, you would have passed.

❏ He died that others might live.

❏ I made him put out the lamp.

❏ He does not need to be helped.

❏ He ought to have worked hard.

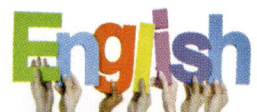

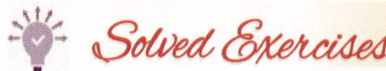

Solved Exercises

I. Fill in the blanks with suitable modals:

1. I _____ speak three languages.
2. You _____ run a marathon.
3. You _____ learn how to drive.
4. You _____ arrive on time for walk.
5. _____ you lock up the office tonight.
6. You _____ try the new medicine.
7. You _____ take as much as you like.
8. Bob _____ swim well.
9. _____ I make an appointment?
10. _____ I borrow your pencil?

II. Fill in the blanks with suitable modals:

1. _____ I carry some of your bags?
2. _____ I have another slice of cake?
3. You _____ go to the doctor.
4. They _____ visit the castle.
5. He _____ play the guitar.
6. When Milan was seven he _____ play the violin.
7. Excuse me, _____ I sit here please?
8. _____ I reserve a table for 8 pm.
9. _____ I open the window?
10. That _____ be lovely.

III. Fill in the blanks with suitable modals:

1. You _____ wear a hat as it is very sunny.
2. You _____ study science in college.
3. You _____ visit the palace. It is beautiful.
4. She _____ take this medicine.
5. They _____ have taken him to other market
6. If I were you I _____ leave early.
7. I don't know if I _____ take this job.
8. You _____ wear a scarf. It's very cold outside.
9. I don't think you _____ go to work today.
10. _____ I have some popcorn.

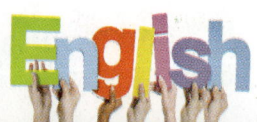

IV. **Fill in the blanks with suitable modals:**

1. Dad, _____ we go swimming today?
2. We _____ obtain a license before we can sell liquor.
3. I wish I _____ go horse riding.
4. If I were a rich man, I _____ build homeless shelters everywhere.
5. You _____ be right.
6. _____ you lift this heavy box?
7. She really _____ find new friends.
8. _____ Our friends join you for lunch?
9. I _____ leave by tomorrow morning.
10. No one _____ play the drums better than john.

V. **Fill in the blanks with suitable modals:**

1. There was a long walk; you _____ be tired.
2. Sorry I was away yesterday. I _____ to go to the hospital.
3. _____ you be able to give some help tomorrow?
4. Do you _____ go now?
5. Peter _____ ride a bike when he was seven.
6. Mary _____ be in her bedroom. The light is on.
7. Students _____ not leave their bicycles near this door. It is forbidden.
8. We _____ to try very hard, but we succeeded in the end.

ANSWERS

I. Can, should, ought to, must, will, could, may, can, may, can.

II. Shall, could, should/ought to, should, can, could, could, may, shall, would.

III. Should, could, must, has to, might, would, should, ought to/should, should, can.

IV. May, must, could, would, might, can, ought to, may, have to, can.

V. Must, had, will, have, could, must, must, had.

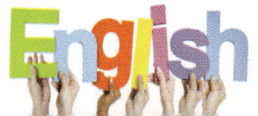

Practice Exercises

I. Fill in the blanks with have to, has to, had to must or need:

1. You _____ come to school in time.

2. The room is not dirty. You _____ not clean it.

3. He _____ be in the house at nine every day.

4. We don't _____ go to school on Sunday.

5. I still have fever. I _____ go to hospital.

6. I _____ pay my fee tomorrow.

7. Rita won a scholarship. She _____ work hard for it.

8. His eyesight is weak. He _____ wear glasses for reading.

9. We _____ not drive fast, we have plenty of time.

10. There was no bus, so we _____ walk home.

II. Fill in the blanks with will, shall, would or should:

1. One _____ keep one's promise.

2. As you sow, so _____ you reap.

3. I _____ stand by you, come what may (promise)

4. Walk carefully lest you _____ fall.

5. We _____ fight to the last man (determination).

6. _____ that my father were alive today !

7. She _____ be seventeen next week.

8. You _____ see a doctor.

9. _____ you go there?

10. _____ I switch on the fan for you?

III. Fill in the blanks with can, may, could, might:

1. I thought it _____ rain.

2. Stop! you _____ not do it.

3. _____ you paint when you were nine?

4. _____ I go out, sir?

5. _____ you read this letter?

6. She _____ pass if she works hard.

7. His officer told him that he _____ make or mar his career

8. He works hard so that he _____ pass.

9. I ran fast so that I _____ catch the train.

10. He _____ swim very well when he was young.

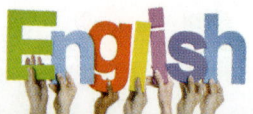

IV. Fill in the blanks with ought to, dare or used to:

1. Everyone _____ love his country.
2. She _____ come late to school every day.
3. We _____ obey our parents.
4. Last year she _____ wear the same dress in every party.
5. He _____ not speak rudely.
6. People _____ think that the sun travelled round the earth
7. You _____ come to school in time.
8. How _____ he oppose me?
9. We _____ help the poor.
10. He has lost your watch and he _____ not tell you.

V. Fill the blanks with mustn't or 'needn't:

1. You _____ scribble on others' books.
2. You _____ enter the kitchen with your slippers on.
3. You _____ run. The train is late by an hour.
4. You _____ worry. Things will be normal
5. You _____ use my towel in future.
6. The boy students _____ enter the girls common room.
7. You _____ light the match. I can see alright.
8. The parents _____ give their children too much liberty.
9. We _____ leave our fan on when we are not using it.
10. I'll do it myself. You _____ come.

VI. Fill in the blanks with appropriate modals:

1. _____ I speak to the principal for a moment.
2. The breeze is cool and fresh; it _____ rain soon.
3. You _____ not enter my class. I forbid it.
4. He has been absent for a fortnight, he _____ be ill.
5. _____ I come in? I am sorry to be late.
6. You _____ respect your elders.
7. _____ you possibly lend me a thousand rupees?
8. I _____ not come yesterday since I was too busy.
9. We _____ go to the station by taxi, it is getting late.
10. I _____ come there even if it rains.

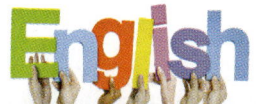

VII. Fill in the blanks with appropriate modals:

1. He _____ be rich, but he is very cruel.
2. We _____ do as we are told.
3. _____ his soul rest in peace.
4. If I were you, I _____ not do it.
5. Hurry up lest you _____ be late for school.
6. He said that he _____ return tomorrow.
7. I was afraid if I asked him again he _____ refuse.
8. It is almost time for the meeting. I _____ leave.
9. You _____ have the money tomorrow.
10. She _____ speak English fluently.

VIII. Fill in the blanks with appropriate modals:

1. I _____ that I had the wings of a dove.
2. You _____ not disobey your father.
3. You_____ take my car if you are in a hurry.
4. It _____ rain in the evening.
5. The children asked if they _____ have ice cream.
6. I _____ help him with money before I leave for London.
7. Don't run because you ____ fall.
8. I still remember my childhood. I ____ play marbles then.
9. The doctor told him that he _____ not smoke anymore.
10. We _____ not borrow any money. We have enough for our needs.

IX. Fill in the blanks with appropriate modals:

1. If I were rich, I ____ help the poor.
2. Who _____ tolerate such an insult?
3. The case is serious. You ____ consult some good doctor.
4. You _____ to serve your aged parents.
5. _____ I smoke here?
6. You have finished your work. You _____ go now.
7. We _____ stand united.
8. We _____ forget our duties.
9. ____ I come again? No, you needn't.
10. Who ____ answer this question? said the teacher.

X. Fill in the blanks with appropriate modals:

1. We have completed our work _____ we go now?
2. I hope she _____ do well in the examination.

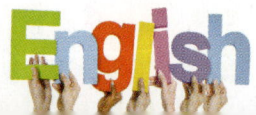

3. He can bowl well, but he _____ bat quite as well.

4. He might pass, but he ____ not get good marks.

5. He_____ drive a car when he was ten.

6. I have brushed my teeth. You __ bring the coffee now.

7. He said that he _____ finish the work in time

8. Sit down. You _____ leave the hall so soon.

9. The principal is busy. You _____ see him just now.

10. You are not a member of the club. You _____ attend its meeting.

11. In a democracy, everyone ____ obey the laws of the country.

12. The patient _____ be shown to the doctor at once.

13. You _____ worry about your son.

14. I _____ help him in every way.

15. _____ we love our country? Of course.

XI. Fill in the blanks with appropriate modals:

1. You ____ do it if he does not help you.

2. You _____ to work very hard this year.

3. I think you _____ succeed if you try.

4. We _____ hurry we are very late.

5. I am afraid I ____ tell you that. It is a secret.

6. Amar is good at shotput but Anant _____ run faster than he.

7. Our team _____ easily beat your team.

8. I _____ lift this box. It is so light.

9. I was afraid lest we _____ be late.

10. It _____ rain tonight.

11. He was sure he _____ win.

12. I _____ like to go to my village during the holidays.

13. _____ you please open the door?

14. A judge _____ be just.

15. _____ heaven protect you.

XII. Fill in the blanks with appropriate modals:

1. Everyone _____ makes mistakes.

2. _____ I sit down, sir?

3. _____ God bless you!

4. _____ you speak English then?

5. I said that it _____ rain.

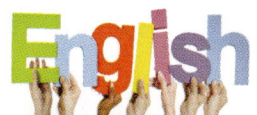

6. _____ he write Hindi now?

7. _____ you lend me your camera?

8. You _____ walk for hours without reaching there.

9. He died so that others _____ live.

10. We work hard so that we _____ succeed.

XIII. **Fill in the blanks with appropriate modals:**

1. You _____ finish this essay before you leave for home.

2. He _____ play hockey when he was a student.

3. You _____ not light a candle, there is enough light yet.

4. You _____ not make a noise, the patient may wake up.

5. You have already informed him _____ I inform him myself?

6. A weak person _____ not oppose strong enemy.

7. We _____ love our country.

8. Things _____ be very cheap in those days.

9. You _____ work hard or fail.

10. Everybody _____ help the needy.

11. You _____ not worry about the result. It is going to be excellent.

12. What you cannot cure you _____ endure.

13. You _____ not drive fast; we have already plenty of time.

14. You _____ not drive so fast; we may meet with an accident.

15. Railway notice : Passengers _____ not smoke in this compartment.

XIV. But now and then, when her husband was at the office, she _____ sit by the window and her thoughts _____ go back to that far away evening, the evening of her beauty and her success. What _____ have been the end of it if she had not lost the necklace? Who _____ say? How strange and various are the chances of life. How small a thing _____ save or ruin you.

XV. Her friend did not recognize her and said : I'm afraid I don't know you. You _____ have made a mistake.

XVI. If the matter is one that _____ be settled by observation, make the observation yourself. Aristotle _____ have avoided the mistake of thinking that women have fewer teeth than men, by the simple device of asking Mrs Aristotle to keep her mouth open while he counted.

XVII. Suresh: _____ you recite a nursery rhyme?

Atul: I _____ when I was in my nursery classes but I _____ not recite it now.

XVIII. Dear Rajan, last year I _____ send you Rs 500 every month. But I'm afraid I _____

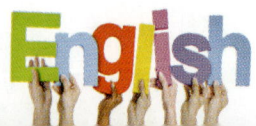

not send you this amount now. You may or _____ not like this but I _____ like to make it clear that I _____ make a cut somewhere if I want to live within my income. However, you _____ not worry about anything.

XIX. I do not suggest that the cultural side of education _____ be ignored. I think, on the contrary, that it is essential to the production of the sort of adult who best fits the modern world. But I think that what is important in cultural education _____ be conveyed, at any rate in the early stages, by methods far more attractive than those now usual. History and geography _____ be taught at first by means of cinema. When taught this way, they _____ give pleasure, attention _____ be spontaneous and therefore the impression _____ be less temporary.

ANSWERS

I.   Have to, need, have to, have to, must, have to, had to, has to, need, had to.

II. Should, shall, will, should, will, would, will, should, will, should.

III. Might, can, could, may, can, might, can, can, could, could.

IV. Ought to, used to, ought to, used to, dare, used to, ought to, dare, ought to, dare.

V.   Mustn't, mustn't, needn't, needn't, mustn't, mustn't, needn't, mustn't, mustn't, needn't.

VI. Can, may, need, might, may, ought to, can, would, have to, shall.

VII. May, should, May, would, should, would, would, must, can, can.

VIII. Would, need, can, might, could, can, might, could, should, need.

IX. Would, can, must, need, may, can, must, shouldn't, should, can.

X.   Should, will, can, can, could, can, would, cannot, cannot, cannot, should, can, needn't, cannot, should.

XI. Cannot, have, can, should, cannot, can, can, can, should, might, could, will, can, has to, May.

XII. Can, may, may, could, might, can, can, cannot, could, can.

XIII. Have to, could, need, should, should, need, ought to, could, have to, can, need, must, need, should, must.

XIV. Could, would, could, could, can.

XV. Must.

XVI. Can, could.

XVII. Can, could, can.

XVIII. Used to, can, may, will, have to, need.

XIX. Should, can, can, can, can, can.

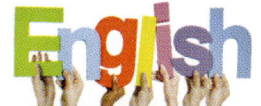

NOTES

Chapter 11

Prepositions

INTRODUCTION

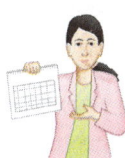

Study the following sentences:

i.   I am angry with you.

ii. I saw my teacher in the school.

iii. He is very kind to us.

iv. We are sitting on the bench.

In sentence (i), the word 'with' shows the relation between the adjective *angry* and the pronoun *you*. In sentence (ii), the word 'in' shows the relation between the noun *teacher* and the noun *school*. In sentence (iii), the word 'to' shows the relation between adjective *kind* and the pronoun *us*. In sentence (iv), the word 'on' shows the relation between the verb *are sitting* and the noun *chairs*. Such words with, in, to, on used in these sentences that establish some relation between two words are called preposition.

DEFINITION

A preposition is a word placed before a noun or a pronoun to show the relation between a noun or pronoun and some other word in a sentence.

A preposition is usually placed before its object. A preposition may have more than one object.

i.   He gave some money to John, Jill and me.

Here *John, Jill* and me are objects of the preposition to.

POSITION OF PREPOSITION

The word "preposition" *(pre + position)* means *that which is positioned (placed) before.* Thus a preposition is usually placed before the noun or pronoun it governs.

A preposition is usually placed before its object but now-a-days it is increasingly being placed at the end of the sentence, especially in the relative clauses and when it governs an interrogative pronoun or adverb.

❑ This is the book (That) you were looking 'for'.

❑ Where are you going 'to'?

Exception

1. The preposition can be placed at the end of a sentence:
    a. When the object of a preposition is a relative pronoun (The relative pronouns could also be sometimes omitted):
        - This is the book (that) I was searching for.
    b. When the object of a preposition is an interrogative pronoun:
        - What are you looking at?
        - Who (m) are you talking about?
2. The Preposition may be placed sometimes in the beginning of a sentence about whom are you talking:
    - In which box did you keep my purse?

KIND OF PREPOSITIONS

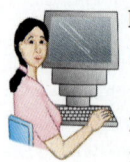

Prepositions are of four different kinds:

1. **Simple prepositions:** In, of, an, off, to, up, with at, by, for, behind, besides, beneath, below, across, between, etc.
2. **Compound prepositions:** Without, within, outside, inside, into, etc.
3. **Double propositions:** Outside of, out of, from out, from behind, from beneath, etc.
4. **Phrase propositions:** By means of, because of, on account of, in opposition to, with regards to, for the sake of, instead of, on behalf of, with a view to, in the event of, etc.

    There are several words which can be used as prepositions as well as adverbs. If the word is used as a preposition, it will have noun or pronoun as its object. (Adverb modifies a verb, adjective or another adverb).

Preposition	Adverb
The lion is in the cage.	Please come in.
He stood before me.	He came here before.
Keep the Book on the table	Let us move on.
He will come after a month	He arrived soon after.

Study the use of some prepositions given below:

About	:	I asked him *about* his health.
Above	:	The water came *above* his shoulders.
		His father is *above* fifty.
		No book in the shop was *above* ₹80.
		This boy weighs *above* seventy pounds.
Across	:	(from one side to the other side of): I Walked *across* the road.
		(on the other side of): My school is just *across* the street.
After	:	I saw him *after* the meeting.
		B comes *after* A

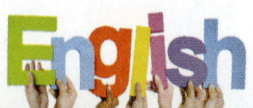

Against	:	We are *against* bad customs.
		He hit his head *against* the tree.
		Place the ladder *against* the wall.
Along	:	We walked *along* the road.
Among	:	He divided his property *among* his five sons.
		New Delhi is *among* the largest cities of India.
		The teacher sat *among* his students.
At	:	I met him *at* the railway station.
		Look *at* the picture.
		He came *at* 5 o'clock.
		He went to school *at* (the age of) five.
		The boys are *at* play.
		He drove *at* full speed.
		I bought bananas *at* ₹8 a dozen.
Before	:	The meeting took place *before* Monday.
		A comes *before* B.
		We sat *before* (in front of) the fire.
Beside	:	(at the side of; close to): She sat *beside* her children.
Besides	:	(in-addition to) We were ten, *besides* Suresh.
Between	:	The son sat *between* his father and mother.
		I shall see him *between* 2 pm and 3 pm.
		Its price is *between* ₹10 and ₹15.
		Divide the mangoes *between* two brothers.
		(Between is used to refer to two persons, things, etc.)
By	:	He sat *by* (near) the tree.
		Our examination begins on Monday, so we must finish the course *by* Sunday.
		Oranges are sold *by* the dozen.
		The work was completed *by* four laborers.
		We can travel *by* land, sea/air/train/car.
During	:	(throughout, the duration of)
		It rained *during* the night.
		(at somepoint of time in the duration):
		Somebody came to see me *during* my absence.
For	:	Is there a train *for* Mumbai now?
		There is a letter *for* you.
		He is preparing *for* the examination.
		We have separate room *for* sleeping in.
		Exercise is good *for* health.
		The score is 150 *for* 6 wickets.
		I paid ₹20 *for* the book.
		He lived here *for* two weeks.

From	:	We travelled *from* Kolkata to Chennai.
		I have started teaching him *from* the first of this month.
		He stayed away *from* home for 3 years.
		I have received a letter *from* my mother.
		She drew water *from* a well.
		Steel is made *from* iron.
		Its price has increased *from* ₹10 to ₹15.
In	:	He lived *in* India for many years.
		Does she live *in* New Delhi?
		He was born *in* a village.
		The children were playing *in* the street.
		He has stick *in* his hand.
		I read it *in* a book.
		This happened *in* 1986.
		It is very cold *in* January.
		He visited me *in* the morning.
		I shall be back *in* a few days.
		She was dressed *in* red.
		(= was wearing red clothes)
Into	:	She came *into* the room.
		Throw it *into* the dustbin.
		The water changed *into* ice.
Of	:	I bought a table *of* wood. (= a wooden table)
		He is a boy *of* eight years.
		He is the master *of* the house.
		A leg *of* the table is broken.
		Give me a piece *of* paper.
		He is the best *of* all the boys.
On	:	There is a jug *on* the table.
		There is a picture *on* the wall.
		They are sitting *on* the grass.
		I went there *on* Sunday.
		He came here *on* first july.
		He hit me *on* the head.
		His house is *on* the main road.
Since	:	I have not seen him *since* 1980.
		The two friends have not met *since* their school days.
Till	:	I shall wait *till* 5 o'clock/next Sunday.
		He worked from morning *till* night.

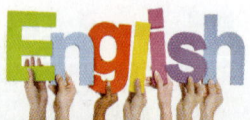

To	:	He went from Chennai *to* Delhi.
		She went from place *to* place.
		The traffic light turned from red *to* green.
		He worked here from Sunday *to* Wednesday.
		We won by four goals to three.
With	:	This is a cup *with* a broken handle.
		She is a girl *with* blue eyes.
		His pockets were filled *with* toffees.
		Cut the apple *with* a knife.
		I did it *with* the help of my brother.
		I went for a walk *with* my friends
		He did not work *with* pleasure.
		Leave the child *with* its nurse.
Up to	:	What have you been *up to* (doing) recently?
		The children are always *up to* some kind of mischief.
		It's *up to* you to deal with the problem.
Along	:	Jack is walking *along* the lake.
		We sailed *along* the canal.
		The cinema is further *along* the street.
		There are bookshelves all *along* the wall.
Among	:	There is a boy *among* the girls.
Amongst	:	She comes from a village high up *among* the mountains.
		Amongst the guests was the new Mayor.
		Amongst can be used interchangeably with where members of group are involved:
		You can relax *amongst* (or among) your friends.

WHICH PREPOSITION TO BE USED AND WHEN?

Sometimes it may be a little difficult to decide which preposition is to be used. Thus the following prepositions need careful handling:

1. **In, at**: 'In' is used with the name of continents, countries, states, sizeable territories and large cities. 'At' is used with towns, villages, etc.
   - He is not 'at' home. He lives 'at' Batala.
   - He lives 'in' Punjab.
   - He lives 'at' Chandarnagar 'in' Bengal.

But when we speak of very large places, we usually say:
   - He lives 'in' England (not at London).
   - He died 'in' Paris 'in' France (not at Paris).

2. **At, on:** Compare the following sentences:
   i. He sat 'at' the table.
   ii. He sat 'on' the table.

'At' in the first sentence, means that he sat with his chair drawn up to the table.

'On' in the second sentence means that he sat on top of the table.

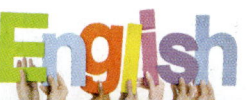

3. **Between, among:** Between is used in speaking of two persons or things:
   Among is used in speaking of more than two persons or things.
   The cat sat *between* Mohan and Rohan.
   Usage: *Between* can also relate to more than two persons or things, when we have a definite number in mind.

4. **Beside, besides:** *Beside* means at or by the side of: 'besides' means in addition to or other than.
   • I live *beside* the stream.
   • *Besides* all this, the corn must be cut.
   • Nobody, *besides* Mohan, could have done it.

5. **In, within:** In means at the end of, within means before the end of.
   • He will return 'in' a week (at the end of week).
   • He will return 'within' a week (before the end of a week).

6. **At, about:** 'At', is used with a fixed moment; 'about' indicates proximity to a certain time.
   • He left work 'at' four o'clock.
   • It is 'about' four now.
   Expression like: 'at about four o'clock', 'at about the time he left work', are therefore wrong.

7. **Till, by:** 'Till' means not earlier than; 'by' means not later than:
   • I was kept waiting till 3 o'clock (up to 3 o'clock).
   • I shall return home by 3 o'clock (not later than 3 o'clock).

8. **Since, for:** 'Since' as a preposition is used before a noun or phrase denoting some point of time:
   For is used to denote a period of time, as:
   • He has been working 'since' morning.
   • I have been doing nothing 'for' two hours.
   • I have been living in Mumbai 'since' 1980.
   Note: 'Since' is preceded by a verb in some perfect tense.

9. **From** is used before noun or phrase denoting some point of time, but unlike since it is used with all the tenses, as:
   • Ram Swarup works 'from' morning to evening.
   • I shall join office 'from' Monday.

10. **Before, for:** Before is used to denote a point of future time. 'for' is used in negative sentences to denote a period of future time, as:
    • I shall finish my work 'before' next month (during this month).
    • I am not resuming duty 'for' week yet (until a week has passed).

11. **On, over:** On denotes actual contact with some object; 'over' does not do so:
    • Put the pen 'on' the table.
    • Thick mist hung 'over' the forest.

12. **To, till/until-till:** Means up to:
    Both are based with 'from' 'to' cannot be used without 'from'. 'till' however can be used alone:
    • We work from 8 am 'to' 4 pm.
    • We work 'till' 4 pm.
    'Until' cannot be used with a negative verb.

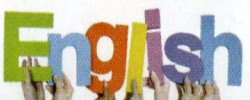

Some Important Distinctions

1. **By and with:** 'By' is used before the doer, 'with' before the name of an instrument with which the action is done. The cake was cut 'by' her 'with' a knife.
2. **Between and among:** 'Between' is used with two persons or things, 'among' is used with more than two persons or things.
   - The father divided the property 'between' his two sons.
   - Sweets were distributed 'among' children.
3. **Beside and besides:** 'Beside' means by the side of; 'besides' means in addition to.
   - The temple stands 'beside' the Gurudwara.
   - 'Besides' food, we gave the beggar some money.
4. **On and upon:** 'On' is used for things at rest, 'upon' for things in motion.
   We sat 'on' the ground.
   - The dog jumped 'upon' the table.
5. **Under and underneath:** 'Underneath' is used for things only.
   - Hide this 'underneath' that box.
   - A captain works 'under' a Major.

Errors in the use of Prepositions

Incorrect Sentences

- You are kind on me.
- I said it upon his face.
- See me behind this period.
- I am searching after my lost book.
- You should not quarrel on traifles.
- He invited me for tea.
- I refrain to tell a lie.
- He sat under the shade of a tree.
- He died from cholera.
- The teacher is angry upon me.
- Open you book on page twenty.
- She meditates her past life.
- Write to me on this address.
- I have been standing here from two hours.
- He fell in the well.
- Chennai is to the South of India.
- She repented for her mistake.
- I am not afraid from you.
- Is there any remedy of this?
- What is the time in your watch?
- I will take revenge from my enemy.

Correct Sentences

- You are kind to me.
- I said it to his face.
- See me after this period.
- I am searching for my lost book.
- You should not quarrel over trifles.
- He invited me to tea.
- I refrain from telling a lie.
- He sat in the shade of a tree.
- He died of cholera.
- The teacher is angry with me.
- Open your book at page twenty.
- She meditates on her past life.
- Write to me at this address.
- I have been standing here for two hours.
- He fell into the well.
- Chennai is in the South of India.
- She repented of her mistake.
- I am not afraid of you.
- Is there any remedy for this?
- What is the time by your watch?
- I will take revenge on my enemy.

Contd...

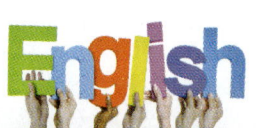

- I am tired with this job.
- She resembles with her mother.
- He does not obey to his teachers.
- I ordered for his dismissal.
- She complained upon me.
- You can depend my word.
- Five prizes were competed.
- He will dispense your services.
- I have signed on that application.
- Will you assist to me in this matter?
- You should not boast your merits.
- The police investigated into the case.
- It is useless to muse the past.
- He recommended for me to the officer.
- You must apply the judge for mercy.
- I have disposed business in hand.
- Eyes are to see.
- Who is knocking the door?
- I looked his face.
- We pray God daily.
- You do not attend your lesson.
- I wrote him yesterday.
- She is averse from smoking.
- Do not shirk from work.
- He is expert to do this.
- She is bent to take revenge.
- I am tired to do nothing.
- We entered into the hall.
- Why do you fear from me?
- A mother loves with her children.
- I told to him to go there.
- We reached at the station in time.
- I shall resign from my post.
- I shall pass in the examination.
- I am intent to win.
- I insisted to go there.
- I am confident to win.

- I am tired of this job.
- She resembles her mother.
- He does not obey his teachers.
- I ordered his dismissal.
- She complained against me.
- You can depend on my word.
- Five prizes were competed for.
- He will dispense with your services.
- I have signed that application.
- Will you assist me in this matter?
- You should not boast of your merits.
- The police investigated the case.
- It is useless to muse upon the past.
- He recommended me to the officer.
- You must apply to the judge for mercy.
- I have disposed off the business in hand
- Eyes are to see with.
- Who is knocking at the door?
- I looked at his face.
- We pray to God daily.
- You do not attend to your lesson.
- I wrote to him yesterday.
- She is averse to smoking.
- Do not shirk work.
- He is expert in doing this.
- She is bent upon taking revenge.
- I am tired of doing nothing.
- We entered the hall.
- Why do you fear me?
- A mother loves her children.
- I told him to go there.
- We reached the station in time.
- I shall resign my post.
- I shall pass the examination.
- I am intent on winning.
- I insisted on going there.
- I am confident of winning.

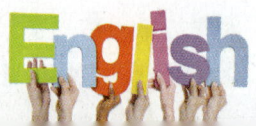

Solved Exercises

I. Fill in the blanks with suitable prepositions:

1. Instead _____ applying for a job, I went _____ college.
2. The cat is _____ the table.
3. There's a sign _____ the door.
4. I leave the house _____ 7 am
5. The dog is sleeping _____ his basket.
6. The library is closed _____ Sundays.
7. It's twenty _____ seven.
8. I have been working _____ 9 am.
9. I work _____ 9 am _____ pm.
10. I will finish work _____ 6 o'clock.

II. Fill in the blanks with suitable prepositions:

1. I want a job _____ a good salary.
2. This was painted _____ a famous artist.
3. I will meet you _____ the beach.
4. My house is _____ a lovely park.
5. She's going to Europe _____ June.
6. I have been working _____ 6 hours.
7. I relaxed _____ my break.
8. Tom ran _____ the room and sat down.
9. He sold the house _____ the family.
10. My garden is _____ the back of the house.

III. Fill in the blanks with suitable prepositions:

1. Have you heard? Pinky is _____ hospital _____ the moment.
2. Excuse me, is George _____ home ?
3. Anu and sonu went to the city centre _____ the bus.
4. Jasmine is tired _____ watching children's shows _____ TV.
5. I have a good relationship _____ my parents.
6. Pests are a serious problem _____ farmers.
7. The demand _____ public buses increases every year.
8. I broke my phone _____ dropping it _____ the floor.
9. Watch TV _____ the weekend.
10. She is hiding _____ the tree.

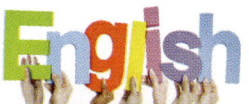

IV. Fill in the blanks with suitable prepositions:

1. Jacky is married _____ Jimmy.
2. Could I please have the dictionary when you are finished _____ it?
3. My car is equipped _____ air conditioning and a sun roof.
4. Gandhi was committed _____ nonviolence.
5. Bunny turned off the TV because he was tired _____ listening to the news.
6. The choices in that restaurant are limited _____ pizza and sandwiches.
7. Their house is always messy _____ newspapers, books, clothes and dirty dishes.
8. Are you interested _____ working with them?
9. They are dedicated _____ helping people in times of crisis.
10. The ground is covered _____ snow.

V. Fill in the blanks with suitable prepositions:

1. She is excited _____ creating toys for children so that they could enjoy.
2. She is known _____ creating high quality toys.
3. She is interested _____ how children play with one another.
4. She is pleased _____ the response to her toys.
5. Her toys are made _____ wood.
6. The materials in her toys are limited _____ wood.
7. She is disappointed _____ many of the popular toys in store today.
8. She worries _____ toys that don't encourage children to use imagination.
9. I am not acquainted _____ that man.
10. A person who is addicted _____ drugs needs medical help.

VI. Fill in the blanks with suitable prepositions:

1. We thought _____ going to the beach.
2. We talked _____ going there.
3. We're interested _____ going there.
4. My family is excited _____ going there.
5. The children insisted _____ going there.
6. They're looking forward _____ going there.
7. The rain prevented us _____ going there.
8. A storm kept up _____ going there.

Answers

I. Of -my, under, above, at, in, on, to, since, from -to, before.

II. With, by, at, near, in, for, during, into, to, at.

III. In-at, at, in, of-on, with, for, for, by-on, on or at, behind.

IV. To, with, with, to, of, to, with, in, to, with.

V. About, for, in, with, of, to, in/with, about, with, to.

VI. About, about, in, about, on, to, from, from.

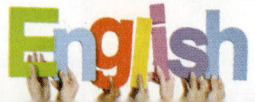

Practice Exercises

I. **Fill in the blanks with appropriate prepositions:**
   (at, in, on, by, to, with, of, after, into, about, from)

   1. The two brothers met _____ a long time.
   2. She asked me_____ my business.
   3. I am coming _____ the railway station.
   4. They live _____ Kolkata.
   5. They marched_____ the room.
   6. There are no books_____ the table.
   7. 'They won _____ four goals _____ nil.
   8. He is an old man_____ white hair.
   9. The chair is made _____ iron.
   10. He reached here _____ 5 pm.

II. **Fill in the blanks with appropriate prepositions:**
   (with, among, at, since, by, till, beside, for, to, from, besides)

   1. They have not visited us _____ 1984.
   2. I have been waiting for her_____ two days.
   3. He divided the money _____ his four children.
   4. I have two other pens _____ this.
   5. Don't disturb me_____ 6 pm.
   6. I sat _____ my friend.
   7. I bought oranges _____ ₹15 a dozen.
   8. I must finish my work _____ Monday.
   9. The crow flew_____ branch_____ branch.
   10. I shall go there _____ my friend.

III. **Fill in the blanks with appropriate prepositions:**
   (along, against, for, above, with, in, before, across, between, of)

   1. How many boys in the class weigh_____ sixty pounds?
   2. His school is situated_____ the road.
   3. Finish this work _____ sunset.
   4. He walked slowly _____ the road.
   5. Don't stand _____ the electric poll.
   6. B comes_____ A and C.
   7. Is there a parcel _____ me?
   8. I read it_____ the newspaper.
   9. I bought a piece _____ cloth.
   10. He filled the cup _____ tea.

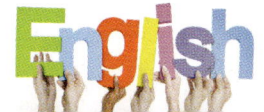

IV.   **Fill in the blanks with appropriate prepositions:**

1. He is not fit_____this job.
2. He took the initiative_____this matter.
3. You are almost mad _____anger.
4. He is obliged_____you_____your kindness.
5. Kalyan is very poor_____English.
6. I shall stand surety_____you.
7. You are not afraid_____him.
8. I am acquainted_____him.
9. You are always busy_____writing letter.
10. This pen is different_____that one.

V.   **Fill in the blanks with appropriate prepositions:**

1. You are quick _____solving sums.
2. Vikram has fondness_____table tennis.
3. I had an interview_____the headmaster.
4. Are we not entitled_____patient hearing?
5. Monika is gifted_____ a sweet voice.
6. We are opposed_____this policy of yours.
7. Songs are proper_____this function.
8. She has no interest_____studies.
9. He has no eagerness_____anything.
10. She is engaged _____my elder brother.

VI.   **Fill in the blanks with appropriate prepositions:**

1. It is foolish to quarrel _____anybody_____a trifle.
2. He is blind_____ one eye.
3. I am sorry I cannot comply_____your request.
4. Why should you be envious_____his riches?
5. She was convinced_____my sincerity?
6. It has been drizzling_____Monday?
7. Tibet is_____the North of India.
8. His sister was married _____a doctor.
9. He warned me_____the danger.
10. Have you disposed _____your goods?

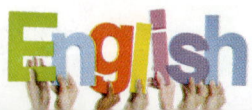

VII. Fill in the blanks with appropriate prepositions:

1. The people listened_____the speaker.
2. He is lavish_____money.
3. I shall look _____the matter.
4. I am interested _____reading novels.
5. He died_____his country.
6. He was very happy_____his success.
7. Women banker is _____money.
8. The Taj is famous_____its beauty.
9. Meenu has no fancy_____books.
10. Let us exchange views_____each other.

VIII. Fill in the blanks with appropriate prepositions:

1. He plotted_____the king.
2. His marriage has broken_____.
3. Pray to God_____mercy.
4. They live _____small salary.
5. The maid-servant made_____with the purse.
6. It is not good to make fun _____one's elders.
7. She kicked_____the offer of marriage.
8. This road is closed_____ repairs.
9. I jumped_____the river and saved the child.
10. He was very happy_____his success.

IX. Fill in the blanks with appropriate prepositions:

1. Shri Nehru lived _____his country.
2. I cannot make_____the meaning of this sentence.
3. Boys and girls freely mingle _____each other.
4. This house is infected _____mosquitoes.
5. Do not interfere_____his work.
6. He informed the police _____the theft.
7. This happened _____long ago.
8. He is innocent_____his crime.
9. I am hunting_____a rare book.
10. I hit _____a plan.

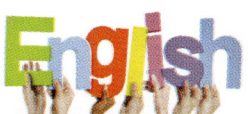

X. Fill in the blanks with appropriate prepositions:

1. He had an advantage_____ me due to my illness.
2. Latif and Subhash were arguing _____ the matter.
3. She disapproved_____my proposal.
4. Mohini is guilty_____cheating me.
5. Sudesh is familiar_____ the state of affairs.
6. Brush your teeth _____ the morning.
7. Sabina is the only heir_____her father's wealth.
8. Ram could not qualify _____ the test.
9. The bridge was blown_____.
10. She should not absent herself_____the class.

XI. Fill in the blanks with appropriate prepositions:

1. They supplied us _____food.
2. She has no taste _____ music.
3. The stain_____her character cannot be washed.
4. My uncle is a stranger_____this city.
5. Children are very quick _____ quarrel.
6. I shall look _____the matter.
7. Don't let your passions rule_____you.
8. I repose my full faith_____you.
9. Death is preferable _____ poverty.
10. She is fond _____ jewels.

XII. Fill in the blanks with appropriate prepositions:

1. He can play_____ a piano.
2. O God! Have mercy_____the sinner.
3. Ali laughed_____him for his foolishness.
4. I have no liking_____meat.
5. He infected me_____his enthusiasm.
6. I have great influence_____the minister.
7. His name was excluded_____the list.
8. He is good _____hockey.
9. We are fighting_____ higher wages.
10. He fell _____the river.

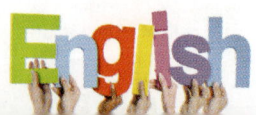

XIII. **Fill in the blanks with appropriate prepositions:**

1. One must save something_____one's bad time.
2. I go_____my school _____foot every day.
3. The guests are sitting _____ both sides.
4. This boy was born_____15th September_____ Patiala.
5. I joined this school _____1987_____Monday.
6. The cat jumped_____the wall.
7. A tree stands just _____the gate of our house.
8. We must return _____this very month.
9. The eggs are lying_____ a basket _____ the table.
10. The Sun looks just _____ our heads _____ noon.

XIV. **Fill in the blanks with appropriate prepositions:**

1. He has no control_____his tongue.
2. She is angry_____me_____nothing.
3. Beware_____cheats and pick-pockets here.
4. Both the friends quarreled _____a triffle.
5. Who does not long_____prosperity and fame?
6. Do remind me_____ my promise in time.
7. Emperor Akbar was very fond_____ music.
8. He was accused_____theft and murder.
9. The patient is slowly recovering_____illness.
10. He apologized_____me_____his mistake.
11. Meena is no match_____Reena in beauty.
12. The wrestlers grappled_____each other in the arena.
13. I congratulated him_____his brilliant success.
14. The hungry fox was roaming_____search_____food.
15. Rana Pratap remained true_____ his pledge all his life.

XV. **Fill in the blanks with appropriate prepositions:**

1. Always live _____ your means.
2. Leaves fall _____ trees in Autumn
3. She has invited us all _____ her birthday party.
4. This table differs _____ that in many ways.
5. You must feel ashamed _____ your folly.
6. Indrani was married with _____ Engineer.
7. I prevented Mohan _____ go there.
8. The children left the ground one _____ one.
9. She is very proud _____ her charms.
10. I cannot depend _____ a friend like you.
11. Are you confident _____ win a scholarship?

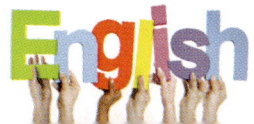

12. The baby was clinging _____ her mother in fear.
13. Compare Jainism _____ Buddhism in detail.
14. He has been complaining about headache _____ morning.
15. Early man lived _____ hunting and food gathering.

XVI. Fill in the blanks with appropriate prepositions:

1. The chocolates are to be divided _____ twenty children.
2. The note books are to be divided _____ Rita and Gita.
3. Three girls _____ Neet were seen in the library.
4. Madhu sat _____ Nidhi.
5. Smriti Parted _____ her father with tearful eyes.
6. She parted _____ her golden necklace.
7. Her father agreed _____ her proposal.
8. My teacher agrees _____ me on this point.
9. My brother lives _____ Delhi.
10. The dustbin is___the table.

XVII. Fill in the blanks with appropriate prepositions:

1. Geeta prayed _____ God _____ his mercy.
2. Miss Pandit is always kind _____ the poor.
3. Everybody is afraid _____ death.
4. The king ruled _____ his country.
5. She is tired _____ the drama of household-chores.
6. A working woman performs double role _____ pleasure.
7. Lazy persons often cry_____split milk.
8. She spoke _____ me in French.
9. Smoking is injurious _____ health.
10. She is different _____ her sister.

XVIII. Fill in the blanks with appropriate prepositions:

1. Her teacher congratulated her _____ her brilliant success.
2. My mother is very anxious _____ my health.
3. They warned him _____ the danger.
4. He insisted _____ her leaving the room at once.
5. Her parents are proud _____ her accomplishments.
6. She felt sorry _____ the poor child.
7. Ramu was obliged _____ his master _____ his kindness.
8. We should listen _____ what our elders say.
9. She quarreled _____ me _____ a trifle.
10. There is a beautiful park _____ my house.

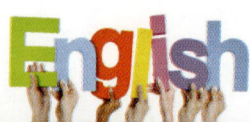

XIX. Fill in the blanks with appropriate prepositions:

1. Fresh air is conducive _____ health.
2. The environment is congenial _____ studies.
3. Your argument is contrary _____ that which your teacher has given.
4. This act of yours is derogatory_____your institution.
5. Her tale of woe is painful _____hear.
6. He appears deficient _____calcium and vitamins.
7. She is confident _____ her success in this venture.
8. He is famous _____ his intelligence.
9. He is angry _____ his friend's behavior.
10. You will be responsible _____ what you do now.

XX. Fill in the blanks with appropriate prepositions:

1. It is all due to his ambition _____ name and fame.
2. She has great conifidence _____ him.
3. She is confident _____ success.
4. He has no desire _____ wealth.
5. She acted according _____ her mother's advice.
6. In accordance _____ his advice I started this work.
7. She has great respect _____ his learning.
8. He is respectful _____ elders.
9. He is ambitious _____ name & fame.
10. He is not desirous _____ wealth.

XXI. Fill in the blanks with appropriate prepositions:

1. Kamal was born _____ 26th February.
2. Vidhu placed the purse _____ the table and came_____the house.
3. She goes to college_____8 o'clock.
4. He dropped his cap _____the well.
5. The cat jumped _____the table.
6. He killed the tiger _____ a gun shot.
7. Her father agreed _____ her proposal.
8. He walked _____the end of the street.
9. She sat _____ Radha.
10. He jumped _____ the canal to save his friend.

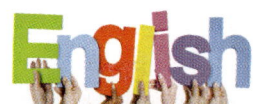

XXII. **Fill in the blanks with appropriate prepositions:**

1. _____ the party's failure, the minister left the party.
2. She apologized _____ her friend _____ the mistake.
3. His father was annoyed _____ his misconduct before his friends.
4. Her song was appropriate _____ the occasion of farewell.
5. We are answerable _____ our deeds.
6. He is proficient _____ spoken English.
7. You should make efforts to bring _____ improvement in the existing social set up.
8. She is a victim _____ circumstances.
9. He cannot tolerate interference _____ his work.
10. He intends _____ complete a Hindi dictionary.

XXIII. **Fill in the blanks with appropriate prepositions:**

1. He believes _____ taking plenty of exercise.
2. Beware _____ imitations.
3. They fought _____ heavy odds.
4. She aspires _____ fame as an author.
5. He hankers _____ fame.
6. Always stick _____ your principles.
7. We were exposed _____ great danger.
8. Her uncle deals _____ motor-cycles.
9. Deal fairly _____ everyone.
10. She persisted _____ her folly.

XXIV. **Fill in the blanks with appropriate prepositions:**

1. Mothers have affection _____ their children.
2. We are thankful _____ God _____ His blessings.
3. I felt no appetite _____ food.
4. We are tired _____ you.
5. He has an easy access _____ his officer.
6. He was true _____ his principles.
7. Pay great attention _____ English.
8. Is he unfit _____ practical work?
9. You are vexed _____ me.
10. I have an advantage _____ my enemy.

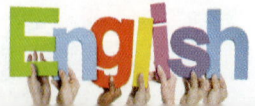

ANSWERS

    I. After, about, from, in, into, on, by-with, with, of, at.

   II. Since, from, among, besides, till, with, at, by, to, with.

  III. Above, across, before, across, against, between, for, in, of, with.

  IV. For, into, with, by-for, in, for, of, with, in, from.

  V. In, of, with, for, with, to, for, in, for, to.

  VI. With-over, by, on, of, with, since, to, with, of, off.

 VII. To, with, into, in, for, with, with, for, for, with.

VIII. Against, off, for, with, off, of, off, for, into, with.

  IX. For, over, with, with, in, about, along, in, for, upon.

  X. Of, in, to, of, with, in, to, in, off, from.

  XI. The, for, an, in, to, into, over, in, to, of.

 XII. On, with, at, for, for, of, from, in, for, into.

XIII. For, to-by, on, on-in, in-on, from, near, in, in-on, on-in.

XIV. On, in-for, of, over, for, of, of, of, from, to-for, for, with, on, in-of, for.

 XV. Within, form, on, from, of, an, to, by, of, on, to, to, with, since, with.

XVI. Among, between, besides, beside, from, from, to, with, in, under.

XVII. To-for, to, of, over, of, for, over, to, for, from.

XVIII. On, for, of, on, of, for, with-for, to, with-over, near.

XIX. To, for, to, for, to, of, of, for, at, for.

 XX. Of, in, of, for, to, to, for, to, for, of.

XXI. On, on-into, at, into, upon, with, to, till, beside, into.

XXII. On, to-for, at, for, to, in, some, of, in, to.

XXIII. In, of, for, of, for, to, to, with, for, to.

XXIV. For, to-for, in, of, to, with, to, for, with, for.

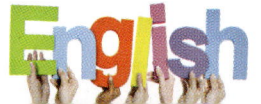

NOTES

Chapter 12

Tenses

INTRODUCTION

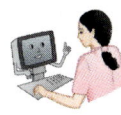

The word 'tense' means full of tension, i.e., stretched. So in English Grammar, the tense means the degree to which a verb can be stretched in terms of:

- Time of its action.
- Continuance of its action.
- Degree of completeness of its action.

The tense of a verb indicates the time reference of the action stated in the sentence present, past or future. The principal tense forms are—simple, continuous, perfect and perfect continuous. Thus, there are total of twelve tense forms. The tense of the verb brings about some changes in the verb form. The functions of these forms may be distinct or overlapping, i.e., in some cases more than one tense form may be used.

Read the following sentences:

1. I write this essay to help you.
2. I wrote this essay in his very presence.
3. I shall write another essay tomorrow.

In sentence 1: The verb *write* refers to present time.
In sentences 2: The verb *wrote* refers to past time.
In sentence 3: The verb *shall write* refers to future time.

Thus a verb may refer:

- To present time
- To past time
- To future time

Let us see the three forms of verb 'Sing':

PRESENT TENSE

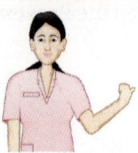

	Singular number	Plural number
1st person	I sing	We sing
2nd person	You sing	You sing
3rd person	He sings	They sing

PAST TENSE

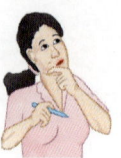

	Singular number	Plural number
1st person	I sang	We sang
2nd person	You sang	You sang
3rd person	He sang	They sang

FUTURE TENSE

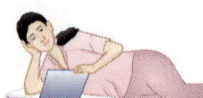

	Singular number	Plural number
1st person	We shall/will sing	We shall/will sing
2nd person	You will sing	You will sing
3rd person	They will sing	They will sing

PRESENT TENSE

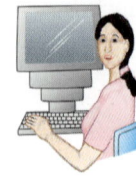

The Present Tense shows the forms of a verb which indicate that the action is done in the present time. But when the continuance and completeness of the action are taken into account, we see that there can be four forms of the Present Tense.

Observe the following sentences:

1. The baby cries for milk.
2. The baby is crying for milk.
3. The baby has cried for milk.
4. The baby has been crying for milk.

In these sentences:

❏ Sentence 1 shows an action which is done in the present time, but its exact time is not definitely known. This time is indefinite. So, this form of the present is called the **Present Indefinite Tense**.

❏ Sentence 2 shows an action in the present time. It is going on just at this time, i.e., continues to be done. So, this form of tense is called **Present Continuous Tense**.

❏ Sentence 3 indicates an action which was going on for some time in the past but has been perfected just in the present tense. So, this form of tense is called **Present Perfect Tense**.

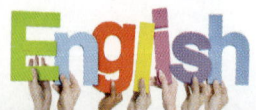

- Sentence 4 indicates an action which was going on in the past and after a partial completeness, is going on in the present time too. So, this form of tense is called the **Present Perfect Continuous Tense**.

Thus there are four forms of the Present Tense:

1. Present Indefinite Tense
2. Present Continuous Tense
3. Present Perfect Tense
4. Present Perfect Continuous Tense

PAST TENSE

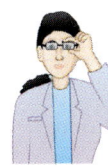

The Past Tense shows the forms of a verb which indicates that the action is done in the time gone by. But when the continuance and completeness of the action are taken into account we see that there can be four forms of the Past Tense just as can be of the Present Tense.

Observe the following sentences:

1. The baby cried for milk.
2. The baby was crying for milk.
3. The baby had cried for milk.
4. The baby had been crying for milk.

In these sentences:

- Sentence 1 shows the action of crying in the past. But the time of this action is Indefinite. So this form of the verb is called **Past Indefinite Tense**.
- Sentence 2 indicates the action of crying in the past. It continued in the past. Nothing has been said about its completeness. So this form of the verb is called **Past Continuous Tense**.
- Sentence 3 shows the action of crying not only done in the past but perfected in the past too. So this form of the verb is called **Past Perfect Tense**.
- Sentence 4 shows the action of crying in the past. It was perfected but only partially and continued to be done in the past. So this form of the verb is called **Past Perfect Continuous Tense**.

Thus there are four forms of the Past Tense:

1. Past Indefinite Tense
2. Past Continuous Tense
3. Past Perfect Tense
4. Past Perfect Continuous Tense

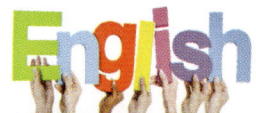

THE FUTURE TENSE

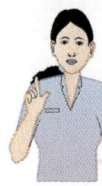

The future tense shows the forms of a verb which indicates that the action is done in the time to come. But when the continuance and completeness of the action are into account we see that there can be four forms of the Future Tense just as can be of the present and past tenses.

Observe the following sentences:

1. The baby will cry for milk.
2. The baby will be crying for milk.
3. The baby will have cried for milk.
4. The baby will have been crying for milk.

In these sentences:

❑ Sentence 1 shows the action of crying in the Future Tense. But the time of the action is indefinite. So, this form of verb is called **Future Indefinite Tense**.

❑ Sentence 2 shows the action of crying in the Future Tense. It will continue in future. Nothing has been said about its completeness. So, this form of the tense is called **Future Continuous Tense**.

❑ Sentence 3 shows the action of crying in the Future Tense. It will be perfected in the future too. So, this form of the verb is in **Future Perfect Tense**.

❑ Sentence 4 shows the action of crying in the Future Tense. It will be partially complete or perfect but will still continue in future. So, this form of the verb is called **Future Perfect Continuous Tense**.

Thus there are four forms of the Future Tense:

1. Future Indefinite Tense
2. Future Continuous Tense
3. Future Perfect Tense
4. Future Perfect Continuous Tense

SIMPLE PRESENT/PRESENT INDEFINITE

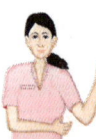

This has the same form as the root form (infinitive without 'to') of the verb 's' or 'es' is added for the third person singular he, she, it. The negative is formed with 'do not' + first form; 'does not' + first form of the verb for the third person singular. The interrogative is formed with do/does subject + first form of the verb.

Affirmative	Negative	Interrogative	Negative Interrogative
I play.	I do not play.	Do I play?	Do I not play?
We play.	We do not play.	Do we play?	Do we not play?
You play.	You do not play.	Do you play?	Do you not play?
He/she/it play.	He/she/it does not play.	Does he/she/it play?	Does he/she/it not play?
They play.	They do not play.	Do they play?	Do they not play?
Ravi plays.	Ravi does not play.	Does Ravi play?	Does Ravi not play?
Boys play.	Boys do not play.	Do boys play?	Do boys not play?

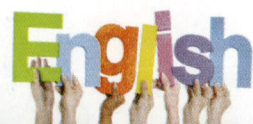

The simple present tense is used:

☐ To express habitual action
  • He smokes.
  • I always take my tea without sugar.

☐ To express general or universal truth
  • The sun rises in the east.
  • Water boils at 100°C.
  • Man is mortal.

☐ To express a fact or something which is true at present
  • All trains stop at this station.
  • She teaches English in a school.

☐ To express future action planned in advance, especially concerning a journey or programme
  • The train leaves at six in the morning.
  • Schools close in May for summer vacation and reopen in June.

☐ To introduce quotation with the verb 'say'
  • The notice says, "No parking".
  • Keats says, "A thing of beauty is a joy forever."

☐ To express a past event in a dramatic manner
  • Alexander raises his hand and salutes Porus.

☐ In exclamatory sentences beginning with 'here' and 'there'
  • There goes the bill !
  • Here comes the rain !

PRESENT CONTINUOUS TENSE

This Present Continuous Tense is formed with is/are/am + (first form + ing). The negative is formed by putting 'not' after is/are/am. The interrogative is formed by placing is/are/am before the subject.

Affirmative	Negative	Interrogative	Negative
I am playing.	I am not playing.	Am I playing?	Am I not playing?
We are playing.	We are not playing	Are we playing?	Are we not playing?
You are playing.	You are not playing.	Are you playing?	Are you not playing?
He/she/it is playing.	He/she/it are not playing.	He/she/it is playing?	He/she/it is not playing?
Ravi is playing.	Ravi is not playing.	Is Ravi playing?	Is Ravi not playing?
They are playing.	They are not playing.	Are they playing?	Are they not playing?
Boys are playing	Boys are not playing.	Are boys playing	Are boys not playing?

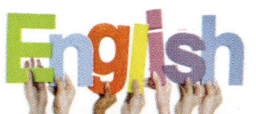

Usage

Present Continuous is used:

❏ To express an action happening now at the time of speaking.
   • I am writing a letter.
   • She is reading a book.
❏ To express an action in progress. But not necessarily at the time of speaking.
   • He is teaching English at the High School.
   • They are building a new house.
❏ To express a definite arrangement in the near future.
   • I am going to London next week.
   • I am meeting her tonight.
      The time of action must be mentioned in this case.
❏ To express an action which begins before a given time and continues after it.
   • At 8 a.m. I am having my breakfast.
❏ To express some undeniable habit.
   • He is always wasting his time in gossips.

PRESENT PERFECT TENSE

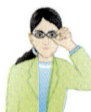

Forms

The Present Perfect Tense is formed with have (has) + Past Participle. The negative is formed by putting 'not' after have (has) the interrogative is formed by placing have (has) before the subject.

Affirmative	Negative
I have played.	I have not played.
We have played.	We have not played.
You have played.	You have not played.
He/she/it has played.	He/she/it has not played.
They have played.	They have not played.
Ravi has played.	Ravi has not played.
Boys have played.	Boys have not played.

Interrogative	Negative Interrogative
Have I played?	Have I not played?
Have we played?	Have we not played?
Have you played?	Have you not played?
Has he/she/it played?	Has he/she/it not played?
Have they played?	Have they not played?
Has Ravi played?	Has Ravi not played?
Have boys played?	Have boys not played?

The Present Perfect Tense is used:

❏ To express a recently completed action
   • I have just finished my work.
   • He has gone to school.
❏ To express past action when the time is not given and not definite
   • I have read the poem but I do not understand it.
   • Have you had your lunch? No, I have not had it yet.

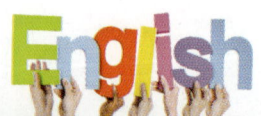

- ❏ To express past action or events the results of which are still present
  - He has had a bad accident (Perhaps he is in hospital).
  - The prisoners have escaped from the jail (They are still at large).
- ❏ To express an action that began in the past and continues up to the present moment
  - l have lived here for ten years (I am still here).
  - We have waited all day (We are still waiting).
  - He has always helped us (He still helps us).

PRESENT PERFECT CONTINUOUS

Affirmative	Negative	Interrogative
I (we, you, they) have been playing.	I (we, you, they) have not been playing.	Have I (we, you they) been playing?
He (she/it) has been playing.	He (she/it) has not been playing.	Has he (she, it) been playing?
Mohan has been playing.	Mohan has not been playing.	Has Mohan been playing?

Usage

- ❏ To express an action which began in the past and is still continuing
  - It has been raining since 6 a.m.
  - They have been playing for two hours.
  - I have been waiting for him for an hour and he still has not come.
- ❏ To express an action which is already finished, but whose effect or result persists
  - He is shivering because he has been bathing for an hour.
  - The boys have been running round the town all day and are now resting.

SIMPLE PAST TENSE

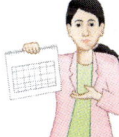

Form

The Simple Past Tense is formed with the past tense second form of the verb. The negative is formed with did not + first form of the verb. The interrogative is formed with did + subject + first form of the verb.

Affirmative	Negative	Interrogative	Negative Interrogative
I played.	I did not play.	Did I play?	Did I not play?
We played.	We did not play.	Did we play?	Did we not play?
You played.	You did not play.	Did you play?	Did you not play?
He/she/it played.	He/she/it did not play.	Did he/she/it play?	Did he/she/it not play?
They played.	They did not play.	Did they play?	Did they not play?
Ravi played.	Ravi did not play.	Did Ravi play?	Did Ravi not play?
Boys played.	Boys did not play.	Did boys play?	Did boys not play?

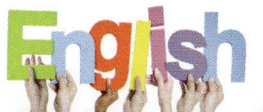

Usage

The Simple Past Tense is used:

- ❑ To express a past event or past action. The action is complete till the present
  - It is therefore, used when the time is given.
  - I met him yesterday.
  - She died in 1987.
- ❑ When the time is not given, but it is implied and definite
  - The train was half on hour late.
  - I bought this pen in Mumbai.
- ❑ When the time is asked for
  - When did you meet him?
  - When did you come here?
- ❑ To express a past habit or regular action in the past
  - Every day he read a chapter of the Gita.
  - He never smoked.
- ❑ To express an action which lasted for a period of time in the past
  - He worked in that office for four years.
  - She lived in Delhi for a long-time.
    'For' in the Simple Past Tense expresses the duration of the past action.

PAST CONTINUOUS TENSE

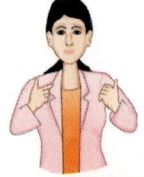

Form

The Past Continuous Tense is formed by was/were + (first form + ing). Negative is formed by putting 'not' after was/were. The interrogative is formed by putting was/were before the subject.

Affirmative	Negative		Interrogative	Negative interrogative
I was playing.	I was not playing.		Was I playing?	Was I not playing?
We were playing.	We were not playing.		Were we playing?	Were we not playing?
You were playing.	You were not playing.		Were you playing?	Were you not playing?
He/she/it was playing.	He/she/it was not playing.		Was he/she/it playing?	Was he/she/it not playing?
They were playing.	They were not playing.		Were they playing?	Were they not playing?
Ravi was playing.	Ravi was not playing.		Was Ravi playing?	Was Ravi not playing?
Boys were playing.	Boys were not playing.		Were boys playing?	Were boys not playing?

Usage

The Past Continuous Tense is used:

- ❑ To express an action that was in progress at some time in the past
  - I was taking my bath at 8 o'clock.
  - I was playing in the garden when he came.

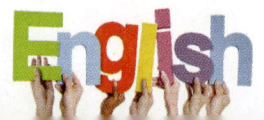

- ❑ To express two or more actions in progress at the same time
  - While I was doing my homework, my brother was playing outside.
  - The students were talking when the teacher was writing on the black-board.
- ❑ To express an often repeated (undesirable) past action
  - She was always taunting him.
  - He was always coming at odd hours.

PAST PERFECT TENSE

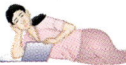

Form

This Past Perfect Tense is formed with had + Past Participle (second form of the verb). The negative is formed by putting 'not' after had. The interrogative is formed by putting had before the subject.

Interrogative	Negative Interrogative	Interrogative	Negative Interrogative
I had played.	I had not played.	Had I played?	Had I not played?
We had played.	We had not played.	Had We played?	Had we not played?
You had played.	You had not played.	Had I Played?	Had I not played?
He/she had played.	He/she had not played.	Had you played?	Had you not played?
They had played.	They had not played.	Had he/she/it played?	Had he/she/it not played?
Ravi had played.	Ravi had not played.	Had they played?	Had they not played?
Boys had played.	Boys had not played.	Had Ravi played?	Had Ravi not played?
		Had boys played?	Had boys not played?

Usage

The Past Perfect Tense is used:

- ❑ To express an action completed before a certain moment in the past
  - At 7 p.m. all the shops had closed.
  - At 16 years she had passed her BA examination.
- ❑ To express action in the past which was completed before another action also in the past
  - We had locked all the rooms before we left the house.
  - I had already known the result when they rang me up.
- ❑ To express unfulfilled desires of the past
  - I wish I had listened to my father's advice (But I did not listen).
  - If only he had not wasted his time (But he wasted).
  - To express impossible (unfulfilled) conditions of the past.
  - If you had worked hard, you would have passed.
  - If he had left earlier, he would have reached in time.

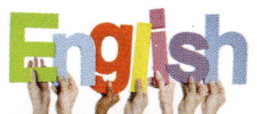

PAST PERFECT CONTINUOUS TENSE

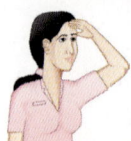

Form

The Past Perfect Continuous Tense is formed with had been + (first form + ing). The negative is formed by putting 'not' after had. The interrogative is formed by putting had before the subject.

Affirmative	Negative
I had been playing.	I had not been playing.
We had been playing.	We had not been playing.
You had been playing.	You had not been playing.
He/she/it had been play- ing.	He/she/it had not been playing.
They had been playing.	They had not been playing.
Ravi had been playing.	Ravi had not been playing.
Boys had been playing.	Boys had not been playing

Interrogative	Negative Interrogative
Had I been playing?	Had I not been playing?
Had we been playing?	Had we not been playing?
Had you been playing?	Had you not been playing?
Had he/she/it been playing?	Had he/she/it not been playing?
Had they been playing?	Had they not been playing?
Had Ravi been playing?	Had Ravi not been playing?
Had boys been playing?	Had boys not been playing?

Usage

The Past Perfect Continuous Tense is used:

❑ To express an action that began before a certain time in the past and continued up to that time or stopped just before it
  • The baby had been crying for ten minutes when the nurse attended to her.
  • Until he reached VIII class, Ravi had been studying in a village school.
❑ To express a repeated action in the past perfect on a continuous action
  • He had tried many times to phone her.
  • He had been trying to phone her.

SIMPLE FUTURE TENSE

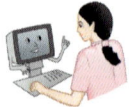

Form

The form of the verb in the Simple Future Tense is shall/will + base form of the verb. To express the Future Tense, shall is used with pronouns of the first person (I, will) with all other subjects.

Affirmative	Negative
I shall go.	I shall not go.
We shall go.	We shall not go.
You will go.	You will not go.
He will go.	He will not go.
They will go.	They will not go.

Interrogative	Negative Interrogative
Shall I go?	Shall I not go?
Shall we go?	Shall we not go?
Will you go?	Will you not go?
Will he go?	Will he not go?
Will they go?	Will they not go?

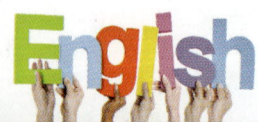

On speech shall and will are usually contracted to 'll in affirmative sentence.

I shall play.	I'll play.
He will play.	He'll play.

In the negative shall not become shan't and will not become won't:

I shall not go.	I shan't go.
He will not go.	He won't go.

Simple Future Tense is used:
- ❑ To express an action that will take place in the future
  - I shall visit Amritsar next week.
  - Our team will play a match tomorrow.
- ❑ To denote the main clause when the other clause is of condition or time
  - If you work hard, you will succeed.
  - When it rains, we shall stop work.

FUTURE CONTINUOUS TENSE

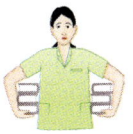

The form of the verb in the Future Continuous Tense is: shall/will + be + verb + ing.

Affirmative	Negative
I shall be waiting.	I shall not (or shan't) be waiting.

Interrogative	Negative Interrogative
Will he be waiting?	Will he not (won't he) be waiting?

The negative is formed by putting not after shall/will. The interrogative is formed by inverting the subject shall/will.

Future Continuous Tense is used:
- ❑ To express an action that will be going on at a given point of time in the future
  - We shall be having a party tomorrow night.
  - When I reach Shimla, it will be snowing.

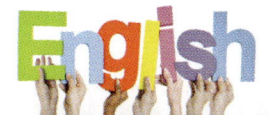

FUTURE PERFECT TENSE

The form of the verb in the Future Perfect Tense is: shall/will + have + past participle. The negative is formed by putting not after shall/will. The interrogative is formed by inverting the subject and shall/will.

Affirmative	Negative	Interrogative	Negative Interrogative
They will have left.	They will not have left.	Will they have left?	Will they not have left?

Future Perfect Tense is used:

- ❑ To express an action that will be completed at some point of time in the future
  - • The film will have started before we reach the cinema hall.
  - • By this time next year he will have become a graduate.

FUTURE PERFECT CONTINUOUS TENSE

The form of the verb in the Future Perfect Continuous Tense is: shall/will + have been + verb + ing.

Affirmative	Negative	Interrogative	Negative Interrogative
He will have been sleeping.	He will not have been sleeping.	Shall we have been sleeping?	Shall we not have been sleeping?

The negative is formed by putting not after shall/will. The interrogative is formed by inverting the subject and shall/will. Future Perfect Continuous Tense is used to express action continuing beyond some given time in the future.

- ❑ By next month I shall have been reaching in this college for 30 years.
- ❑ They will have been waiting for an hour when we reach there.

Errors in the use of Tenses

Incorrect Sentences

- ❑ The rain has ceased yesterday.
- ❑ Babar founded the Mughal Empire.
- ❑ I has been to Paris.
- ❑ I have gone there in 1987.
- ❑ I have passed my examination.
- ❑ I have passed it two years ago.
- ❑ I learn that my friend has failed.
- ❑ I have finished my letter last evening.
- ❑ The parrot has died of cold last night.
- ❑ The judge declared that he is guilty.
- ❑ I said that it was easier to talk than to act.
- ❑ If you had played the piano, I would sing.

Correct Sentences

- ❑ The rain ceased yesterday.
- ❑ Babar found the Mughal Empire.
- ❑ I have been to Paris.
- ❑ I went there in 1987.
- ❑ I passed my examination.
- ❑ I passed it two years ago.
- ❑ I learnt that my friend has failed.
- ❑ I finished my letter last evening.
- ❑ The parrot died of cold last night.
- ❑ The judge declared that he was guilty.
- ❑ I said that it is easier to talk than to act.
- ❑ If you had played the piano, I would have sung.

Contd...

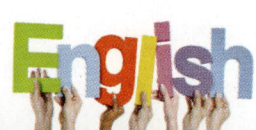

- If you played the piano, I will sing.
- The patient died before the doctor came.
- Look! The smoke comes out of the window.
- I saw her as I passed by her house yesterday.
- He came into my room while I wrote.
- If you will play the piano, I will sing.
- I solved all the questions before the time was over.
- He was ill for two days when the doctor was sent for.
- The boat was sunk by a storm which suddenly sprang up.
- You will be hearing this news already, so I need not to repeat it.

- If you had played the piano, I would sing.
- The patient had died before the doctor came.
- Look! The smoke is coming out of the window.
- I saw her as I was passing by her house yesterday.
- He came into my room while I was writing.
- If you play the piano. I will sing.
- I had solved all the questions before the time was over.
- He had been ill for two days when the doctor was sent for.
- The boat was sunk by a storm which had suddenly sprung up.
- You will have heard this news already, so I need not repeat it.

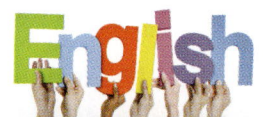

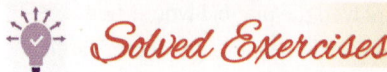

Solved Exercises

I. **Complete each sentence with a suitable tense of the verb in brackets:**

1. Peter _____ (not go) to the cinema last night.
2. Sorry, I _____ (forget) to do my homework yesterday.
3. What _____ (you see) on TV last night?
4. Sonia _____ (leave) Italy and travelled to France last month.
5. _____ (they enjoy) their holiday in Greece last year?
6. While I _____ (eat) my dinner, the phone _____ (ring)
7. Richard _____ (always, get up) before 7 am.
8. Hurry up; the bus _____ (wait) for us.
9. Where _____ (we, go) _____? This is the wrong road.
10. My friends _____ (not believe) my story.
11. Please be quiet; I _____ (read) a very interesting book.
12. Marie _____ (usually, sit) at the front of the class.
13. Carol cannot talk to you at the moment. He _____ (have) a shower.
14. Please wait for a moment, Alka. I _____ (talk) to Swati.
15. This car _____ (cost) a lot of money.

II. **Complete the sentences with the past form of the verb in brackets:**

1. The last lesson _____ (begin) at 2.30.
2. Johnny _____ (feel) ill after lunch.
3. Suddenly a bird _____ (fly) in the window.
4. I think you _____ (do) the wrong thing.
5. Babita _____ (get) ready very quickly.
6. We _____ (know) the answer.
7. The students _____ (stand) up when the teacher arrived.
8. It was cold, but I _____ (wear) two pullovers.
9. Anudeep _____ (eat) two plates of noodles.
10. Richa _____ (tell) us the time.

III. **Complete the sentences with the perfect form of the verbs in brackets:**

1. Harish _____ (do) the housework.
2. Kitty and Bimla _____ (find) a new flat.
3. Neeru _____ (send) an email.
4. I _____ (decide) to learn Spanish.
5. Sarla and Diana _____ (eat) all the sandwiches.
6. Francis _____ (buy) a dog.

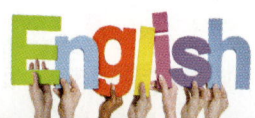

7. Meera and Radha _____ (start) at a new school.
8. Farida _____ (break) her cup.
9. I _____ (Lose) my umbrella.
10. Manish _____ (take) the dog for a walk.

IV. Complete the sentences with the past simple or present perfect form of the verbs in brackets:

1. Where _____ (you go) for your holidays last year?
2. I cannot play anymore. I _____ (just hurt) my foot.
3. Jennifer is a famous writer, and _____ (write) over fifty books.
4. Sorry, I _____ (not finish) my letters yet.
5. We had a great party last week. Who _____ (you invite)?
6. Where _____ (you, meet) Sonia? Was it at the sports centre?
7. Pradeep _____ (not play) basketball for a month.

V. Complete each sentence with the past simple or the present perfect form of the verbs in brackets:

1. Tina is not here. She _____ (just go) to school.
2. What time _____ (you get up) this morning?
3. Parveen _____ (have) a bad car accident three years ago.
4. I (live) in the same house since 2015.
5. What _____ (you do) last night?
6. Betty _____ (not finish) his work yet.
7. Tina _____ (arrive) here in 2018.
8. _____ (you see) my watch? I cannot find it.

VI. Complete each sentence using the present continuous form of the verb in brackets:

1. What _____ (you do) this evening?
2. I _____ (not come) to school tomorrow.
3. Tiny _____ (go) to Italy next week.
4. _____ (you have) a party this week.
5. We _____ (not go) home on the bus after school.
6. Mrs Mangat _____ (teach) us this afternoon.
7. Ora and Gulu _____ (not come) to the meeting.
8. _____ (Jack go) to the football match tomorrow?
9. Annie _____ (not work) on Friday.
10. _____ (you leave) this afternoon.

VII. Put each verb in brackets into either the past simple or past continuous:

1. When Harry _____ (wake up), we _____ (tell) him the news.
2. Everyone _____ (wait) for the concert to begin when a message _____ (arrive).
3. Charlie _____ (want) a relaxing holiday, so she _____ (choose) to stay on a small island.
4. When Romy _____ (study) in America, his parents _____ (phone) him every week.

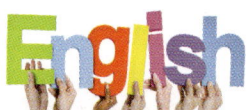

5. I _____ (find) my pen while I _____ (look for) my bag.

6. Anil _____ (watch) a film on television when Jane _____ (arrive).

7. When the lights _____ (go out), I _____ (lie) in bed reading.

8. When you _____ (go) to the new restaurant, what _____ (you eat)?

VIII. Put each verb in brackets into either the present perfect, past simple or present simple:

1. Last week I _____ (lose) my scarf, and now I _____ (lose) my gloves.

2. I _____ (work) for BLC Bank now but I _____ (decide) to change job.

3. We _____ (be) here for hours. Are you sure we _____ (come) to the right place?

4. _____ (you see) my mobile? I am sure I _____ (leave) it here earlier.

5. We _____ (have) some coffee and then _____ (catch) the bus home.

6. I _____ (never eat) Octopus, but once on holiday I _____ (eat) some squid.

7. I _____ (hope) you are not a vegetarian. I _____ (cook) you some lamb chops.

8. Recently a lot of young people _____ (take up) charity work.

9. When we _____ (reach) the cinema, there _____ (not be) any tickets left.

10. Please come quickly; Nick _____ (have) an accident, and he _____ (go) to hospital.

IX. Put each verb in brackets into the present simple or continuous, or the past simple or continuous:

1. What _____ (you do)? I am an engineer.

2. The door was open so the dog _____ (run) into the living room.

3. When we arrived home, John _____ (sit) outside the door.

4. Can you help me? I _____ (did) not understand Spanish.

5. At the beginning of the film I _____ (realize) I'd seen it before.

6. I am sorry, I cannot talk long. I _____ (study) for an examination.

7. At the moment of the earthquake Pintoo _____ (read) in bed.

8. I will phone you as soon as I _____ (know) the results.

9. I _____ (stay) at the hotel Taj. Why do not you call me?

10. What _____ (you do) when you saw the snake?

X. Complete each sentence with a suitable form of the verb in brackets:

1. I am soaked to the skin; if only I _____ (bring) an umbrella.

2. This pullover was really cheap. I wish I _____ (buy) two of them.

3. I like your school. I wish I _____ (go) there too.

4. I must get in touch with Sophia. If only I _____ (know) her phone number.

5. This bus is really slow; I wish we _____ (take) the train.

6. I am disappointed with this camera. I wish I _____ (not buy) it.

7. I answered three questions well. If only I _____ (finish) the whole test.

8. I cannot understand Maria; I wish I _____ (speak) Spanish.

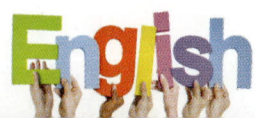

Answers

I. Didn't go, forgot, did you see, left, did they enjoy, was eating, rang, always gets up, is waiting, are we going, don't believe, am reading, usually sits, is having, am talking, costs.

II. Began, felt, flew, did, got, knew, stood, wore, ate, told.

III. Has done, have found, has sent, have decided, have eaten, has brought, have started, has broken, have lost, has taken.

IV. Did you go, have just hurt, has written, haven't finished, did you invite, did you meet, hasn't played.

V. Has just gone, did you get up, had, have lived, did you go, hasn't finished, arrived, have you seen.

VI. Are you doing, am not coming, is going, are you having, are not going, is Mrs Mangat teaching, are not coming, Is Jack going, is not working, are you leaving.

VII. Woke up, told; was waiting, arrived; wanted, chose; was studying, phoned; found, was looking for; was watching, arrived; went out, was lying; went, did you eat.

VIII. Lost, have just lost; work, have decided; have been, have come; have you seen, left; had, caught; have never eaten, ate; hope, have cooked; have taken up; reached, weren't; has had, has gone.

IX. Do you do, ran, was sitting, do, realised, am studying, was reading, know, am staying, did you do.

X. Had brought, had bought, went, knew, had taken, hadn't bought, had finished, spoke/could speak.

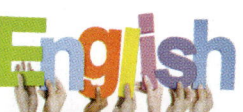

Practice Exercises

I. Fill in the blanks with the simple present tense of the verbs given in brackets:

1. He who _____ (stand) first will get the prize.
2. As soon as the referee _____ (whistle) the match will start.
3. Do in Rome as the Romans _____ (do).
4. If it _____ (rain) hard, she will cancel her tour.
5. When they are here, they often _____ (visit) me.
6. Please tell him what you _____ (want).
7. There is a saying that nothing _____ (Succeed) like success.
8. If she _____ (try) she can win the race.

II. Put the verbs in brackets into the present continuous tense:

1. The train _____ (arrive).
2. She _____ (stand) by the fire.
3. They cannot come because they _____ (suffer) from fever.
4. What you _____ (do) here?
5. You cannot see her now; she _____ (have) a bath.
6. I am _____ (write) a letter at the moment.
7. He _____ (wear) a warm coat today because it is very cold.
8. Please take an umbrella with you. It _____ (rain).

III. Fill in the blanks with the present perfect tense of the verbs given in brackets:

1. You _____ enough food. (eat)
2. Khursheed Ahmed _____ the examination. (pass)
3. I _____ here for four years. (live)
4. How long _____ you _____ her? (know)
5. He _____ me to lunch twice. (ask)
6. We _____ a new house. Come and look at it. (buy)
7. She _____ just _____ her father's letter. (receive)
8. They _____ not _____ the electricity bill yet. (pay)

IV. Fill in the blanks, using the present perfect continuous tense of the verb in brackets:

1. He _____ from fever since Friday. (suffer)
2. I _____ this house since Christmas. (build)
3. How long _____ you _____ English? (learn)
4. It _____ for two days now. (snow)
5. We _____ strange noises since evening. (hear)
6. I _____ for five years. (drive)
7. They _____ only milk for the last two days. (take)
8. _____ You _____ for a long time? (wait)

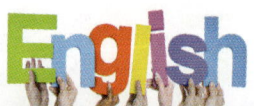

V. Fill in the blanks with the simple past tense of the verbs given below:

1. I _____ the play very much. (like)
2. They _____ their mistake at last. (realize)
3. He was taking tea when I _____ him. (visit)
4. He was very careless. He _____ his time. (waste)
5. I _____ him for his bad ways. (hate)
6. As he was getting into the car, it _____ suddenly. (start)
7. He always _____ this identity card with him. (carry)
8. My servant _____ the fire. (light)

VI. Put the verbs in brackets in the continuous form of the past tense:

1. She _____ (sing) when someone knocked at her door.
2. He _____ (clean) his gun when it accidently went off.
3. He found his broken toy as he _____ (dig) in the garden.
4. While he _____ (make) his speech he forgot it.
5. When I last saw her she _____ (wear) an attractive dress.
6. When I _____ (look) the other way someone picked my pocket.
7. We could not go out as a strong wind _____ (blow).
8. He _____ (talk) to a close friend when the servant entered the room.

VII. Put the verbs in brackets in the past perfect tense:

1. Santa Singh _____ (live) in Kolkata for five years when we met.
2. I _____ (see) him only once before he left for Europe.
3. She _____ (never see) such a huge building before.
4. If I _____ (know) your address, I would have written to you.
5. When he _____ (finish) his speech, he sat down.
6. If I _____ (take) care of my health, I would not have fallen ill.

VIII. Put the verbs in brackets in the past perfect continuous tense:

1. She _____ (write) a novel for two months when she came across a good publisher.
2. I _____ (read) in that school for three years when it had a new principal.
3. The school bell _____ (ring) for some time before I heard it.

IX. Add 'will' or 'shall' to these sentences:

1. The match _____ begin at 5 pm.
2. Nobody _____ go without permission.
3. It _____ rain today.
4. _____ We have a house of our own? We have enough money.
5. Tomorrow _____ be a holiday.
6. Some friends _____ visit me next week.
7. Tea _____ be ready soon.
8. You _____ not steal again.

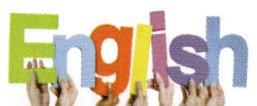

X. Answer the following questions, using the future continuous tense:

1. What will you be doing when he comes here?

   _____

2. Where will he be living next year?

   _____

3. When will they be arriving here?

   _____

4. How will you be helping him?

   _____

5. What will Rajan be learning in London?

   _____

XI. Put the verbs in brackets in the future perfect tense:

1. He _____ (reach) the railway station when the train arrives.
2. I _____ (take) tea when he comes.
3. The guests _____ (leave) before 8 p.m.
4. They _____ (catch) the thief before the arrival of the police.
5. He _____ (make) many attempts before he succeeds.

XII. Put the verbs in brackets in the future perfect continuous tense:

1. You _____ (talk) for a long time before the teacher warns you.
2. They _____ (build) the house for a year when they get a loan.
3. He _____ (use) the scooter for a few years when he buys a new one.
4. The post _____ (lie) vacant for three months before they appoint a new man.
5. The tap _____ (run) for some time before that careless boy turns it off.

XIII. Fifty years from now we will _____ (live) in multi-storied buildings. That will happen because there _____ (be) no land left to build houses on. We _____ probably _____ (move) around in vehicles all the time because it _____ (be) quite impossible to walk along roads. No plants or trees _____ (grow) anywhere because there _____ (be) no soil for them to grow on. We _____ (eat) not natural but synthetic food, and our children _____ (drink) not cow's but artificial milk.

XIV. It was not until she _____ (arrive) at her relative's house in Panchkula that Meenu _____ (realize) she _____ (lose) her purse, containing some money, jewellery and important documents. Desperate to get it back, she even _____ (race) up to Kalka to see if she _____ (leave) it behind on the train she _____ (travel) by. But in vain next morning as she was about to leave the house, she _____ (see) a boy coming up to the door with her purse in his hand. His name _____ (be) Aman and he _____ (live) next door. He _____ (spot) the purse lying on a pile of garbage near the house.

XV. The storm didn't break, but in the evening a strong wind _____ (start) blowing. The ship _____ (rock) to and fro, rocking and rolling to the music of the wind _____ waves _____ (dash) against it. Even though there _____ (be) slippery, I _____ (run) around. That's when

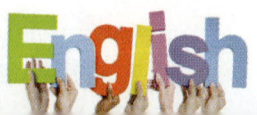

I _____ (notice) uncle leaving over the railings. I _____ (run) up to him, thinking he too, _____ (enjoy) the experience, "good morning, uncle, _____ (be not) it lovely?". I _____ (ask) him.

XVI. It _____ (be) however, not easy to convince others. People _____ (hold) on to their old beliefs and _____ (not like) to change them. Base _____ (suggest) that the animal, vegetable and mineral kingdoms _____ (be) one and have a good deal in common. He _____ (say) that plants and metals _____ (have) a life of their own and _____ (can) become tired depressed or happy. People _____ (laugh) at him. They _____ (not take) him seriously.

XVII. All of a sudden there was a noise. A man in Kurta pyjama (a) _____ (stand) in the middle of the playfield. His Turkish cap (b) _____ (be) on the ground upside down. The gulli (c) _____ (seem) to have hit the cap on its way to me. The Wonder of it all (d) _____ (be) that the gulli (e) _____ (land) inside the cap. The man (f) _____ (be) furious. "You naughty boys I see what you (g) _____ (do). I (h) _____ (teach) you a lesson," he (i) _____ (shout).

XVIII. Suddenly I heard Safdar's cry, Ajay! Lokesh! Run, run! The watchman (a) _____ (come). Perched on top of a branch, I (b) _____ (see) the tall sinister looking figure of the watchman approaching. He (c) _____ (wave) a staff in his hand. Safdar & Ajay (d) _____ (be) already on the ground, and (e) _____ (start) running. The watchman (f) _____ (wave) his staff and ran after them, shouting. "Thieves! Thieves! See they (g) _____ (not escape). I (h) _____ (lose) no time. I (i) _____ (jump) down from the tree and (j) _____ (take) to my heels. Safdar and Ajay (k) _____ (be) far ahead and I (l) _____ (run) faster. As I (m) _____ (leap) over ditches and boulders in the orchard, the guavas (n) _____ (begin) to fall out of my pockets.

XIX. When I got home my dog (a) _____ (sit) at the door, waiting for me. I (b) _____ (feel) very bad, for I (c) _____ (delay) by the traffic jam. He (d) _____ (wag) his tail and I knew that he was annoyed. In order to please him, I (e) _____ (pat) him on the back and then (f) _____ (give) him a dog biscuit, thus removing his annoyance.

XX. Name the *"Tense of the Verb"* in each sentence:

1. The school shall remain closed tomorrow.
2. It is raining cats and dogs outside.
3. Ram has stood first in the test.
4. She will have finished her home-work by 4 p.m.
5. We shall have Diwali in early November.
6. Your mother has been looking for you since morning.
7. She is going to join this school on Monday.
8. The cook lights a match-stick.
9. She has cut her little finger while mending her pencil.

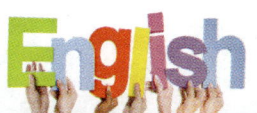

10. Ravana abducted Sita to his kingdom.
11. The earth revolves round the sun.
12. I have helped him for a long time.
13. Did you ever smoke in your life?
14. Does she run this primary school?
15. The cowherd had run a thorn into his foot.
16. Will you be bringing my book tomorrow?
17. Shall we not have completed this job by dusk?
18. Meena has been ill with fever since Monday.
19. The church bells had not been ringing since dawn.
20. She cut her finger in the kitchen.

XXI. **Fill each blank with the correct form of the Verb given in brackets:**

1. Prices _____ up very high. (go)
2. We _____ Agra a day before the earthquake. (leave)
3. The scissors _____ blunt, not sharp. (be)
4. To fear men _____ the biggest sin. (be)
5. How many eggs has your hen _____ today? (lay)
6. The train _____ when I reached the station. (arrive)
7. Your message _____ me yesterday. (reach)
8. Your message _____ me today morning. (reach)
9. Your message _____ me by then. (reach)
10. The match _____ on for an hour. (go)

XXII. **Choose the correct alternative out of those given in brackets:**

1. The principal _____ to see you. (wants, is wanting)
2. I _____ a new bike yesterday. (bought, have bought)
3. She _____ a lot of work today. (did, has done)
4. I _____ here since 1980. (am working, have been working)
5. We _____ our lunch at 1 pm. (had, had had)
6. The train _____ before we reach. (has left, will have left)
7. I _____ him with a single hit. (fell, felled)
8. I _____ ill for two weeks. (am, have been)
9. He _____ his lesson when you return. (will learn, will be learning)

XXIII. **Correct the following sentences:**

1. He left for the school before I reached his house.

_____

2. I have been for Agra yesterday.

_____

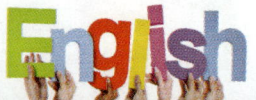

3. You look sad for some days.

   _____

4. The sheep ran away before the wolf came.

   _____

5. I had sent him his books in the morning.

   _____

6. Children are playing in the park since morning.

   _____

7. I am in Delhi for more than a week.

   _____

8. Pt. Jawaharlal Nehru had been born in 1889.

   _____

9. They are living in this house since 1982.

   _____

10. I told you I have no money in my pocket.

    _____

11. Reading always made people wiser.

    _____

12. He never has and will never help you.

    _____

13. He was so proud that nobody likes to talk to him.

    _____

14. An idle man will not work in my office.

    _____

15. I had bought this hat at a fair.

    _____

16. I am reading the Bible every day since 1987.

    _____

17. Did you not go to the bank as yet?

    _____

18. The sun rose in the east every day.

    _____

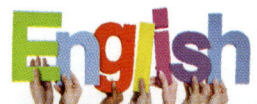

Answers

I. Stands, whistles, do, rains, visit, want, succeeds, tries.

II. Is arriving, is standing, are suffering, are doing, is having, writing, is wearing, is raining.

III. Have eaten, has passed, have lived, have-known, has asked, have bought, has-received, have-paid.

IV. Has been suffering, have been building, have-been learning, has been snowing, have been hearing, have been driving, have been taking, Have-been waiting.

V. Liked, realized, visited, wasted, hated, started, carried, lighted.

VI. Was singing, was cleaning, was digging, was making, was wearing, was looking, was blowing, was talking.

VII. Had lived, had seen, had never seen, had known, had finished, had taken.

VIII. Had been writing, had been reading, had been ringing.

IX. Will, shall, shall, Will, will, shall, will, will.

X. I will be studying when he comes here, He will be living in Delhi next year, They will be arriving here in the evening, I will be helping him with money, Rajan will be learning.

XI. Will have reached, will have taken, will have left, will have caught, will have made.

XII. Will have been talking, will have been building, will have been using, will have been lying, will have been running.

XIII. Be living, will be, will, be moving, will be, will be grown, will be, will eat, will be drinking.

XIV. Arrived, realized, had lost, raced, had left, travelled, saw, was, lived, spotted.

XV. Started, rocked, with, dashing, was, ran, noticed, ran, enjoyed, is not, asked.

XVI. Is, hold, do not like, suggests, are, says, have, can, laugh, do not take.

XVII. Stood, was, seemed, was, landed, was, have done, will teach, shouted.

XVIII. Is coming, saw, waved, were, started, waved, should not escape, lost, jumped, took, were, ran, leapt, began.

XIX. Was sitting, felt, was delayed, wagged, patted, gave.

XX. Future indefinite, present continuous, present perfect, future perfect, future perfect, present perfect continuous, present continuous, present indefinite, present perfect continuous, present indefinite, present indefinite, present perfect, past indefinite, present indefinite, past indefinite, future continuous, future perfect, past perfect continuous, past continuous, past indefinite.

XXI. Have gone, left, are, is, laid, had arrived, reached, will reach, had reached, went.

XXII. Is wanting, bought, did, have been working, had, will have left, fell, have been, will be learning.

XXIII. He had left for the school before I reached his house, I have been to Agra yesterday, You look sad from some days, The sheep had run away before the wolf came, I sent him his books in the morning, Children have been playing in the park since morning, I am in Delhi from more than a week, Pt. Jawahar Lal was born in 1889, They have been living in this house since 1982, I told you that I have no money in my pocket, Reading always makes people wiser, He has never and will never help you, He is so proud that nobody likes to talk to him, An idle man cannot work in my office, I had bought this hat at a fair, I have been reading the Bible everyday since 1987, Have you not gone to the bank yet?, The sun rises in the east every day.

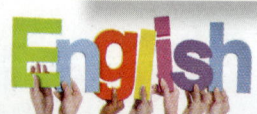

Chapter 13

Active and Passive Voice

ACTIVE AND PASSIVE VOICE

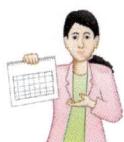

When a verb represents its subject as doing the action, it is said to be in the active voice. When a verb represents its subject as being acted upon, it is said to be in passive voice.

e.g., *Sheela* wrote a *letter* – Active

(Subject) (Object)

A letter was written by *Sheela* – Passive

In the first sentence (i.e., active voice), the stress is on the subject.

In the second sentence, the object occupies the important position.

CHANGE OF VOICE

The most important rule for change of a sentence from the active voice to the passive voice is:

❏ The object of the verb in the active voice becomes the subject of the verb in the passive. In addition to this, the agent, when mentioned is preceded generally by the preposition 'by' in the passive voice.

An interrogative sentence continues to remain interrogative when changed from the active to the passive form.

$$NP_1 \; Aux\text{-}V\text{-}NP_2 \Rightarrow Np_2 - Aux\text{-}be\text{-}en - V\text{-}by\text{-}Np_1$$

Sheela - past-write - *a letter* $\Rightarrow$ A letter – past – be – en – write – by Sheela

$$\begin{bmatrix} be + past = was \\ write + en = written \end{bmatrix}$$

RULES FOR CHANGE OF VERBS

Tenses

1. Present Indefinite

Rule:

First form of verb
First form of verb+s or es
Do - Ist form
Does - IInd form
→
is
am
are
third form

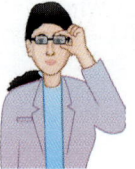

Do not lose the focus

Active	Passive
1. Ram plays a match.	A match is played by Ram.
2. She likes singing.	Singing is liked by her.
3. We do not like pictures.	Pictures are not liked by us.
4. He does not abuse me.	I am not abused by him.
5. Do you play a match?	Is a match played by you?

2. Past Indefinite

Rule:

Second form of verb
Did–first form
→
was
were
third form

Active	Passive
1. Jesus saved the child.	The child was saved by Jesus.
2. They struck his name off.	His name was struck off by them
3. Did they help you in time?	Were you helped by them in time?
4. We did not see the books.	The books were not seen by us.
5. I opened an account.	An account was opened by me.

3. Future Indefinite

Rule:

will
shall
– 1st form
will be
shall be
third form

Active	Passive
1. You will select him.	He will be selected by you.
2. She will punish me.	I shall be punished by her.
3. I shall not read a book.	A book will not be read by me.
4. You will catch him copying.	He will be caught copying by you.

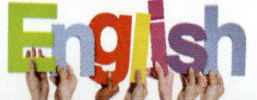

4. **Present Continuous**

Rule: $\left.\begin{array}{c} \text{is} \\ \text{am} \\ \text{are} \end{array}\right\}$ first form + ing $\rightarrow$ $\left.\begin{array}{c} \text{is} \\ \text{am} \\ \text{are} \end{array}\right\}$ behind third form

Active	Passive
1. She is milking the cow.	The cow is being milked by her.
2. The children are plucking flowers.	Flowers are being plucked by the children.
3. Are they writing a book?	Is a book being written by them?
4. She is collecting stamps.	Stamps are being collected by her.
5. Is he using the right words?	Are the right words being used by him?

5. **Past Continuous**

Rule: $\left.\begin{array}{c} \text{was} \\ \text{were} \end{array}\right]$ 1st form + ing $\rightarrow$ $\left.\begin{array}{c} \text{was} \\ \text{were} \end{array}\right]$ being + third form

Active	Passive
1. I was solving the sums.	The sums were being solved by me.
2. You were reading books	Books were being read by you.
3. Were they seeing a picture?	Was a picture being seen by them?
4. Was he laughing at you?	Were you being laughed by him?
5. Was she following him?	Was he being followed by her?

6. **Present Perfect**

Rule: $\left.\begin{array}{c} \text{has} \\ \text{have} \end{array}\right]$ third form $\rightarrow$ $\left.\begin{array}{c} \text{has been} \\ \text{have been} \end{array}\right]$ third form

Active	Passive
1. You have seen this.	This has been seen by you.
2. I have drawn this picture.	This picture has been drawn by me.
3. I have not abused him.	He has not been abused by me.
4. Has he made a noise?	Has a noise been made by him?
5. She has not bought these pens.	These pens have not been bought by her.

7. **Past Perfect**

Rule: had – third form $\rightarrow$ had been – third form

Active	Passive
1. I had heard the story.	The story had been heard by me.
2. He had already read the books.	The books had already been read by him.
3. Had he learnt this lesson?	Had his lesson been learnt by him?
4. He had stolen my pen.	My pen had been stolen by him.
5. Had he told you the truth.	Had you been told the truth by him?

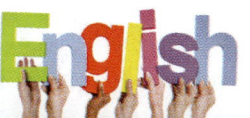

8. Future Perfect

Rule: $\left.\begin{array}{l}\text{will have}\\ \text{shall have}\end{array}\right]$ third form → $\left.\begin{array}{l}\text{will have been}\\ \text{shall have been}\end{array}\right]$ third form

Active	Passive
1. I shall have written a letter.	A letter will have been written by me.
2. She will have sent me a book.	A book will have been sent to me by her.
3. Will she have written a book?	Will a book have been written by her?
4. Mohan will not have killed a snake before you go there.	A snake will not have been killed by Mohan.
5. She will have sung a song by now.	A song will have been sung by her now.

Summary of rules for change of voice (in tenses)

1. $\left.\begin{array}{l}\textit{first form, + s, es}\\ \textit{do, does – first form}\end{array}\right]$ → *is, am, are – third form*

2. $\left.\begin{array}{l}\textit{second form,}\\ \textit{did – first form}\end{array}\right]$ → $\left.\begin{array}{l}\textit{was}\\ \textit{were}\end{array}\right]$ *– third form*

3. $\left.\begin{array}{l}\textit{will}\\ \textit{shall}\end{array}\right]$ *– 1st form* → $\left.\begin{array}{l}\textit{will be}\\ \textit{shall be}\end{array}\right]$ *– third form*

4. $\left.\begin{array}{l}\textit{is}\\ \textit{am}\\ \textit{are}\\ \textit{was}\\ \textit{were}\end{array}\right]$ *– first form + ing* → $\left.\begin{array}{l}\textit{is}\\ \textit{am}\\ \textit{are}\\ \textit{was}\\ \textit{were}\end{array}\right]$ *being + third form*

5. $\left.\begin{array}{l}\textit{has}\\ \textit{have}\\ \textit{had}\\ \textit{will have}\\ \textit{shall have}\end{array}\right]$ *– third form* → $\left.\begin{array}{l}\textit{has}\\ \textit{have}\\ \textit{had}\\ \textit{will have}\\ \textit{shall have}\end{array}\right]$ *been + third form*

ACTIVE/PASSIVE VOICE

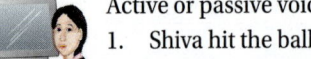

Active or passive voice is a verb form. Read the following sentences:

1. Shiva hit the ball.
2. The ball was hit by Shiva.

In sentence 1, the 'doer' of the activity (hitting the ball) is Shiva. Here, we give prominence to the 'doer' of the action. This type of sentence is in the active voice.

In sentence 2, the subject 'ball' is acted upon. The receiver or the subject 'ball' becomes prominent here. This type of sentence is in the passive voice.

It is important to remember that we use active voice when we want to highlight the subject of an action, and passive voice when we want to highlight the receiver of an action.

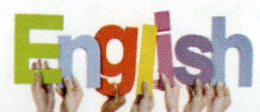

CHANGE OF ACTIVE TO PASSIVE VOICE

1. The object of the verb in active voice is turned to subject.
2. The passive form of the verb (be + V3) is used.
3. The subject of the verb is used as object, preceded by the preposition 'by' or any other.

Note the following diagrams:

a.
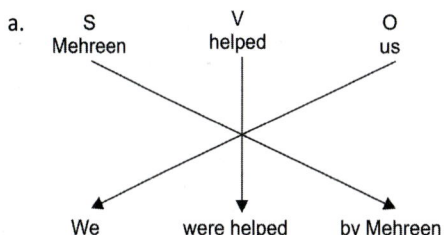

b.
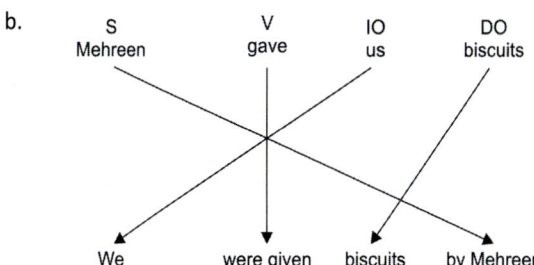

c.
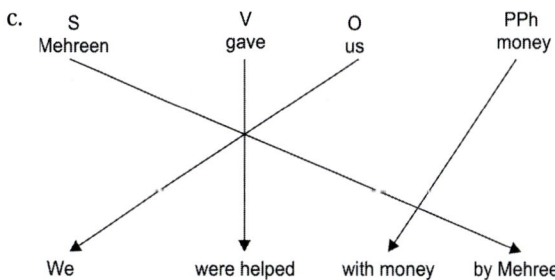

(S = subject; V = verb; O = Object; IO = Indirect Object; DO = Direct Object; PPh = Prepositional Phrase)

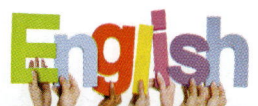

4. **The tense-wise changes that are made in the forms of verbs are as follows:**

Active Voice	Passive Voice
1. Present Indefinite (V_1/V_1 + s or es)	is/am/are + V_3
2. Past Indefinite (V_2)	was/were + V_3
3. Future Indefinite (will/shall + V_1)	will/shall + be + V_3
4. Present Continuous (is/am/are + V_1 + ing)	is/am/are + being + V_3
5. Past Continuous(was/were + V_1 + ing)	was/were + being + V_3
6. Present Perfect (has/have + V_3)	has/have + been + V_3
7. Past Perfect (had + V_3)	had been + V_3
8. Future Perfect (will/shall + have + V_3)	will/shall + have been + V_3

Note

1. Intransitive verbs (verbs which do not take objects) appear only in the active voice. (There can be no passive construction with these verbs).

Examples:

- Tears came into her eyes (no passive voice).
- She smiled at the child (no passive voice).

2. Some transitive verbs (verbs which take objects) do not have passive forms.

Examples:

- Sophia resembles her mother (no passive voice).
- Arun has a bike (no passive voice).

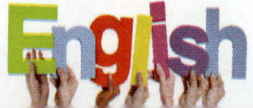

VOICE OF SENTENCES INVOLVING TENSES

Present Indefinite

> **Rule:**
> **Active:** V_1 or V_1 + 's' or 'es'
> **Passive:** Is/am/are + V_3

Rule: V_1 = First forms of verb.
V_3 = Third form of verb.

Active	Passive
1. I play chess.	Chess is played by me.
2. You miss your classes.	Your classes are missed by you.
3. We respect our elders.	Our elders are respected by us.
4. She does not deliver a letter.	A letter is not delivered by her.
5. They do not love us.	We are not loved by them.
6. Do you tell a lie?	Is a lie told by you?
7. Does she attend her classes?	Are her classes attended by her?
8. What do you play?	What is played by you?
9. Why does he make a noise?	Why is noise made by him?
10. Who hurts your feet?	By whom is your feet hurt?

EXERCISE 1

Change the voice:

1. Arun likes sweets.
2. Rima writes a poem.
3. Farmers sow seeds.
4. You do not abuse her.
5. He does not obey his teachers.
6. Does Manu sing a song?
7. Do you like new books?
8. How does Harpreet solve the sum?
9. Where do you keep your money?
10. When do you meet her?

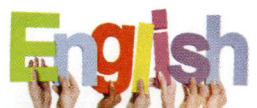

Past Indefinite

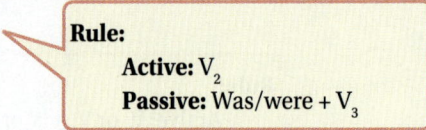

> **Rule:**
> **Active:** V_2
> **Passive:** Was/were + V_3

Rule: V_2 = Second forms of verb
V_3 = Third form of verb

Active	Passive
I. India won the match.	The match was won by India.
2. She watched the television.	The television was watched by her.
3. I did not steal the money.	The money was not stolen by me.
4. We did not like the color.	The colour was not liked by us.
5. Did she not pay her fee?	Was her fee not paid be her?
6. Didn't she help you?	Were you not helped by her?
7. Who disturbed the boy?	By whom was the boy disturbed?
8. How did you manage the match?	How was the match managed by you?
9. Why you did not inform them?	Why were they not informed by you?
10. What did they do?	What was done by them?

EXERCISE 2

Change the voice:

1. She lost all the books.
2. The host kept his promise.
3. You did not attempt all the questions.
4. She did not pay her dues.
5. Did you like the dish?
6. Didn't you play chess?
7. Where did you spend the night?
8. When did he buy a new car?
9. Who broke my mobile?
10. Why did Dr Amit hide the truth?

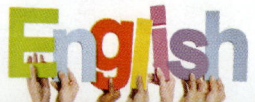

Future Indefinite

> **Rule:**
> **Active:** Shall/will + V$_1$
> **Passive:** Shall be/will be + V$_3$

Rule: V$_1$ = First form of verb
  V$_3$ = Third form of verb

Active	Passive
1. The law will protect you.	You will be protected by law.
2. We shall celebrate the victory.	The victory will be celebrated by us.
3. I shall not attend the meeting.	The meeting will not be attended by me.
4. They will not spare you.	You will not be spared by them.
5. Will Tarzan start his work?	Will his work be started by Tarzan?
6. Shall we accompany them?	Will they be accompanied by us?
7. Who will pay the tax?	By whom will the tax be paid?
8. What will you do now?	What will be done by you now?
9. When will they open the shop?	When will the shop be opened by them?
10. How will they feel?	How will be felt by them?

EXERCISE 3

Change the voice:

1. You will sign the bond.
2. I shall accept his proposal.
3. We will not be visited.
4. Jyoti will not take rest.
5. WIll the maid prepare tea?
6. Shall we meet them again?
7. When will they fly kites?
8. Where will you spend the night?
9. Who will drive the car?
10. Which game will you play?

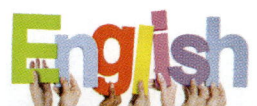

Present Continuous

> **Rule:**
> **Active:** Is/are/am + V_1 + ing
> **Passive:** Is/are/am + being + V_3

Rule: V_1 = First form of verb.
V_3 = Third form of verb.

Active	Passive
1. The people are enjoying the match.	The match is being enjoyed by the people.
2. She is teasing the dog.	The dog is being teased by her.
3. You are not making a noise.	A noise is not being made by you.
4. I am not blowing whistles.	Whistles are not being blown by me.
5. Are you favoring him?	Is he being favored by you?
6. Is he not serving the country?	Is the country not being served by him?
7. When are you visiting us?	When are we being visited by you?
8. Who is attending him?	By whom is he being attended?
9. Why are you cheating him?	Why is he being cheated by you?
10. What are you doing these days?	What is being done by you these days?

EXERCISE 4

Change the voice:

1. They are polishing the shoes.
2. The gardener is watering the plants.
3. The police is not chasing the thief.
4. You are not saving money.
5. Is Mukesh singing sad songs?
6. Are the boys learning their lesson?
7. What is Tom doing here?
8. Who is ironing my clothes?
9. How are you solving the sum?
10. Why are you wasting the time?

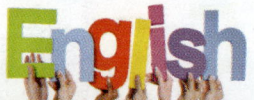

Past Continuous

> **Rule:**
> **Active:** Was/Were + V_1 + ing
> **Passive:** Was/Were + being + V_3

Rule: V_1 = First form of verb

V_3 = Third form of verb

Active	Passive
I. The peon was ringing the bell.	The bell was being rung by the peon.
2. The Prime Minister was addressing the nation.	The nation was being addressed by the Prime Minister.
3. He was not doing his duty.	His duty was not being done by him.
4. We were not plucking flowers.	Flowers were not being plucked by us.
5. Were they reading novels?	Were novels being read by them?
6. Was she celebrating her birthday?	Was her birthday being celebrated by her?
7. What were you eating?	What was being eaten by you?
8. Why were they joining the army?	Why was the army being joined by them?
9. Where were they holding the conference?	Where was the conference being held by them?
10. Who was disturbing us?	By whom were we being disturbed?

EXERCISE 5

Change the voice:

1. The police was searching Meera's house.
2. He was running a race.
3. They were not selling their goods.
4. He was not hitting the ball hard.
5. Was he doing nothing?
6. Were not they taking test?
7. When were you changing your school?
8. Whom was Jaspreet inviting home?
9. Why were they selling their bike?
10. Who was digging the earth?

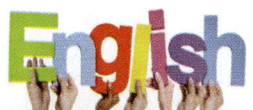

Future Continuous

Note: This tense has no passive voice.

Present Perfect

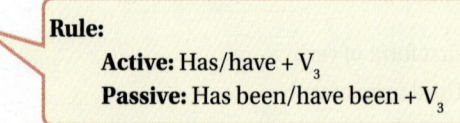

Rule:

Active: Has/have + V$_3$

Passive: Has been/have been + V$_3$

Note: V$_3$ Third form of verb

Active	Passive
1. He has shut the window.	The window has been shut by him.
2. She has washed my clothes.	My clothes have been washed by her.
3. We have not painted the pictures.	The pictures have not been painted by us.
4. The teacher has not scolded me.	I have not been scolded by the teacher.
5. Have you received her message?	Has her messaged been received by you?
6. Has he returned the notes?	Have the notes been returned by him?
7. Who has damaged the car?	By whom has the car been damaged?
8. Why have you discontinued studies?	Why have studies been discontinued by you?
9. What have you finally decided?	What was finally been decided by you?
10. How many moves have you seen?	How many moves have been seen by you?

EXERCISE 6

Change the voice:

1. Somebody has stolen the scooter.
2. He has just finished his work.
3. You have not spoken truth.
4. I have not harmed her.
5. Have you posted the letter?
6. Has he left this place for ever?
7. When have you seen the Taj?
8. Why have they left you alone?
9. Who has blamed you?
10. Where have you kept my books?

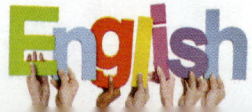

Past Perfect

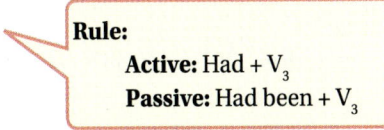

Rule:
Active: Had + V$_3$
Passive: Had been + V$_3$

Active	Passive
1. She had made several mistakes.	Several mistakes had been made by her.
2. I had heard it before.	It had been heard by me before.
3. We had not bought the car.	The car had not been bought by us.
4. Pradeep had not changed his profession.	His profession had not been changed by Pradeep.
5. Had she rejected your offer?	Had your offer been rejected by her?
6. Had you hidden the bat?	Had the bat been hidden by you?
7. Who had broken the table?	By whom had the table been broken?
8. Why had you abused my brother?	Why had my brother been abused by you?
9. Where had they built their house?	Where had their house been built by them?
10. When had you seen this play?	When had this play been seen by you?

EXERCISE 7

Change the voice:

1. Parth had done nothing wrong.
2. He had already completed the work.
3. You had not cast your vote before 11 am.
4. He had not consulted the doctor.
5. Had Columbus discovered America?
6. Had Mrs Rama dismissed her servant?
7. Whom had the principal fined?
8. How had you managed the programme?
9. Why had you disbelieved him?
10. Who had torn these pages?

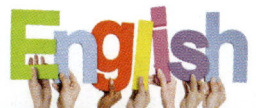

Future Perfect

> **Rule:**
> **Active:** Will have/shall have + V_3
> **Passive:** Will have been/shall have been + V_3

Active	Passive
1. You will have read this poem.	This poem will have been read by you.
2. We shall have visited many places.	Many places shall have been visited by us.
3. He will not have missed the train.	The train will not have been missed by him.
4. She will not have told a lie.	A lie will not have been told by her.
5. Will they have taken coffee.	Will coffee have been taken by them?
6. Shall I have attended the lecture?	Shall the lecture have been attended by me?
7. Who will have misunderstood you?	By whom will you have been misunderstood?
8. Why will they have rejected your proposal?	Why will your proposal have been rejected by them?
9. How will you have settled the issue?	How will the issue have been settled by you?
10. Where will they have held the meeting?	Where will the meeting have been held by them?

EXERCISE 8

Change the voice:

1. The police will have caught the thief.
2. He will have kept his promise.
3. Mohini will not have attended the class.
4. The teacher will not have punished us.
5. Will she have painted the picture?
6. Will he have arranged his son's marriage?
7. When will he have passed his graduation?
8. Who will have won the match?
9. Whose notes will he have stolen?
10. Why will they have sold their car?

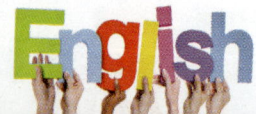

VOICE OF SENTENCES WITH PREPOSITIONAL VERBS

Rule: Prepositions attached to the verbs in the active form continue to be attached in the passive form.

Active	Passive
1. He laughs at you.	You are laughed at by him.
2. I objected to his remarks.	His remarks were objected to by me.
3. They will wait for you.	You will be waited by them.
4. We have seen through his trick.	His trick has been seen through by us.
5. They are praying to God.	God is being prayed to by them.
6. He was looking into the matter.	The matter was being looked into by him.
7. Who has knocked at the door?	By whom has the door been knocked at?
8. The mother has brought up the child.	The child has been brought up by the mother.
9. Why don't you listen to me?	Why am I not listened to by you?
10. He had agreed to my views.	My views had been agreed to by him.

EXERCISE 9

Change the voice:

1. He wasted away his time.
2. We laid out in a small garden.
3. He does not agree with me.
4. Have you set up a new business?
5. I shall write to you.
6. Who asked for water?
7. Is he searching for a job?
8. Why had you put out the candle?
9. He played upon my weaknesses.
10. Did he not care for you?

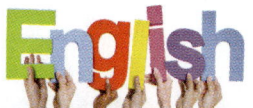

VOICE OF SENTENCES IN WHICH PREPOSITION 'BY' IS NOT USED

Rule:

Verb		Preposition used
1. Known	⟶	to
2. Contained	⟶	in
3. Surprised, astonished, alarmed, offended, shocked, wondered, frightened	⟶	at
4. Displeased, pleased (conduct/behavior)	⟶	at
5. Displeased, pleased (person)	⟶	with
6. Satisfied, disgusted, lined, filled, crowded, grown	⟶	with

Active	Passive
1. I know you very well.	You are known to me very well.
2. This jug contains water.	Water is contained in this jug.
3. His behavior surprised us.	We were surprised at his behavior.
4. The people crowded the platform.	The platform was crowded with the people.
5. You have greatly pleased them.	They have been greatly pleased with you.
6. The news alarmed us.	We were alarmed at the news.
7. The people lined the roads.	The roads were lined with the people.
8. His failure shocked me.	We were shocked at his failure.
9. His performance satisfied the teacher.	The teacher was satisfied with his performance.

EXERCISE 10

Change the voice:

1. Do you know his sister?
2. This book contains much information.
3. Did your work please the boss?
4. His success astonished us.
5. The students lined the play ground.
6. Will you satisfy your parents?
7. You have annoyed him.
8. His rude behavior will upset you.
9. The loud sound alarmed the people.
10. Wild flowers grow over the lawn.

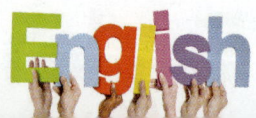

VOICE OF SENTENCES HAVING MODALS

Can, could, may, might, will, would, shall, should, dare,
must, ought to, used to, need

Rule:

$$\text{Modal} + \text{be} + V_3$$
$$V_3 = \text{Third form of Verb}$$

Active	Passive
1. I can help you.	You can be helped by me.
2. May I take your glass?	May your glass be taken by me?
3. You should respect your elders.	Your elders should be respected by you.
4. The rich must help the poor.	The poor must be helped by the rich.
5. Could I take your pen?	Could your pen be taken by me?
6. We ought to serve our country.	Our country ought to be served by us.
7. He may win a scholarship.	A scholarship may be won by him.
8. Who can bell the cat?	By whom can the cat be belled?
9. I dare not disobey you.	You dare not be disobeyed by me.
10. They might win the match.	The match might be won by them.

EXERCISE 11

Change the voice:

1. I must sign the will.
2. May I ask someone to tea?
3. Could Preety finally solve the sum?
4. Would you repeat it?
5. You should not disobey your teacher.
6. I can't solve this sum.
7. He might deceive her friend.
8. What can I do for you?
9. You needn't bring your bags.
10. He may not join the army.

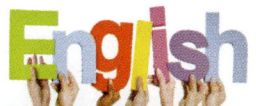

VOICE FOR IMPERATIVE SENTENCES

Rule:

(i) Let + be + V_3
    or
    Subject + should be + V_3

(ii) In sentences beginning with 'kindly' or 'please'.
    We make use of 'You are requested to'.

Active	Passive
1. Serve your country.	Let your country be served. Or Your country should be served.
2. Do it.	Let it be done. Or It should be done.
3. Pray to God daily.	Let God be prayed to daily. Or God should be prayed to daily.
4. Never tell a lie.	A lie should never be told. Or You are advised never to tell a lie.
5. Never waste your time.	Your time should never be wasted. Or You are forbidden to waste your time.
6. Don't pluck flowers.	Let not flowers be plucked. Or Flowers should not be plucked.
7. Kindly grant me leave.	You are requested to grant me leave.
8. Please help me.	You are requested to help me.
9. Respect your elders.	Let your elders be respected. Or Your elders should be respected.
10. Post this letter.	Let this letter be posted. Or This letter should be posted.

EXERCISE 12

Change the voice:

1. Open the door.
2. Never hurt others.
3. Show the guest in.
4. Learn it by heart.
5. Don't make a noise.
6. Please sit down.
7. Speak the truth.
8. Pay your fee in time.
9. Never shout so loudly.
10. Let me do it.

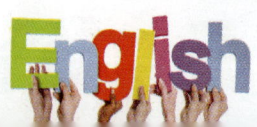

VOICE OF INFINITIVE (i.e. to + v$_1$)

Rule: To + be + V$_3$

Active	Passive
1. You should do it.	It has to be done by you.
2. It is time to say our prayer.	It is time for our prayer to be said.
3. You will have to leave this place.	This place will have to be left by you.
4. He likes his subordinate to respect him.	He likes to be respected by his subordinate.
5. You may have to give up your studies.	Your studies may have to be given up by you.
6. I wish to help you.	I wish you to be helped.
7. We propose to start a business.	A business is proposed to be started by us.
8. I want you to recite this poem.	I want this poem to be recited by you.
9. He likes others to admire him.	He likes to be admired by others.
10. You have to attend on her.	She has to be attended on by you.

EXERCISE 13

Change the voice:

1. I have to obey him.
2. It is time to revise our lesson.
3. Women like men to flatter them.
4. I shall have to exclude his name.
5. I want to buy this book.
6. We wish to give him a fair trial.
7. We propose to build a new house.
8. He is sure to win a prize.
9. He does not like to take bath daily.
10. Shall I have to punish him?

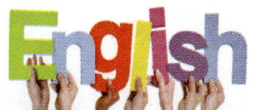

VOICE OF SENTENCES WITH DOUBLE OBJECT

Rule: In some sentences, there are two objects. Either of the two objects can be made the subject in passive voice. However, it is more common to make indirect object (which comes immediately after the verb in active voice) the subject of the passive voice.

Active	Passive
1. He gave me this book.	I was given this book by him.
2. I presented him a mobile.	He was presented a mobile by me.
3. Who teaches you English?	By whom are you taught English?
4. You have written him a letter.	He has been written a letter by you.
5. The teacher will give us a test.	We shall be given a test by the teacher.
6. Who gave you this money?	By whom were you given this money?
7. Has Ram told you the truth?	Have you been told the truth by Ram?
8. They do not give him good food.	He is not given good food by them.
9. My uncle had sent me a present.	I had been sent a present by my uncle.
10. You will have sent him a message.	He will have been sent a message by you.

EXERCISE 14

Change the voice:

1. He gave me hundred rupees.
2. Who gave you this letter?
3. Are you giving the beggar money?
4. You have done me much harm.
5. He will give you a pleasant surprise.
6. Have they sent you many gifts?
7. He has done me a favor.
8. Will you show us your photograph?
9. Why have you given him my book?
10. They named the child Manik.

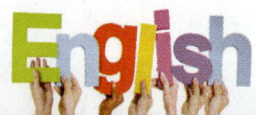

VOICE OF SENTENCES WITH QUASI-PASSIVE VERBS

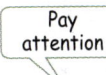
Pay attention

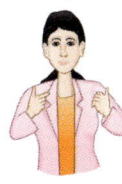

Active	Passive
1. This mango tastes sweet.	This mango is sweet when tasted.
2. I do not like his staring at me.	I do not like being stared at by him. Or His staring is not liked by me.
3. She likes helping others.	She likes others being helped by her.
4. This carpet needs dusting.	This carpet needs to be dusted. Or Dusting is needed by this carpet.
5. I found him laughing at you.	I found you being laughed at by him.
6. This book is selling like hot cakes.	This book is being sold like hot cakes.
7. Do you mind my opening this window.	Do you mind this window being opened by me?
8. He is fond of making such remarks.	He is fond of such remarks being made by him.
9. I can't recall having met him before.	I can't recall he having been met by me before.
10. I remember having heard this story.	I remember this story having been heard by me.

EXERCISE 15

Change the voice:

1. The milk tasted sour.
2. Quinine tastes bitter.
3. Rose smells sweet.
4. This novel is selling well.
5. I like children doing their work.
6. Sea-water tastes saltish.
7. I do not like people shirking their duty.
8. Does this exercise need correcting?
9. Does honey taste sweet?
10. I do not mind doing your work here.

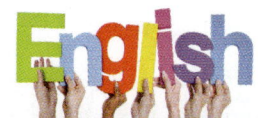

VOICE OF SENTENCES WITH SUBJECT IMPLIED

Rule: In some sentences (generally in the passive form), the subject has to be supplied. Then the sentence has to be changed into the active voice.

Active	Passive
1. Duty must be done.	(You) must do duty.
2. The matter is being looked into.	(They) are looking into the matter.
3. He has been released on bail.	(They) have released him on bail.
4. The city was destroyed.	(The enemy) destroyed the city.
5. The murderer was sentenced to death.	(The judge) sentenced the murderer to death.
6. My note-book has been checked.	(The teacher) has checked my note book.
7. Trespassers will be prosecuted.	(They) will prosecute trespassers.
8. Your case will be discussed tomorrow.	(We) shall discuss your case tomorrow.
9. The thief will have been arrested.	(The police) will have arrested the thief.
10. He has been made the monitor.	(The teacher) has made him the monitor.

EXERCISE 16

Change the voice:

1. He has been dismissed.
2. A meeting is to be held tomorrow.
3. They were refused admission.
4. The bond was signed.
5. The college will be closed.
6. He was forced to resign.
7. Promises must be kept.
8. They have been informed.
9. What can't be cured must be endured.
10. He will have been marked absent.

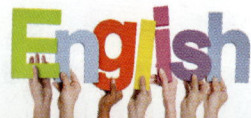

TRANSFORMATION OF ACTIVE INTO PASSIVE VOICE

Statements

Active	Passive
1. We burn wood to get energy.	Wood is burnt by us to get energy.
2. I do not like city life.	City life is not liked by me.
3. She told me a story.	I was told a story by her.
4. The accused denied the charges.	The charges were denied by the accused.
5. The box did not contain sweets.	Sweets were not contained in the box.
6. Rakesh will help you.	You will be helped by Rakesh.
7. We will not share the blame.	The blame will not be shared by us.
8. They are eating nice things.	Nice things are being eaten by them.
9. She is not waiting for you.	You are not being waited by her.
10. Anita was doing something.	Something was being done by Anita.
11. The maid was not using the cooker.	The cooker was not being used by the maid.
12. They have sent us a message.	We have been sent a message by them.
13. She has not scored good marks.	Good marks have not been scored by her.
14. They had built the dam by 2008.	The dam had been built by 2008 by them.
15. They had not done their work by then.	Their work had not been done by them by then.

(*Imperative Sentences*)
Active: Shut the door.
Passive: Let the door be shut.
Active: Obey your parents.
Passive: Let your parents be obeyed.

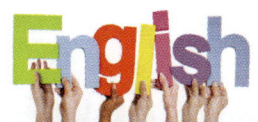

Practice Exercises

I. Change the voice:

1. The doctor treats the patients.

   _____

2. My classmates respect me.

   _____

3. People light lamps on Diwali nights.

   _____

4. Columbus discovered America.

   _____

5. We did not beat them.

   _____

6. The servant killed a snake.

   _____

7. Everybody was praising you.

   _____

8. We were taking a test.

   _____

9. The washerman is washing the clothes.

   _____

10. They have insulted you.

    _____

II. Change the voice:

1. I do not tell a lie.

   _____

2. We sing prayers every morning.

   _____

3. The teacher corrected our notebooks.

   _____

4. They missed the train.

   _____

5. The teacher will teach a new lesson today.

   _____

6. She will help us.

   _____

7. You are doing this exercise.

   _____

8. The students are singing the national anthem.

   _____

9. The grandmother was telling a story.

   _____

10. The magician was showing interesting tricks.

    _____

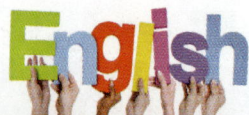

III. Change the voice:

1. She submits her assignments daily.

   _____

2. We wish our teacher in the morning.

   _____

3. Ashutosh reads a novel.

   _____

4. Geeta sings a song.

   _____

5. The labourers are constructing a house.

   _____

6. The students are making a noise.

   _____

7. They are holding a general body meeting this week.

   _____

8. The students are reviewing their lessons.

   _____

9. They have accomplished their desired goals.

   _____

10. She has done her home task.

    _____

IV. Change the voice:

1. Madhu will write a letter.

   _____

2. She will sing a song.

   _____

3. Ritu will paint a picture.

   _____

4. Madhvi will win a prize.

   _____

5. Geetanjali will write a book.

   _____

6. He will have executed his plans.

   _____

7. Manisha will have accomplished her task.

   _____

8. Neeta will have written her question.

   _____

9. Raina will have prepared her notes on Wordsworth.

   _____

10. She will have reached her destination.

    _____

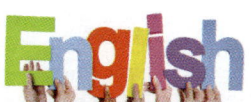

V. Change the voice:

1. Is he reading this novel?

   _____

2. Does he play cricket?

   _____

3. Are you planning your budget?

   _____

4. Is she attending the refresher course?

   _____

5. Is she researching on the Indian women novelists in English?

   _____

6. Where did Natayala find this casio?

   _____

7. Has anyone satisfied my query?

   _____

8. Who will help you?

   _____

9. Who broke the jug?

   _____

10. Were they extended a warm welcome by you?

    _____

VI. Change the voice:

1. We refused them admission.

   _____

2. I forgave him for his fault.

   _____

3. He watched the sports.

   _____

4. Sohrab gave Rustum a brave fight.

   _____

5. They took no notice of me.

   _____

6. Did Sita paint this picture?

   _____

7. Who taught you French?

   _____

8. The dentist pulled out one of my teeth.

   _____

9. The policeman caught the thief.

   _____

10. The postman gave me two letters.

    _____

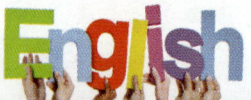

VII. Change the voice:

1. The boys are learning their lessons.

   _____

2. The washerman is washing the clothes.

   _____

3. The teacher is not calling the roll.

   _____

4. The boys are making much noise.

   _____

5. He is speaking the truth.

   _____

6. Is the peon ringing the bell?

   _____

7. The labourers are cutting down the trees.

   _____

8. That man is repairing our transistor.

   _____

9. Are these boys beating the donkey?

   _____

10. He is driving a motor car.

   _____

VIII. Change the voice:

1. Carry it to home.

   _____

2. Let him play the match.

   _____

3. Please bring me a glass of water.

   _____

4. Lower the boats.

   _____

5. Send him to school.

   _____

6. Please help me in my hour of need.

   _____

7. Carry out my orders.

   _____

8. Tell him to leave the room.

   _____

9. Do not hate the poor.

   _____

10. Don't disturb me.

   _____

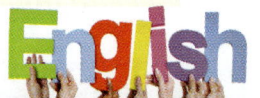

IX. Change the voice:

1. You are wanted outside.

   _____

2. The thief has been arrested.

   _____

3. The telephone wires were cut.

   _____

4. This matter will be discussed tomorrow.

   _____

5. He was elected member of Parliament.

   _____

6. He has been killed.

   _____

X. Change the voice:

1. She recites a poem.

   _____

2. The principal delivered a lecture.

   _____

3. People all over the world know Newton.

   _____

4. Mrs Sharma teaches us English.

   _____

5. Do it.

   _____

6. I made him do this work.

   _____

7. It is time to take lunch.

   _____

8. Can it ever be done by me alone?

   _____

9. The rich often laugh at the poor.

   _____

10. She will have taken the test.

    _____

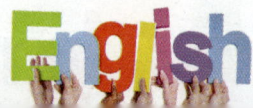

XI. Change the voice:

1. Why has he been abused by his friend?
   _____

2. The thief has been arrested at last.
   _____

3. All his property has been sold.
   _____

4. We have not been invited to her birthday party.
   _____

5. The speaker has been warmly cheered.
   _____

6. Many people have been ruined by gambling.
   _____

7. Haven't several mistakes been made by her?
   _____

8. Why have all the biscuits been eaten by you?
   _____

9. By whom has the box been locked?
   _____

10. My slate must have been used in my absence.
    _____

XII. Change the voice:

1. Nobody has ever taken me for a policeman before.
   _____

2. This pen has been used by me only once so far.
   _____

3. We have been treated by ice-cream.
   _____

4. Has anybody even taught you how to behave?
   _____

5. The fire has destroyed many valuable paintings.
   _____

6. I have been lent this book by one of my friends.
   _____

7. Have we contacted her during this week?
   _____

8. Who has drunk milk out of this cup?
   _____

9. A new company has taken over the business.
   _____

10. Nothing has been done by them till now.
    _____

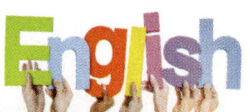

XIII. Change the voice:

1. Where have you kept the bunch of keys?
   _____

2. The principal has fined him two rupees.
   _____

3. The traders have hoarded the grains.
   _____

4. Some body has stolen my watch.
   _____

5. She has done much to help me.
   _____

6. No one has opened the lock.
   _____

7. Nobody has appointed him the captain.
   _____

8. A friend has told me this news.
   _____

9. Somebody has left the tap running after use.
   _____

10. Has anyone answered your question?
    _____

XIV. Change the voice:

1. He was promised all help by us.
   _____

2. May God bless you with success.
   _____

3. The strike has been called off.
   _____

4. No one can understand him so soon.
   _____

5. They will not agree to this proposal.
   _____

6. The rose smells sweet.
   _____

7. It is time to close the shops.
   _____

8. The teacher is calling the roll.
   _____

9. She is milking the cow.
   _____

10. He will have taken tea.
    _____

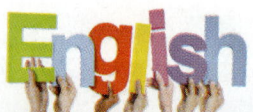

XV.   Change the voice:

1. They elected him their leader.

    _____

2. Who did this?

    _____

3. I have to help my cousin.

    _____

4. One must do one's duty.

    _____

5. Who broke the window pane?

    _____

6. My friend gifted me a book.

    _____

7. Don't pluck flowers.

    _____

8. It is time to ring the bell.

    _____

9. Promises must be kept.

    _____

10. Where did the dog hide the bone?

    _____

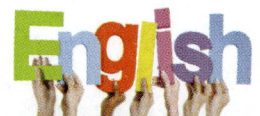

ANSWERS

EXERCISE 1

1. Sweets are liked by Arun.
2. A poem is written by Rima.
3. Seeds are sown by farmers.
4. She is not abused by you?
5. His teachers are not obeyed by him.
6. Is a song sung by Manu?
7. Are new books liked by you?
8. How is the sum solved by Harpreet?
9. Where is your money kept?
10. When is she met by you?

EXERCISE 2

1. All the books were lost by her.
2. His promise was kept by the host.
3. All the questions were not attempted by you.
4. Her dues were not paid by her.
5. Was the dish liked by you?
6. Was the chess not played by you?
7. Where was the night spent by you?
8. When was a new car bought by him?
9. By whom was my mobile broken?
10. Why was the truth hidden by Dr Amit?

EXERCISE 3

1. The bond will be signed by you.
2. His proposal will be accepted by me.
3. We will not be visited.
4. Rest will not be taken by Jyoti.
5. Will the tea be prepared by the hostess?
6. Will they be met again by us?
7. When will the kites be flown by them?
8. Where will the night be spent by you?
9. By whom will the car be driven?
10. Which game will be played by you?

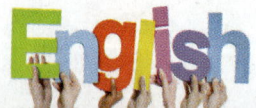

EXERCISE 4

1. The shoes are being polished by them.
2. The plants are being watered by the gardener.
3. The thief is not being chased by the police.
4. Money is not being saved by you.
5. Are sad songs being sung by Mukesh?
6. Is their lesson being learnt by the boys?
7. What is being done here by Tom?
8. By whom are my clothes being ironed?
9. How is the sum being solved by you?
10. Why is the time being wasted by you?

EXERCISE 5

1. Meera's house was being searched by the police.
2. A race was being run by him.
3. Their goods were not being sold by them.
4. The ball was not being hit hard by him.
5. Was nothing been done by him?
6. Was rest not been taken by them?
7. When was your school changed by you?
8. Who was being invited home by Jaspreet?
9. Why was their bike being sold?
10. By whom was the Earth being dug?

EXERCISE 6

1. The scooter has been stolen by someone.
2. His work has been just finished by him.
3. Truth has been spoken by you.
4. She has not been harmed by me.
5. Has the letter been posted by you?
6. Has this place been left forever by him?
7. When has the Taj been seen by you?
8. Why have you been left alone by them?
9. By whom have you been blamed?
10. Where have my books been kept by you?

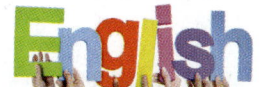

EXERCISE 7

1. Nothing had been done wrong by Parth.
2. The work had been already completed by him.
3. Before 11 am your vote had not been cast.
4. The doctor had not been consulted by him.
5. Had America been discovered by Columbus?
6. Had her servant been dismissed by Mrs Rama?
7. Who had been fined by the Principal?
8. How had the programme been managed?
9. Why had he been disbelieved by him.
10. By whom had these pages been torn?

EXERCISE 8

1. The thief will have been caught by the police.
2. His promise will have been kept by him.
3. The class will not have been attended by Mohini.
4. We will not have been punished by the teacher.
5. Will the picture have been painted by her?
6. Will his son's marriage have been arranged by her?
7. When his graduation will have been passed by him?
8. By whom will have the match been won?
9. Whose notes will have been stolen by him?
10. Why their car will have been sold by them?

EXERCISE 9

1. His time was wasted away by him.
2. A small garden was laid out by us.
3. I am not agreed to by him.
4. Has a new business been settled by you?
5. You shall be written to by me.
6. By whom were you asked for water?
7. Is a job being searched for by him?
8. Why had the candle been put out by him?
9. My weaknesses were played upon by him.
10. Were you not cared for by him?

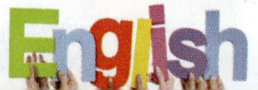

EXERCISE 10

1. Is his sister known to you?
2. Much information is contained in this book.
3. Was the boss pleased with your work?
4. We were astonished at his success.
5. The playground was lined by the students.
6. Will your parents be satisfied by you?
7. He has been annoyed by you.
8. You will be upset at his rude behavior.
9. The people were alarmed by the loud sound.
10. Over the lawn wild flowers are grown.

EXERCISE 11

1. The will must be signed by me.
2. May someone be asked to tea by me?
3. Could the sum be finally solved by Preety?
4. Would it be repeated by you?
5. Your teacher should not be disobeyed by you.
6. This sum cannot be solved by me.
7. Her friend might be deceived by him.
8. What can be done for you by me?
9. Your bags needn't be brought by you.
10. The army may not be joined by him.

EXERCISE 12

1. Let the door be opened.
2. Others should never be hurt.
3. Let the guests be shown in.
4. It should be learnt by heart.
5. You are forbidden to make noise.
6. You are requested to sit down.
7. You are advised to speak the truth.
8. You are advised to pay your fee in time.
9. You are forbidden to shout loudly.
10. Let it be done by me.

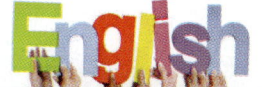

EXERCISE 13

1. He should be obeyed by me.
2. It is time for our lesson to be revised.
3. Women like to be flattered by men.
4. His name will have to be excluded by me.
5. I want this book to be bought by me.
6. We wish a free trial to be given to him.
7. We propose a new house to be built.
8. A prize is surely to be won by him.
9. Taking bath daily is not liked by him.
10. Should he have to be punished by me?

EXERCISE 14

1. Hundred rupees were given to me by him.
2. By whom was this letter given to you?
3. Is the money been given to beggar by me?
4. Much harm has been done to you by me.
5. A pleasant surprise will be given to you by him.
6. Have many gifts be sent to you by them?
7. A favor has been done to me by him.
8. Will your photograph be shown to us by you?
9. Why has my book been given to you by me?
10. The child was named Manik by them.

EXERCISE 15

1. The milk was sour when tasted.
2. Quinine is bitter when tasted.
3. Sweet is the smell of rose.
4. They are selling this novel well.
5. Children doing their work is liked by me.
6. Sea water is saltish when tasted.
7. People shirking their duty are not liked by me.
8. Does this exercise need to be corrected?
9. Is the honey sweet when tasted?
10. Doing your work here is not minded by me.

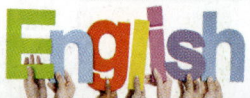

EXERCISE 16

1. They have dismissed him.
2. Tomorrow a meeting is to be held.
3. Admission was refused to by them.
4. They signed the bond.
5. The authorities will close the college.
6. The management forced him to resign.
7. You must keep the promises.
8. He has informed them.
9. Endure what all can't be cured.
10. They will have marked him absent.

NOTES

Chapter 14

Speech— Direct and Indirect

INTRODUCTION

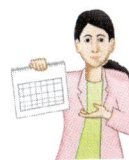

Whatever we speak is called our Speech.

We use our speech to report the ideas that are our own. Also, we speak to report the speech of a person to another person. This job of reporting can be done in two ways - directly or indirectly.

Let us try to understand now in detail.

DIRECT REPORT OF A SPEECH

Observe the following sentences

- ❏ I say, 'I am a player of cricket.'
- ❏ You said to me 'My sister is a doctor.'
- ❏ Shreen says, 'My mother is in Mumbai.'
- ❏ The teacher said, 'Manat is always in time.'
- ❏ He said, 'I go to temple every Sunday.'

Each sentence has two distinct parts:

1. *The part outside the quotation marks, i.e., inverted commas:*

   It has a **subject and a verb**. This verb makes a report in each sentence. So, it is called the **reporting verb**.

2. *The part within the quotation marks:*

   It has the actual words of the person whose speech is reported. So, it is called the reported speech.

As in each sentence, the speech (words) of the person has been reported exactly as it has been heard said. No change has been made in any part of the report. So, this report is called the **direct report or direct speech**.

Note the following facts about Direct Speech:

- ❏ The reporting verb is **followed by a comma** (,)
- ❏ The reported speech is **placed within inverted commas**.
- ❏ The first word of the reported speech begins with a **capital letter**.

INDIRECT REPORT OF A SPEECH

Observe the following sentences:
- ❑ I say that I am a player of cricket.
- ❑ You told me that your sister was a doctor.
- ❑ Shreen says that her mother is in Mumbai.
- ❑ The teacher said that manat was always in time.
- ❑ He said that he went to temple every Sunday.

Each sentence clearly shows that speech of another person has not been reported exactly as it was. Its substance has been reported in the words of the reporter. In other words, the report is indirect. So it is called an **indirect report** or **indirect speech**.

Note the following facts about the indirect speech:
- ❑ The subject and the verb are not followed by a comma but by a **conjunction** (that etc).
- ❑ The reported speech is not placed within inverted commas.
- ❑ The reported speech is changed such that its **pronouns**, **tenses** and **some other words** suit the reporter.

Rules for Changing Direct Speech into Indirect

The following rules will help you in changing direct speech into indirect:

Rule 1

If the reporting verb is in the present or future tense, the verb in reported speech is not changed at all.

Direct	Peter says, 'There is no ink in the ink-pot.'
Indirect	Peter says that there is no ink in the inkpot.
Direct	The teacher *says*, 'The girl was lazy.'
Indirect	The teacher says that the girl was lazy.
Direct	The principal says, 'Meenu will fail.'
Indirect	The principal says that Meenu will fail.
Direct	Ashok *will say*, 'Dinner is ready.'
Direct	Ashok *will say* that dinner is ready.
Indirect	John *will say*, 'Nobody *was* in the room.'
Direct	John *will say* that nobody *was* in the room.
Indirect	The teacher *will Say*, 'Ashok *will* pass.'
Direct	The teacher *will* say that Ashok *will* pass.

If the *introductory verb* is in the past tense, the tense in the direct speech is changed into the past tense:

- (i) '*will*' is changed into 'would.'
- (ii) '*shall*' is changed into 'should' or 'would.'
- (iii) '*can*' is changed into 'could.'
- (iv) '*may*' is changed into 'might.'

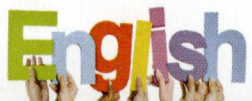

   (v)   The 'simple present' is changed into the 'simple past tense'.
  (vi)   The 'present continuous' is changed into the 'past continuous tense'.
 (vii)   The 'present perfect' is changed into the 'past perfect tense'.
(viii)   The 'present perfect continuous' is changed into the 'past perfect continuous tense'.
  (ix)   The 'simple past' is changed into the 'past perfect tense'.
   (x)   The 'past continuous' is changed into the 'past perfect continuous tense'.
  (xi)   The 'past perfect' and 'past perfect continuous' tenses do not change.

Rule 2

If the reporting verb is in the past tense, the verb in the reported speech is also changed in the past tense.

To work out this rule smoothly, note the following special rules:

1.   The *simple present* becomes the *simple past:*

Direct	Miss Green said, 'Susan works very hard.'
Indirect	Miss Green said that Susan *worked* very hard.
Direct	John said, 'Tom *swims* daily.'
Indirect	John said that Tom *swam* daily.

2.   The *present continuous* becomes the *past continuous.*

Direct	He said, 'Anand *is working* hard.'
Indirect	He said that Anand *was working* hard.
Direct	He said, 'The children *are playing* in the park.'
Indirect	He said that the children *were playing* in the park.

3.   The *present perfect* becomes the *past perfect.*

Direct	Jack said, 'Tom *has done* his work.'
Indirect	Jack said that Tom *had done* his work.
Direct	She said, 'Kamala *has written* the letter.'
Indirect	She said that Kamala *had written* the letter.

4.   *May* is changed into *might* and can is changed into *could.*

Direct	The teacher said, 'The boy *may pass*.'
Indirect	The teacher said that the boy *might pass*.
Direct	I said, 'I *can do* the sum.'
Indirect	I said that I *could do* the sum.

5.   The *simple past* becomes the *past perfect.*

Direct	Bali said, 'Raman *returned* at noon.'
Indirect	Bali said that Raman *had returned* at noon.
Direct	He said, 'Sheila *came* at night.'
Indirect	He said that Sheila *had come* at night.

6.   The *past continuous* becomes the *past perfect continuous.*

Direct	He said, 'All *were laughing* at the beggar.'
Indirect	He said that all *had been laughing* at the beggar.
Direct	Raman said, 'All the boys *were singing*.'
Indirect	Raman said that all the boys *had been singing*.

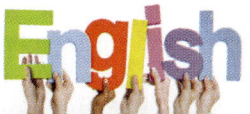

7. 'Shall' is changed into 'should'; 'will' is changed into 'would'

Direct	The teacher said, 'Ashok *will not pass*.'
Indirect	The teacher said that Ashok *would not pass*.
Direct	I said, 'I *shall try* to help her.'
Indirect	I said that I *should try* to help her.

Rule 3 (Exception to Rule 2)

If the reported speech contains some universal or habitual fact, then the simple present in the reported speech is not changed into the corresponding simple past, but remains unchanged.

Direct	The teacher said, 'Honesty is the best policy.'
Indirect	The teacher said that honesty is the best policy,
Direct	He said, 'The earth moves round the sun.'
Indirect	He said that the earth moves round the sun.
Direct	She said, 'God loves all things below.'
Indirect	She said that God *loves* all things below.

If the direct speech states a *past historical fact*, the simple past tense remains unchanged.

Direct	The teacher said, 'India *became* free in 1947.'
Indirect	The teacher said that India *became* free in 1947.

If the direct speech states *two actions that took place at the same time*, the simple past tense or the past continuous tense is not changed:

Direct	She said, 'Manoj *sat* idle while it *rained*.'
Indirect	She said that Manoj *sat* idle while it *rained*.
Direct	I said, 'Sudha *was singing* while Radha *was dancing*.'
Indirect	I said that Sudha *was singing* while Radha *was dancing*.

Changes in Pronouns and Possessive Adjectives

Rule 4

Pronouns of the first person in direct speech are changed in indirect speech to the same person as the subject of the introductory verb.

Direct	John Said, '*I am* busy.'
Indirect	John said that *he was* busy.
Direct	She said, '*I* have done *my* work.'
Indirect	She said that *she* had done *her* work.
Direct	He said, 'I *shall* do *my* best.'
Indirect	He said that *he* would do *his* best
Direct	I said, 'I *will* not go there.'
Indirect	I said that *I* would not go there.
Direct	I said, 'The teacher *likes me*.'
Indirect	I said that the teacher *liked me*.

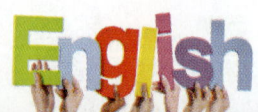

Rule 5

Pronouns of the second person in direct speech are changed in indirect speech to the same person as the noun or pronoun which comes after the introductory verb.

Direct	Henry said to *me*, '*You* are wrong.'
Indirect	Henry told *me* that *I* was wrong.
Direct	Anil said to *Ashok*, *You* are a good boy.'
Indirect	Anil told *Ashok* that *he* was a good boy.
Direct	Sheila said to *Kamala* '*You* are a good girl
Indirect	Sheila told *Kamala* that *she* was a good girl.
Direct	John said to *him*, 'You have not done *your* work.'
Indirect	John told him *he* had not done *his* work.
Direct	James said to *her*, 'You have done *your* duty.'
Indirect	John told *her* that *she* had done *her* duty.'

Rule 6

Pronouns of the third person in direct speech remain the same in indirect speech'

Direct	Harry said to me, '*He* is ill.'
Indirect	Harry told me that *he* was ill.
Direct	He said to me, '*She* is right.'
Indirect	He told me that *she* was right.

But no change of person is made when the speech is reported to the person to whom it was first addressed.

Direct	Harry said to *you*, '*You* are wrong.'
Indirect	Harry told *you* that *you* were wrong.

Note: ln all the above examples the verb *'said'* in *direct speech* becomes *'told'* in *indirect*, and the proposition *'to'* is omitted.

Rule 7

When turning a sentence from direct into indirect speech, words showing nearness are changed into words showing distance. Thus:

- ❑ Now becomes then
- ❑ This becomes that
- ❑ These becomes those
- ❑ Here becomes there
- ❑ Ago becomes before
- ❑ Today becomes that day
- ❑ Tomorrow becomes the next day
- ❑ Yesterday becomes the day before (or the previous day)
- ❑ Last night becomes the night before (or the previous night)

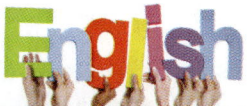

Direct	John said, 'I am busy *now*.'
Indirect	john said that he was busy *then*.
Direct	He said, 'I have seen *this* girl.'
Indirect	He said that he had seen *that* girl.
Direct	I said, '*These* mangoes are sweet.'
Indirect	I said that *those* mangoes were sweet.
Direct	He said to me, 'I finished the work long *ago*.'
Indirect	He told me that he had finished the work long *before*.
Direct	Harry said, 'The boy is *here*.'
Indirect	Harry said that the boy was *there*.
Direct	He said, 'Tony may come *tomorrow*.'
Indirect	He said that Tony might come *the next day*.
Direct	Peter said, '*Today* is a fine day.'
Indirect	Peter said that *that day* was a fine day.
Direct	Mary said, 'I shall go to Poona *tomorrow*.'
Indirect	Mary said that she would go to Poona the *next day*.
Direct	Abraham said, 'l went to the cinema *last night*.'
Indirect	Abraham said that he had gone to the cinema *the night before*.
Direct	Susan said, '*This* happened *yesterday*.'
Indirect	Susan said that *that* had happened *the day before*.

Turn the following sentences into indirect speech:

1. He said, 'There was a big fire here last night.'
2. He said to Pinky, 'You may come with me tomorrow.'
3. He said, 'Mary, l am going to the picture tonight.'
4. The teacher said to the boys, 'If you do your best you will surely pass.'
5. She said, 'l had a wonderful dream last night.'
6. She said, 'l will answer the letter when l have time.'
7. Peter said to john, 'I'm sorry l've broken your pen.'
8. 'My sister and l are leaving shortly,' answered james.
9. 'l have been studying English for five years,' said Pinky.
10. 'l can't see any point in talking to you,' the girl said to me.

CONVERSION OF ASSERTIVE SENTENCES

Direct to Indirect

While reporting assertive sentences indirectly, observe the following rules:

1. The reporting *verb* 'say' is changed into **'tell'** if there is an object after it, otherwise it remains unchanged.
2. Remove the *comma* and the inverted commas and start the reported speech with the conjunction **'that'**.
3. Nouns or pronouns in the *vocative case* are treated as objects of their verbs.

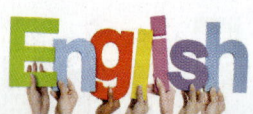

4. Changes of tenses, pronouns and the words showing nearness are carried on.
5. Other general rules are to be observed.

Observe the following examples:

Direct	The teacher said, 'Rehman you are a lazy boy.'
Indirect	The teacher told Rehman that he was a lazy boy.
Direct	He said to me, 'I do not like your habits.'
Indirect	He told me that he did not like my habits.
Direct	The teacher said, 'I shall not take my class today.'
Indirect	The teacher said that he would not take his class that day.
Direct	Mother said to me, 'You are just like your father.'
Indirect	Mother told me that I was just like my father.

Indirect to Direct

While changing assertive sentences from indirect *form to direct form* of speech, the rules given above are reversed.

Observe the following examples:

Indirect	He told his father that he would become a brave general one day
Direct	He said, 'I shall become a brave general one day.'
Indirect	I told Mahreen that I would see her the following day.
Direct	I said to Mahreen, 'I shall see you tomorrow.'
Indirect	You told her that you had done it.
Direct	You said to her, 'I have done it.'
Indirect	The Angel told Abu that his name was not there in that book.
Direct	The Angel said, 'Abu, your name is not there in this book.'

EXERCISE 1

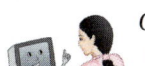

Change each sentence to **indirect form of speech:**
1. The labourer said, 'I do not work on Sundays.'
2. Sita said to Rama, 'I shall accompany you.'
3. The boys shouted, 'We have won the match.'
4. The patient said, 'I have been down with fever for a week.'
5. 'I shall help you, O king, someday,' said the mouse to the lion.
6. The teacher said, 'Your answer does not deserve more marks.'
7. The mother said, 'Always speak the truth, my son.'
8. The teacher said to Mohan, 'I shall take you to the principal, if you misbehave.'
9. The citizens said to the king,' It is your duty to protect us.'
10. The child said, 'I am very hungry, mother.'

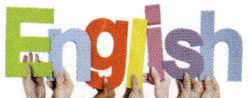

CONVERSION OF INTERROGATIVE SENTENCES—
BEGINNING WITH AUXILIARY VERBS

Direct to Indirect

While reporting interrogative sentences, beginning with auxiliary verbs, indirectly, observe the following rules:

1. The reporting verb 'say' is changed into 'ask' or **'inquire'**. If there is an object after the reporting verb.
2. Remove the *comma* and the *inverted commas* and start the reported speech with the conjunction **'if' or 'whether'**.
3. Change the interrogative form of the reported speech into assertive form.
4. Nouns or pronouns in the vocative case are treated as objects of their verbs.
5. Other general rules are observed too.

Observe the following examples:

Direct	The visitor said to me, 'Is your mom at home?'
Indirect	The visitor asked me if my mom was at home.
Direct	Netaji said to his men, 'Are you ready to die for your country?'
Indirect	Netaji asked his men if they were ready to die for their country.
Direct	The host said to the guest, 'Would you like to have a cup of coffee?'
Indirect	The host asked the guest if he would like to have a cup of coffee.
Direct	Sahil said, 'May I use your pen, Avish?'
Indirect	Sahil asked Avish if he might use his pen.
Direct	The clerk said to his officer, 'Shall I type this letter again, Sir?'
Indirect	The clerk asked his officer respectfully if he would type that letter again.
Direct	The crow said, 'Are the grapes sour, Mr Fox?'
Indirect	The crow asked the fox if the grapes were sour.

Indirect to Direct

While changing this type of interrogative sentences from Indirect to direct form of speech, the rules given above are reversed.

Observe the following examples:

Indirect	He asked me if he should open the door
Direct	He said to me, 'Should I open the door?'
Indirect	The traveller asked the man if he could tell him the way to the nearest market
Direct	The traveller said to the man, 'Can you tell me the way to nearest market.?'
Indirect	I asked Rakesh if he would go with us for a movie.
Direct	I said, 'Will you go with us for a movie, Rakesh?'

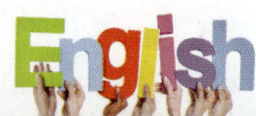

EXERCISE 2

Change each sentence to **indirect form of speech:**

1. Mohan said to me, 'Do you have a bike?'
2. The judge said to the accused, 'Can you prove your innocence?'
3. The shopkeeper said to the customer, 'Will you listen to me or not?'
4. The husband said to his wife, 'Are you not ashamed of your impertinence?'
5. The innkeeper said to me, 'Did you have a sound sleep at night?'
6. The doctor said to the patient, 'Are you still running temperature?'
7. Jim said to Job, 'Didn't you call me a dog last week?'
8. The king said to the slave, 'Can you explain the whole story?'
9. The traveller said to the villager, 'Will you show me the way to the nearest inn?'
10. The villager said to the traveller, 'Do you want to pass the night?'

CONVERSION OF INTERROGATIVE SENTENCES

Direct to Indirect

While reporting interrogative sentences, starting with *What, Why, How, When,..... etc.* indirectly, observe the following rules:

1. The reporting verb 'say' is changed into **'ask'** or **'inquire'** if there is an object after the reporting verb.
2. Remove the **comma** and the **inverted commas** and start the reported speech with the **interrogative word** itself.
3. Change the interrogative form of the reported speech into **assertive form.**
4. Nouns and pronouns in the **vocative** case are treated as objects of their verbs.
5. Other general rules are to be observed too.

Observe the following examples:

Direct	The teacher said to Parth, 'Why are you late?'
Indirect	The teacher asked Parth why he was late.
Direct	Golu said to Molu 'Why did you break my slate?'
Indirect	Golu asked Molu why he had broken her slate.
Direct	He said to me, 'How have you done this question?
Indirect	He asked me how I had done that question.
Direct	Raju said to the policeman, 'Which is the short-cut to the airport?'
Indirect	Raju asked the policeman which was the short-cut to the airport.

Indirect to Direct

Observe the following examples:

Indirect	She asked me what my name was.
Direct	She said to me, 'What is your name?'
Indirect	Ritu asked her where she lived.
Direct	Ritu said to her, 'Where do you live?'

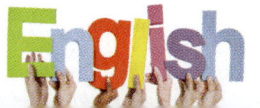

Indirect   The lady asked Sajal when he had met her brother.

Direct   The lady said to Sajal, 'When did you meet my brother?'

EXERCISE 3

Change each sentence to **indirect form of speech:**

1. I said to the miller, 'How can a rope be used to bind flour?'
2. The policeman said to the pick-pocket, 'What were you doing with his pocket?'
3. Mohan said to Sohan, 'What help can I give you?'
4. The mother said to her daughter, 'When can you find time to prepare tea?'
5. The stranger said to me, 'What is your name?'
6. The judge said to the thief, 'What is your name and where do you live?'
7. The inspector said to the lady, 'Why is the door always locked?'
8. The innkeeper asked the traveller, 'When will you go back?'
9. The father said to his wife, 'Why is the baby crying?'
10. The people said the minister, 'How many more taxes shall we pay?'

CONVERSION OF IMPERATIVE SENTENCES

While reporting imperative sentences indirectly, observe the following rules:

1. The reporting verbs 'says', etc. are changed into **'order**, **request, warn, advise or propose'** etc.
2. The commas and the reported speech is put into infinitive form.
3. Nouns and pronouns in the vocative case are treated as objects of their verbs.
4. Changes of pronouns, tenses and the words showing nearness are carried on.
5. Other general rules are observed too.

Observe the following examples:

Direct to Indirect

Direct   The servant said to his master, 'Pardon me this time'.

Indirect   The servant **requested** his master to pardon him that time.

Direct   The mistress said to the maid, 'Make my bed.'

Indirect   The mistress **ordered** the maid to make her bed.

Direct   The doctor said to the patient, 'Take only liquid food for three days at least.'

Indirect   The doctor **advised** the patient to take only liquid food for three days at least.

Direct   Kapil said to me, 'Let us go for a river-bath'

Indirect   Kapil **proposed** to me that we should go for a river bath.

Direct   Shan said to Shavan, 'Let him not deceive you.'

Indirect   Shan **warned** Shavan not to let him deceive her.

Direct   The father said to his son, 'Don't do like that.'

Indirect   The father **forbade** his son to do like that.

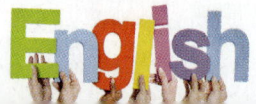

Indirect to Direct

Indirect	The lawyer directed the witness to say as he told him.
Direct	The lawyer said to the witness, 'Say as I tell you.'
Indirect	He proposed to his friends that they should have an outing.
Direct	He said to his friends, 'Let us have an outing.'
Indirect	The father advised his son not to waste time.
Direct	The father said, 'Don't waste your time, my son.'
Indirect	Shiva ordered his servant to fetch him water.
Direct	Shiva said to his servant, 'Fetch me water'
Indirect	He requested him to lend him his book.
Direct	He said to him, 'Lend me your book, please.'
Indirect	Mithu begged his friend to let him go home.
Direct	Mithu said to his friend, 'Let me go home.'

EXERCISE 4

Change each sentence to **indirect form of speech:**

1. The teacher said to the students, 'Don't waste your time in idle gossip.'
2. The principal said to the peon, 'Let pupil come in.'
3. I said to the cheat, 'Be away at once.'
4. The father said to the son, 'Be off and never show me your face again.'
5. The mother said to her son, 'Go to the market and fetch me some vegetables.'
6. The saint said to the widow, 'Trust in God and do the right.'
7. The teacher said to the students, 'Open your book and read the third lesson.'
8. I said to my servant, 'Go and call in the doctor.'
9. The father said, 'Never get up late, my son.'
10. Sunita said to me, 'Please help me do this sum.'

CONVERSION OF OPTATIVE SENTENCES

While reporting optative sentences indirectly, observe the following rules:

1. Change the reporting verb **say** into **wish** or **pray**, etc.
2. Change the optative form into **assertive form**.
3. Introduce the reported speech with the conjunction **'that'**.
4. Change the tenses and pronouns according to rules.
5. Change the vocatives into objects of their verbs.
6. Other general rules are observed too.

Direct to Indirect

Observe the following sentences:

Direct	The old mother said to her son, 'May you live long and prosper!'
Indirect	The old mother wished that her son might live long and prosper.

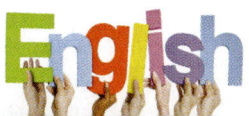

Direct	'God save the king,' said the people.
Indirect	The people prayed that God might save the king.
Direct	'Would that I were rich, said the poor beggar'.
Indirect	The poor beggar wished that he had been rich.
Direct	He said to me, 'Good evening, sir.'
Indirect	He wished me Good evening respectfully.

Indirect to Direct

Indirect	The saint prayed that God might pardon the sinner.
Direct	The saint said, 'May God pardon the sinner.'
Indirect	They wished that her soul might rest in peace.
Direct	They said, 'May her soul rest in peace.'
Indirect	The poor little girl wished that she had been a princess
Direct	The poor little girl said. 'If I were a princess'.
Indirect	He bade his friends **good-bye**.
Direct	He said, '**Good-bye**, friends.'

EXERCISE 5

Change each sentence to **indirect form of speech:**
1. May God bless you with a son! said the beggar to the lady.
2. The priest said to the king, May you live long!
3. The old lady said to me, May you prosper and live long!
4. The goddess said to him, May you win success!
5. He said to me, I were here then!
6. 'O that I had wings!' said she.
7. 'O for a glass of water!' said the wounded soldier.
8. He said, 'If I were a king!'
9. Mala said, 'Good morning daddy.'
10. Geeta said, 'Good night, friends.'

CONVERSION OF EXCLAMATORY SENTENCES

While reporting Exclamatory Sentences indirectly, observe the following rules:
1. Change the reporting verb 'say' into 'exclaim, regret, scold, applaud, confess', etc. according to the feeling expressed in the sentence.
2. Change the exclamatory form into assertive form/declarative form.
3. Omit all Interjections and use the conjunction 'that' to introduce the Reported speech.
4. Observe the rules for changes of pronouns and tenses etc.
5. Complete the sentence if it is incomplete.
6. Exclamation with 'What' how, etc. are changed into He said that it was.

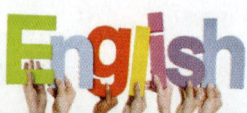

Direct to Indirect

Observe the following examples:

Direct   She said, 'What a beautiful flower it is.'

Indirect   She exclaimed with wonder that it was a very beautiful flower.

Direct   Suraj said, '**Good bye**, my friends.'

Indirect   Suraj bade his friends **good bye**.

Direct   The young lady said,' **Alas! my husband is no more.**'

Indirect   The young lady exclaimed with sorrow that her husband was no more.

Direct   They said. 'Hurrah! we have won the match.'

Indirect   They exclaimed joyfully that they had won the match.

Direct   She said, 'Good morning, Liza. How are you?'

Indirect   She wished Liza good morning and asked her how she was.

Reporting Wishes

Read the following examples:

Direct   She said to me, 'May you live long!'

Indirect   She *wished* that I might live long

Direct   We said, 'May God help you!'

Indirect   We *prayed* that God might help him.

Direct   The boy said to the teacher, 'Good morning, sir.'

Indirect   The boy *respectfully* wished the teacher good morning

Direct   I said, '**Good-bye**, my friends.'

Indirect   I *bade* my friends **good-bye**.

EXERCISE 6

Change the following sentences **into indirect speech**:

1. My friend said to me, 'May you win the prize!'
2. She said, 'May God grant you a long life!'
3. He said, 'May we meet again!'
4. He said to me, 'Good evening.'
5. I said, 'Farewell, my friends.'
6. The children said, 'Hurrah! We have won the match.'
7. She said, 'Alas! We are ruined.'
8. 'What a beautiful fairy!' said the cobbler.
9. 'Bravo! a fine hit!' said the onlookers.
10. 'How foolish I have been!' said the gambler.
11. We said, 'Oh, what a tall building !'
12. 'How clever I am!' said the fox.
13. 'Hurrah! Daddy has come,' said the children.
14. 'How sweet the cuckoo sings!' said she.
15. 'Ah me! What a bloody act!' said the queen.

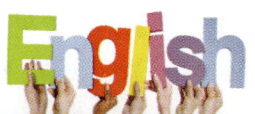

CONVERSION OF SOME TYPICAL SENTENCES

Observe the following examples:

Direct	The pupil said to the teacher, 'May I come in, sir?'
Indirect	The pupil respectfully asked the teacher if he could go in.
Direct	The beggar said to him, 'A lot of thanks for the help.'
Indirect	The beggar thanked him a lot for the help.
Direct	Saira said to me, 'No, I haven't found your pen.'
Indirect	Saira denied having found my pen.
Direct	Sheetal said to me, 'Hello! are you here?'
Indirect	Sheetal cried out in wonder to see me there.
Direct	The accused said, 'By Heavens! I am innocent.'
Indirect	The accused exclaimed on oath that he was innocent.
Direct	She said, 'Yes, 1 am mistaken.'
Indirect	She confessed that she was mistaken.
Direct	He said to me, 'Rest assured! I will stand by you.'
Indirect	He assured me that he would stand by me.
Direct	The king said to them, 'You cowards! You will soon be put to death.'
Indirect	The king called them cowards and threatened them that they would soon be put to death.
Direct	He said, 'God knows I never abused him.'
Indirect	He called upon God to witness that he had never abused him.

Some Typical Sentences

Note the change of the following sentences into the indirect form of speech:

Direct	He said, 'Good morning.'
Indirect	He wished me good morning He greeted me.
Direct	She said to me, 'Thank you for the help.'
Indirect	She thanked me for the help.
Direct	He said, 'May I go out?'
Indirect	He sought my permission to go out.
Direct	I said, 'Shall I lend you a book?'
Indirect	I offered to lend him a book.
Direct	He said,' Happy Christmas.'
Indirect	He wished me happy Christmas.
Direct	She said, 'Congratulations on your success.'
Indirect	She congratulated me on my success
Direct	I said to him, 'Are you happy?' He said, 'yes.'
Indirect	I asked him if he was happy. He replied that he was (happy).
Direct	The doctor said, 'Has the medicine suited you?'. 'No.' I said.
Indirect	The doctor asked if the medicine had suited me. I replied that it hadn't (suited me).

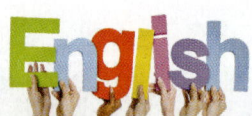

Change each sentence to **indirect form of speech**:

1. The patient said, 'Thanks a lot, doctor.'
2. I said to her, 'Rest assured, I shall help you.'
3. Sohan said, 'By Heavens! I never abused her.'
4. 'May we come in, sir,' said the pupils to the teacher.
5. My father said to me, 'I hope you will get through.'
6. The conductor said to me, 'Beware of pick-pockets.'
7. I said to Anil, 'Cheer up, friend! Don't lose heart.'
8. The servant said to his master, 'Yes, I am at fault, sir.'
9. The general said to soldiers, 'You cowards! I will shoot you all.'
10. Manish said, 'No, I shall not do like that.'

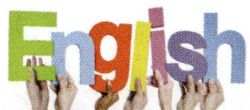

Practice Exercises

I. Change the narration:

1. He says, 'I am working hard.'

   _____

2. He has told you, 'I am coming.'

   _____

3. Raman will say to you, 'I am tired of this work.'

   _____

4. Kittu says, 'I have a toy for you.'

   _____

5. The magician says, 'I will show you a new trick.'

   _____

6. I said to this teacher, 'Sir, I need your help.'

   _____

7. He said, 'My cow died last week.'

   _____

8. Sheeba said to me, 'You may stay here.'

   _____

9. Mohan said to me, 'I will come if I can.'

   _____

10. He said, 'I have been very ill, but am now better.'

    _____

II. Change the narration:

1. He said, 'God is great.'

   _____

2. The boy said, 'I take exercise daily.'

   _____

3. The teacher said, 'The First Battle of Panipat was fought in 1526.'

   _____

4. My friend said to me, 'Might is right.'

   _____

5. The priest said, 'Truth wins in the long run.'

   _____

6. The sage said, 'God helps those who help themselves.'

   _____

7. He said to me, 'When I was teaching, Sohan was dozing.'

   _____

8. She said to me, 'No sooner did I reach the station then the train steamed off.'

   _____

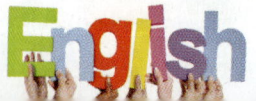

III. Change the narration:

1. The teacher said to me, 'Are you feeling well today?'
   _____

2. He said to the old man, 'What do you want?'
   _____

3. He said to me, 'Have you lost your pen?'
   _____

4. Mohan asked his driver, 'Is the car ready?'
   _____

5. 'Do you know Hindi?' the teacher asked the boy.
   _____

6. She said to me, 'Where are you going?'
   _____

7. He said to me, 'What is the shortest way back?'
   _____

8. I said to him, 'Why did you not tell me the truth earlier?'
   _____

IV. Change the narration:

1. The father said, 'My son, do not waste your time.'
   _____

2. He said, 'Let me play in your garden.'
   _____

3. He said to his servant, 'Do as I tell you.'
   _____

4. I said to him, 'Wait here till I return.'
   _____

5. He said to his friend, 'Please lend me your book.'
   _____

6. The teacher said to the students, 'Do not sit here.'
   _____

7. He said to her servant, 'Get out of my room at once.'
   _____

8. I said to you, 'Wait here till I return.'
   _____

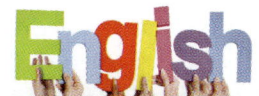

V. Change the narration:

1. The teacher says, 'Ram is an intelligent boy.'
   _____

2. She says, 'Priyanka is a good girl.'
   _____

3. He said, 'Ritu works very hard.'
   _____

4. Mother said, 'Geeta is very obedient.'
   _____

5. Anu said, 'I am painting a natural scenery.'
   _____

6. He said, 'I have an urgent message for you.'
   _____

7. He said, 'I went to Delhi yesterday.'
   _____

8. I said, 'The gardener was watering the plants.
   _____

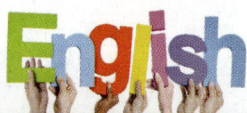

ANSWERS

EXERCISE 1

1. The laborer said that he did not work on Sundays.
2. Sita told Rama that she would accompany him.
3. The boys shouted that they had won the match.
4. The patient told that he had been down with fever.
5. The mouse addressed the lion as king and said that he would help him someday.
6. The teacher said that his answer did not deserve more marks.
7. The mother advised his son to speak the truth always.
8. The teacher told Mohan that he would take him to the Principal if he misbehaved.
9. The citizens told the king that it was his duty to protect them.
10. The teacher told his mother that he was very hungry.

EXERCISE 2

1. Mohan asked me if I had a bike.
2. The judge asked the accused if he could prove his innocence.
3. The shopkeeper asked the customer if he would listen to him or not.
4. The husband asked his wife if she was not ashamed of her impertinence.
5. The innkeeper asked me if I had a sound sleep at night.
6. The doctor asked the patient if he was still running temperature.
7. Jim asked job that didn't he call him a dog the previous week.
8. The king asked the slave if he could explain the whole story.
9. The traveller requested the villager if he would show him the way to the nearest inn.
10. The villager asked the traveler if he wanted to pass the night.

EXERCISE 3

1. I asked miller that how could a rope be used to bind flour.
2. The policeman asked the pick-pocket.that what was he doing with his pocket.
3. Mohan asked Sohan that what help could he give him.
4. The mother asked her daughter that when could she find time to prepare tea.
5. The stranger asked me my name.
6. The judge asked the thief his name and where did he live.
7. The inspector asked the lady that why was the door always locked.
8. The innkeeper asked the traveler that when would he go back.
9. The father asked his wife that why was the baby crying.
10. The people asked the minister that how many more taxes should they pay.

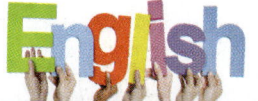

EXERCISE 4

1. The teacher suggested the students not to waste their time in idle gossip.
2. The Principal told the peon to let the pupil in.
3. I told the cheat to be away at once.
4. The father told his son to be off and never show him his face again.
5. The mother requested her son to go to the market and Fetch her some vegetables.
6. The saint advised the widow to trust in God and do the right.
7. The teacher directed her students to open their books and read the third lesson.
8. I ordered my servant to go and call in the doctor.
9. The father advised his son to never get up late.
10. Sunita requested me to help her do that sum.

EXERCISE 5

1. The beggar prayed that God might bless the lady with a son.
2. The priest prayed that the king might live long.
3. The old lady wished that I might prosper and live long.
4. The goddess wished that he might win success.
5. He wished that he was there then.
6. She wished that she had wings.
7. The wounded soldier requested for a glass of water.
8. He wished that he was a king.
9. Mala wished good morning to her daddy.
10. Geeta bade good night to her friends.

EXERCISE 6

1. My friend wished that I might win the prize.
2. He prayed that God might grant him a long life.
3. He wished that we might meet again.
4. He wished me good evening.
5. I bid farewell to my friends.
6. The children exclaimed with joy that they had won the match.
7. She exclaimed with sorrow that they were ruined.
8. The cobbler exclaimed with wonder that it was a beautiful fairy.
9. The onlookers exclaimed with joy that it was a fine hit.
10. The gambler said regretfully that he had been foolish.
11. We exclaimed with a surprise what a tall building it was.
12. The fox exclaimed that how clever it was.

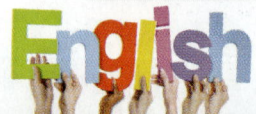

13. The children exclaimed with joy that their daddy had come.

14. The girl exclaimed that how sweet the cuckoo sang.

15. The queen sighed that what a bloody act it was.

EXERCISE 7

1. The patient thanked the doctor.

2. I assured to help her.

3. Sohan swore that he had never abused her.

4. The pupils asked the teacher if they could come in.

5. My father hoped that I would get through.

6. The conductor warned me of pick pockets.

7. I encouraged Anil to cheer up and not to lose heart.

8. The servant admitted his fault before his master.

9. The general addressing his soldiers as cowards said that he would shoot them all.

10. Manish refused and said that he would not do like that.

EXERCISE I

1. He says that he is working hard.

2. He has told me that he is coming.

3. Raman will say me that he is tired of that work.

4. Kittu says that she has a toy for him.

5. The magician says that he would show them a new trick.

6. I told the teacher that I needed his help.

7. He said that his cow died the previous week.

8. Sheeba told me that I might stay there.

9. Mohan told me that he would come if he could.

10. He said that he had been very ill, but was better then.

EXERCISE II

1. He said that God is great.

2. The boy said that he took exercise daily.

3. The teacher told that the first battle of Panipat was fought in 1526.

4. My friend told me that might is right.

5. The priest said that Truth wins in the long run.

6. The sage said that God helps those who help themselves.

7. He told me that when he was teaching, Sohan was dozing.

8. She told me that as soon as he reached the station the train steamed off.

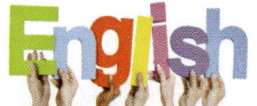

EXERCISE III

1. The teacher asked me if I was feeling well that day.
2. He asked the old man what he wanted.
3. He asked me if I had lost my pen.
4. Mohan asked his driver if the car was ready.
5. The teacher asked the boy if he knew Hindi.
6. She asked me where I was going.
7. He asked me the shortest way back.
8. I asked him why he did not tell me the truth earlier.

EXERCISE IV

1. The father advised his son not to waste his time.
2. He asked for permission to play in his garden.
3. He told his servant to do as he was told.
4. I asked him to wait there till I returned.
5. He requested his friend to lend him his book.
6. The teacher told the students not to sit there.
7. He ordered his servant to go out of his room at once.
8. I told him to wait there till I returned.

EXERCISE V

1. The teacher says that Ram is an intelligent boy.
2. She says that Priyanka is a good girl.
3. He said that Ritu worked very hard.
4. Mother said that Geeta was very obedient.
5. Anu said that she was painting a natural scenery.
6. He said that he had an urgent message for him.
7. He said that he went to Delhi the previous day.
8. I said that the gardener was watering the plants.

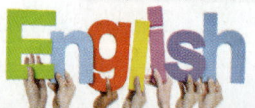

Chapter 15

Building Vocabulary— Antonyms and Synonyms

ANTONYMS

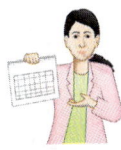

A word opposite in meaning or sense to a given word is called its Antonym. Antonyms are of three types:

1. Words without any prefix or suffix. Such words are called Direct Antonyms.
   Study the following examples:

Word	Antonyms
Abundance	Dearth
Abject	Elevated
Zenith	Nadir

2. Antonyms can be formed by using a prefix before a word. Some important prefixes are: In, Un, Dis. Mark the following examples:

Word	Antonyms
Ability	Inability
Well	Unwell
Advantage	Disadvantage

3. Some antonyms can be formed by changing the suffix of a given word.
   Mark the following examples:

Word	Antonyms
Careful	Careless
Faithful	Faithless

In this part, all types of antonyms are of real importance and their actual uses have been given.

Word	Antonym	Word	Antonym
Ability	Inability	Bitter	Sweet
Abandon	Retain	Blunt	Sharp
Abuse	Praise	Blame	Applaud
Above	Below, beneath	Blessing	Curse
Absent	Present	Bold	Timid
Absurd	Relevant	Borrow	Lend
Accept	Reject	Bottom	Top
Advance	Retreat	Boastful	Modest
Alive	Dead	Bright	Dull
Adversity	Prosperity	Bravery	Cowardice
Active	Passive	Broad	Narrow
Advantage	Disadvantage	Benediction	Malediction
Angel	Devil	Beneficial	Harmful
Affirmative	Negative	Bow	Stern
Agree	Disagree	Buy	Sell
Always	Never	Care	Neglect
All	None	Cheap	Dear, expensive
Appear	Vanish	Cheerful	Sad
Attack	Protect	Calm	Turbulent
Analysis	Synthesis	Clever	Stupid
Appoint	Dismiss	Cruel	Kind
Arm	Disarm	Create	Destroy
Arrival	Departure	Coarse	Fine
Artificial	Natural	Common	Rare
Angry	Pleased	Conquest	Defeat
Ascent	Descent	Comfortable	Uncomfortable
Attract	Repel	Confusion	Simple
Abundance	Scarcity	Cool	Warm
Ally	Enemy	Contract	Expand
Assemble	Disperse	Correct	Incorrect
Audible	Inaudible	Collect	Disperse
Barren	Fertile	Contrast	Comparison
Beautiful	Ugly	Concord	Discord
Begin	End	Comedy	Tragedy
Belief	Doubt, disbelief	Expand	Contract
Conceal	Reveal	Eager	Reluctant

Contd...

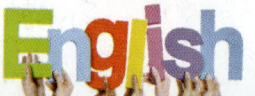

Word	Antonym	Word	Antonym
Compulsory	Optional	Exact	Inaccurate
Connect	Disconnect	Excess	Shortage
Competent	Incompetent	Exterior	Interior
Decrease	Increase	Exhale	Inhale
Deep	Shallow	Eligible	Ineligible
Delay	Haste	Enemy	Friend
Death	Birth	Eternal	Transitory
Dry	Wet	Examiner	Examinee
Dead	Alive	Explicit	Implicit
Difficult	Easy	Expatriate	Repatriate
Decent	Indecent	Exports	Imports
Defensive	Offensive	External	Internal
Dense	Sparse	Far	Near
Deposit	Withdraw	Firm	Shaky
Destructive	Constructive	For	Against
Despair	Hope	Fact	Fiction
Distance	Near	False	True
Discount	Premium	Free	Bound
Divide	Multiply	Failure	Success
Dream	Reality	Fall	Rise
Down	Up	Foreign	Native
Different	Same	Fat	Thin
East	West	Fail	Pass
Edible	Inedible	Fresh	Stale
Enjoy	Dismiss	Famous	Notorious
Encourage	Discourage	Fortunate	Unfortunate
Empty	Full	Freedom	Slavery
Early	Late	Futile	Fruitful
Emigrant	Immigrant	Friend	Foe
East	West	Friendly	Hostile
Easy	Difficult	Folly	Wisdom
Entrance	Exit	Front	Rear
Equal	Unequal	Import	Export
Fickle	Steadfast	Inside	Outside
Fictitious	Genuine	Idle	Active
Forget	Remember	Inferior	Superior
Favor	Disfavor	Inhale	Exhale

Contd...

Word	Antonym	Word	Antonym
Frequent	Occasional	Interesting	Dull, boring
Farewell	Welcome	Ignorance	Knowledge
Gain	Loss	Industrious	Sloth
Give	Take	Insolent	Meek
Gather	Scatter	Improve	Deteriorate
Gay	Grave	Intentional	Accidental
Giant	Dwarf	Immortal	Mortal
Guilty	Innocent	Illegitimate	Legitimate
Gaiety	Melancholy	Innocent	Guilty
Graceful	Hideous	Ingenious	Insincere
Grateful	Ungrateful	Illusive	Real
Generous	Selfish	Individual	Joint
Great	Small	Initial	Final
General	Particular	Insult	Respect
Guest	Host	Include	Exclude
Gentle	Unkind, rough	Junior	Senior
Grieve	Rejoice	Joy	Sorrow
Growth	Decline	Join	Disjoin
Grant	Refuse	Justice	Injustice
Govern	Obey	Kind	Unkind
Head	Tail	Keen	Dull
Heaven	Hell	Knowledge	Ignorance
High	Low	Like	Dislike
Hit	Miss	Lend	Borrow
Hill	Valley	Lawful	Unlawful
Harmony	Discord	Legal	Illegal
Hostile	Friendly	Literate	Illiterate
Hide	Show	Living	Dead
Hate	Love	Loyal	Disloyal
Hollow	Solid	Loud	Soft
Hero	Villain	Limited	Unlimited
Heavy	Light	Liberty	Slavery
Honest	Dishonest	Last	First
Hope	Despair	Lenient	Strict
Heedful	Heedless	Loose	Tight
Holy	Unholy	Long	Short
Huge	Tiny	Leader	Follower

Contd...

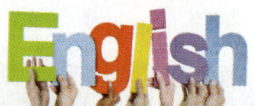

Word	Antonym	Word	Antonym
Healthy	Unhealthy	Light	Dark
Harm	Benefit	Liquid	Solid
Humble	Proud	Lofty	Low
Honour	Dishonour	Maximum	Minimum
Hypocrite	Sincere	Movable	Immovable
Illegible	Legible	Permanent	Temporary
Malice	Good-will	Please	Displease
Mild	Stern	Peace	War
Masculine	Feminine	Profit	Loss
Material	Spiritual	Public	Private
Make	Mar	Pure	Impure
Major	Minor	Poison	Antidote
Master	Servant	Prosperity	Adversity
Moral	Immoral	Partial	Impartial
Majority	Minority	Pleasant	Unpleasant
Merit	Demerit	Plenty	Scarcity
Memory	Forgetfulness	Poetry	Prose
Mortal	Immortal	Pleasure	Pain
Motion	Rest	Penalty	Reward
Notorious	Famous	Perfect	Imperfect
Numerous	Sparse	Poor	Rich
Naked	Covered	Pretty	Ugly
Now	Then	Proud	Humble
Natural	Artificial	Predecessor	Successor
Negative	Positive	Prologue	Epilogue
New	Old	Prose	Verse
Noble	Ignoble	Prolific	Sterile
Neat	Untidy	Powerful	Feeble
Near	Far	Question	Answer
Next	Previous	Quiet	Noisy
Optional	Compulsory	Quick	Slow
Outward	Inward	Quote	Unquote
Optimist	Pessimist	Quiver	Rest
Opponent	Supporter	Queer	Normal
Own	Disown	Quit	Hold
Obligatory	Optional	Quarrelsome	Friendly
Obstruct	Assist	Raise	Lower

Contd...

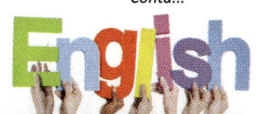

Word	Antonym	Word	Antonym
Obey	Disobey	Real	Unreal
Odd	Even	Regular	Irregular
Oral	Written	Remember	Forget
Off	On	Right	Wrong
Old	Young	Rough	Smooth
Order	Disorder	Rear	Front
Open	Shut	Raw	Ripe
Oppose	Yield	Rise	Fall
Obedient	Disobedient	Round	Flat
Pardon	Punish	Rejoice	Grieve
Praise	Condemn, blame	Rural	Urban
Part	Whole	Rigid	Flexible
Pedestrian	Passenger	Repulsive	Attractive
Peculiar	Normal	Remote	Near
Proper	Improper	Revolution	Evolution
Preserve	Destroy	Retreat	Advance
Prejudiced	Unprejudiced	Top	Bottom
Ruthless	Merciful	Tragedy	Comedy
Remarkable	Ordinary	Thick	Thin
Remove	Restore	Tolerant	Intolerant
Reduce	Increase	Trust	Distrust
Resist	Admit	Truth	Falsehood
Respect	Insult	Tame	Wild
Rival	Supporter	Tear	Repair
Rogue	Saint	Timid	Bold
Revere	Forgive	Torture	Comfort
Rude	Polite	Tough	Soft
Rumour	Fact	Transparent	Opaque
Safe	Unsafe	Trained	Untrained
Safety	Danger	Triumph	Defeat
Sure	Doubtful	Typical	Unusual
Slow	Fast	Torment	Soothe
Sink	Swim	Take	Give
Solid	Liquid	Teach	Learn
Sane	Insane	Theory	Practical
Steady	Unstable	Tie	Unite

Contd...

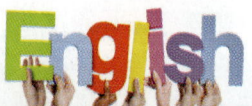

Word	Antonym	Word	Antonym
Suppress	Provoke	Union	Split/diversity
Suspicious	Trustful	Uniform	Variable
Savage	Civilised	Utter	Recall
Sea	Land	Uphold	Oppose
Sensible	Insensible	Use	Misuse
Single	Double	Waive	Demand
Sleep	Wake	Wicked	Virtuous
Straight	Curved	Win	Lose
Secret	Open	Weak	Strong
Satisfaction	Dissatisfaction	Urge	Discourage
Severe	Mild	Unique	Common
Scanty	Sufficient	Universal	Local
Scatter	Gather	Usual	Unusual
Systematic	Unsystematic	Unfair	Fair
Scold	Praise	Victory	Defeat
Slender	Plump, stout	Virtue	Vice
Spacious	Limited	Verbal	Written
Stable	Unstable	Visible	Invisible
Synonym	Antonym	Vulgar	Refined
Surplus	Deficit	Visible	Invisible
Shy	Confident, imprudent	Valour	Cowardice
Simple	Complex	Vacant	Occupied
Similar	Different	Valid	Invalid
Skilled	Unskilled	Vulnerable	Invulnerable
Shocking	Pleasant	Voluntary	Compulsory
Shallow	Deep	Vivid	Unclear, vague
Soft	Hard	Versatile	Steady
Soothe	Irritate	Valuable	Invaluable
Wise	Foolish	Warm	Cool
Woeful	Cheerful	Wrangle	Agree
Wild	Civilized	Yield	Resist
Weep	Laugh	Youth	Aged
War	Peace	Young	Old
Weary	Unweary	Yoke	Liberty
Woe	Joy	Zeal	Indifference
Wax	Wane	Zenith	Lowest
Want	Abundance		

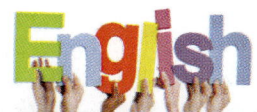

MORE ANTONYMS

Word	Antonym	Word	Antonym
Appreciate	Condemn	Assurance	Doubt
Audience	Speaker	Appropriate	Improper, inappropriate
Adopt	Reject		
Aristocrat	Commoner	Applaud	Condemn, hoot
Ancient	Modern	Acquisition	Loss
Armament	Disarmament	Association	Dissociation
Attraction	Repulsion	Aristocracy	Democracy
Approve of	Reject	Asleep	Awake
Advantage	Disadvantage	Affluence	Poverty
Accord	Disaccord	Agile	Weak, inert
Acceptance	Refusal	Aware	Unaware
Admiration	Condemnation	Activity	Passivity
Action	Inaction	Agony	Joy
Attach	Detach	Acute	Obtuse
Amateur	Professional	Accelerate	Retard
Alienate	Endear	Ambiguous	Unambiguous
Beauty	Ugliness	Benevolent	Malevolent
Barbarism	Civilization	Bare	Covered
Birth	Death	Brotherhood	Enmity
Bitter	Sweet	Brutality	Humanity
Boon	Bane	Beginning	End
Busy	Idle	Better	Worse
Black	White	Bow	Stern
Bashful	Bold	Big	Small
Buoyant	Dejected	Cleanliness	Untidiness, dirt
		Confidence	Distrust, diffidence
Cheerfulness	Cheerlessness, gravity, dejection	Creation	Destruction
Combatant	Noncombatant	Courage	Timidity
Credit	Debit, discredit	Confess	Deny
Continue	Stop	Cowardly	Brave, courageous
Commend	Condemn	Contrast	Similarity
Concave	Convex	Conquest	Defeat
Conventional	New, modern	Conflict	Compromise
Comfort	Discomfort	Complicated	Simple
Cease	Continue	Cruelty	Kindness

Contd...

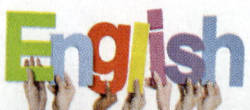

Word	Antonym	Word	Antonym
Comic	Tragic	Certitude	Doubt, skepticism
Confide	Hide	Crafty	Simple
Coward	Brave	Cordial	Rude
Counterfeit	Genuine, original	Combine	Separate
Command	Obey	Clash	Amity, friendship
Constant	Changing, inconstant	Coarse	Smooth
Criticism	Praise	Civil	Uncivil
Confident	Diffident	Competent	Incompetent
Certain	Uncertain	Complicated	Simple
Classification	Declassification	Cold	Hot
Complex	Simple	Cloudy	Clear
Clean	Dirty	Confine	Release
Complainant	Defendant	Compulsory	Optional
Celestial	Terrestrial	Concurrent	Consecutive
Convict(V)	Acquit	Colleague	Antagonist
Caution	Recklessness	Cheerful	Gloomy
Climax	Anticlimax	Distress	Comfort, joy
Debit	Credit	Despair	Hope
Dwarf	Giant	Delight	Displeasure, sorrow
Disease	Health	Diligence	Idleness, indolence
Day	Night	Deficit	Surplus
Danger	Safety	Distinct	Vague
Defeat	Victory	Divine	Human
Dispute	Amity, unity	Discrimination	Indiscrimination
Diverted	Undiverted	Dictate	Obey, follow
Denounce	Praise	Decorate	Disfigure
Domestic	Foreign	Desperate	Confident
Descent	Ascent	Discard	Accept, embrace
Dazed	Calm	Dull	Bright
Do	Undo	Disarrange	Arrange
Doubt	Sure	Dawn	Dusk
Deep	Shallow	Deface	Decorate, repair
Dynamic	Static	Detention	Freedom
Demoralise	Encourage, boost	Deficient	Proficient
Dubious	Clear	Enthusiasm	Indifference
Diligent	Lazy	Examiner	Examinee

Contd...

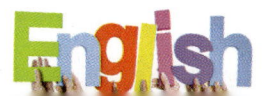

Word	Antonym	Word	Antonym
Economy	Extravagance	End	Beginning
Earning	Spending	Equality	Inequality
Elevation	Depression	Elegance	Ugliness
Enmity	Friendship	Expensive	Cheap
Exterior	Interior	Ever	Never
Experience	Inexperience	Enslave	Free
Enormous	Small, tiny	Exaggerate	Minimise, shorten
Extinguish	Kindle	Eminent	Ordinary
Exception	Rule	Eccentric	Normal
Endowed	Deprived	Early	Late
Exclude	Include	Emigrant	Immigrant
Everywhere	Nowhere	Ecstasy	Boredom
Extravagance	Thrift, economy	Enrage	Pacify
Employ	Dismiss	Fame	Infamy
Enrage	Pacify	Futility	Utility
Exultation	Depression, mourning	Foreigner	Native
Faith	Doubt	Free	Bonded
Fortune	Misfortune	Familiarity	Unfamiliarity
Frankness	Reservedness	Fatal	Life-saving
Freeze	Melt	Find	Lose
Fast	Slow	Fresh	Stale
Flourish	Ruin	First	Last
Final	First, initial	Future	Past
Friend	Enemy, foe	Fidelity	Infidelity
Fat	Thin, lean	Fragile	Strong, tough
Former	Latter	Gaily	Sadly
Force	Persuade	Gigantic	Small, tiny
Formidable	Weak, trivial	Good	Bad
Gratitude	Thanklessness	Happiness	Sorrow
Glorious	Dull	Humanitarian	Beastly, inhuman
Gradually	Quickly	Hasten	Slow down, retard
Hopeless	Hopeful	Hit	Miss
Humility	Pride, vanity	Harmony	Discord
Humorous	Dull, tragic	Happy	Sad
Hygienic	Dirty, unhealthy	Hill	Valley

Contd...

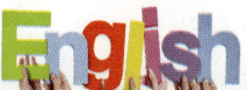

Word	Antonym	Word	Antonym
Hard	Soft	Height	Depth
Health	Sickness, disease	Haughty	Humble, modest
Here	There	Imagination	Reality
Help	Hinder	Intelligence	Foolishness
Hideous	Beautiful	Intimate	Stranger
Hybrid	Pure, unmixed	Incredible	Credible
Interest	Indifference	Inconvenience	Convenience
Invest	Disinvest	Inflict	Suffer
Important	Ordinary, unimportant	Intense	Weak, dim
Inflexible	Flexible, elastic	Immense	Small
Imaginative	Unimaginative, dull	Indifferently	Keenly
Inadequate	Sufficient, adequate	Initial	Final
Immunity	Infection	Inflate	Deflate
Imperial	Ordinary, plebian	Ignorance	Knowledge
Invalid	Valid	Junior	Senior
Interior	Exterior	Juvenile	Adult, mature
Include	Exclude	Knotty	Simple, easy
Inert	Active, brisk	Lack	Plenty
Justice	Injustice	Latent	Patent
Join	Separate	Legendry	Modern, recent
Joy	Sorrow, sadness	Life	Death
Kindle	Extinguish	Least	Most
Landlord	Tenant	Lethargic	Active
Likeness	Difference	Lead	Follow
Laudable	Deplorable	Lazy	Industrious
Lovable	Hateful	Luster	Dullness
Loathing	Liking	Marriage	Divorce
Lucky	Unlucky	Moderation	Excess
Levity	Seriousness	Multiply	Divide
Licentious	Sober, chaste	Merry	Sad
Lawful	Illegal, unlawful	Movement	Stability
Latitude	Longitude	Modest	Proud
Melancholy	Gaiety	Mar	Make
Miser	Spendthrift	Meet	Part
Master	Servant	Monogamy	Polygamy

Contd...

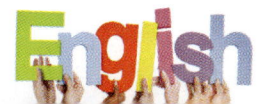

Word	Antonym	Word	Antonym
Move	Stop	Mountain	Plain
Modernity	Traditional	Meagre	Ample
Miniature	Enlargement	Mature	Immature
Mental	Physical	Morbid	Sound, incentive
Masculine	Feminine	Mistress	Maid
Misery	Joy, happiness	Nationalize	Privatise
Monotony	Variety	Noise	Silence
Morning	Evening	Natural	Artificial
Modern	Ancient	Night	Day
Malignant	Benign	Original	Duplicate copy
Mute	Vocal, loud	Official	Unofficial
Native	Stranger	Owner	Tenant
Nowhere	Everywhere	Ordinary	Extraordinary
North	South	Organic	Inorganic
Neutral	Committed	Obscene	Decent, pure
Optimism	Pessimism	Pros	Cons
Obvious	Obscure, latent	Permission	Prohibition
Oppressive	Inoppressive	Patriotism	Cosmopolitanism
Outstanding	Common	Pursuit	Avoidance
Orthodox	Unorthodox	Patience	Impatience
Odious	Pleasant, lovable	Pity	Cruelty
Omission	Commission	Precede	Succeed
Patriot	Traitor	Properly	Improperly
Presence	Absence	Passionate	Dispassionate
Poverty	Richness	Profound	Shallow
Pride	Humility	Permanent	Temporary
Paradise	Hell	Perpetuate	Discontinue
Passion	Coolness	Public	Private
Pathetic	Comic, happy	Pardon	Punish
Particular	General	Prosperous	Indigent
Prestige	Insult	Premature	Overdue
Partial	Impartial	Practical	Dreamy
Probably	Certainly	Quash	Uphold
Perfect	Imperfect	Quick	Slow
Paralyse	Activate	Ruler	Subject, ruled
Polite	Rude, saucy	Roar	Whisper

Contd...

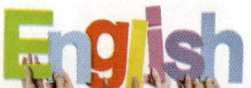

Word	Antonym	Word	Antonym
Pugnacious	Peaceful	Recede	Increase
Prospective	Retrospective	Ruin	Construct
Palatable	Disagreeable	Reverence	Insult, disrespect
Quaint	Common place	Receive	Give
Quell	Excite, fan(V)	Refuse	Accept
Repute	Disrepute	Remedy	Malady
Relief	Aggravation	Rhythmic	Unrhythmic
Recklessness	Prudence	Robust	Feeble, delicate
Regular	Irregular	Regularly	Periodically
Resident	Nonresident	Radiant	Dull, depressed
Renown	Notoriety	Repeal, Revoke	Endorse, enact
Ridicule	Praise	Repugnant	Attractive, pleasant
Resemblance	Difference	Rival	Supporter
Repel	Attract	Ruthless	Merciful, tender
Raise	Suppress	Security	Peril, risk, danger
Right	Left, wrong	Servant, slave	Master
Rapture	Pain, agony	Savagery	Kindness
Relent	Persist	Saint	Sinner
Replenish	Exhaust, waste	Service	Disservice
Resolute	Irresolute, weak	Synthesis	Analysis
Rustic	Urbane	Stubborn	Flexible
Recovery	Relapse, loss	Survive	Succumb, pass away
Smile	Frown	Stiff	Elastic
Sympathy	Antipathy	Superiority	Inferiority
Sorrow	Joy	Splendour	Dullness
Silence	Noise	Selfless	Selfish
Success	Failure	Solitary	Crowded, popular
Sin	Virtue	Sooth	Harass
Silly	Intelligent	Sparse	Populated
Stereotyped	Unique, individual	Sacred	Profane
Scholar	Foolish, illiterate	Spacious	Limited
Serene	Turbulent	Singular	Plural
Sentimental	Unsentimental	Straight	Crooked
Significance	Insignificance	Zig Zag	Straight
Spongy	Hard	Foolish	Clever
Shun	Open	Sweet	Sour, bitter

Contd...

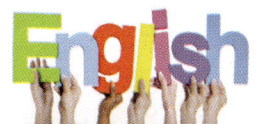

Word	Antonym	Word	Antonym
Stoop	Rise	Serpentine	Straight, direct
Slim	Chubby, stout	Sombre	Gay, bright
Sober	Intoxicated	Tyranny	Benevolence
Stationary	Moving	Tender	Hard
Summer	Winter	Want(N)	Abundance
Smart	Stupid	Worthless	Valuable
Start	Finish	Wither	Grow
Secular	Religious	Wide	Narrow
Shallow	Deep	Tiny	Big
Symmetrical	Asymmetrical, irregular	Tortuous	Direct, straight
Tyrant	Affectionate	Tranquil	Disturbed, upset
Tumult	Calmness	Tarnish	Brighten
Twist	Straighten	Utility	Harmfulness
Terrestrial	Heavenly	Uplift	Downgrade
Transverse	Longitudinal	Vital	Weak
Tolerance	Intolerance	Vicious	Virtuous
Unfortunately	Luckily	Vanity	Humility
Undaunted	Afraid	Wisdom	Folly
Upper	Lower	Work	Rest
Venture	Hesitate	Weep	Laugh
Vehement	Feeble	Whole	Part
Vogue	Disuse		

ANTONYMS (MISCELLANEOUS)

Word	Antonym	Word	Antonym
Brilliant	Dull	Blurred	Dull
Agile	Sluggish	Rapid	Slow
Envy	Generosity	Sparkling	Dull
Chilly	Hot	Panting	Dislike
Anxious	Indifferent	Terrified	Unmoved
Stall	Ignore	Nimble	Sluggish
Precious	Worthless	Grave	Trivial
Concocted	Natural	Incontrovertible	Untrue
Dispute	Harmony	Cease	Continue
Prostrate	Standing	Worthy	Useless

Contd...

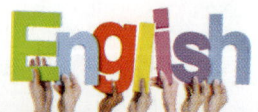

Word	Antonym	Word	Antonym
Array	Disarray	Tender	Worthless
Skill	Inability	Delight	Sadness
Rear	Front	Strew	Collect
Twilight	Daylight	Humbly	Defiantly
Appreciate	Criticize	Strong	Weak
Punish	Praise	Wild	Tamed, civilized
Rest	Stir	Wisdom	Foolishness
Learned	Simple	Strength	Weakness
Ancient	Modern	Peace	Turbulence
Grassy	Sandy	Sorrowful	Joyful
Rejoice	Mourn	Ascent	Descent
Infirmity	Strength	Console	Trouble, torment
Substantial	Meager	Accost	Avoid, shun
Acquaintance	Stranger	Perpetual	Occasional
Mortify	Honour	Invidious	Pleasant, fair
Exclusive	General	Privilege	Prohibition
Obnoxious	Loveable	Patent	Covert, hidden
Countenance	Disapproval	Single	Married
Sneer	Love	Pretend	Exhibit
Vicious	Honourable	Insolent	Respectful
Assume	Prove	Appoint	Dismiss
Caress	Rebuke	Untreatable	Controllable
Morose	Social	Boisterous	Calm
Snap	Join	Makeshift	Permanent
Indifferent	Caring	Fancy	Reality
Amiable	Unpleasant	Appendage	Deleted
Dainty	Ugly, rough	Fast	Unfirm
Precarious	Safe	Authentic	False
Marked	Unmarked	Queer	Usual
Excrescence	Normal	Consort	Desert
Esteem	Disdain	Infinite	Finite
Riveted	Free	Trifling	Important
Candid	Secretive	Discovered	Lost
Excited	Calm	Blockhead	Smart
Assistance	Hindrance	Dumbfounded	Stable
Repress	Free	Gorgeously	Simply

Contd...

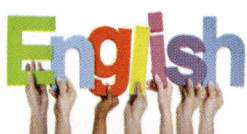

Word	Antonym	Word	Antonym
Swamp	Drought	Appropriate	Insufficient
Mongrel	Pedigree	Settled	Shaky, unsettled
Continual	Irregular	Throb	Sink
Tag	Push	Inherit	Disinherit
Peasant	Aristocrat	Own	Disown
Favor	Disapprove	Peculiar	General
Rage	Patience	Snort	Inhale
Monster	Angel	Skinny	Brawny
Distinct	Vague	Flatter	Criticize
Faint	Clear	Humiliate	Honour
Robes	Rags	Bow	Stand
Radiant	Dull	Holy	Evil
Reckless	Calm	Taint	Clean
Boundless	Limited	Trespass	Resistance
Defile	Purify	Sought	Ignore
Commence	End	Contest	Concede
Wisdom	Foolishness	Generosity	Miserliness
Swift	Sluggish	Diligence	Lethargy
Delight	Sorrow	Realize	Misunderstood
Probable	Improbable	Endowed	Deprived
Toiling	Resting, lazy	Mortal	Immortal
Unwearied	Wearied	Require	Avoid
Superiority	Inferiority	Assurance	Denial
Companion	Enemy	Stigma	Laurel
Impart	Take	Self-centered	Benevolent
Odd	Even	Egotism	Modesty
Handicap	Compensation	Confide	Mistrust
Immunity	Exposure	Exclusively	Ordinarily
Notorious	Famous	Just	Unjust
Audience	Performer	Pleasant	Unpleasant
Rapid	Slow	Blurred	Clear
Faded	Polished	Varnished	Worn out
Disgust	Liking	Complement	Criticism
Sufficient	Insufficient	Jolly	Sulking
Perceived	Ignored	Essential	Inessential
Definite	Indefinite	Intellectual	Illiterate

Contd...

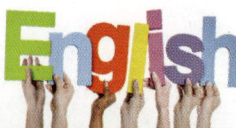

Word	Antonym	Word	Antonym
Certain	Uncertain	Conform	Rebel, revolt
Initiate	Conclude	Antitype	Modern
Reverie	Reality	Ethical	Immoral
Far	Near	Abstract	Concrete
Dialogue	Silence	Vital	Unimportant
Soliloquy	Dialogue	Fashionable	Outdated
Frank	Introvert, shy	Acute	Obtuse
Discreet	Tactless	Please	Displease, annoy
Prudently	Tactlessly	Recall	Forget
Secretive	Open	Delicate	Rough

SYNONYMS

1. A synonym is a word that has almost the same meaning as another word. For example, a synonym for beautiful is stunning.
    - She is a beautiful girl.
    - She is a stunning girl.

    Learning synonyms is a great way of improving your vocabulary and can make your writing and speaking more exciting or interesting. In the UK, it is a known fact that teachers hate to see the word 'nice' in an essay! Can you think of some synonyms for nice?

2. There is a certain skill involved in choosing the most appropriate synonym, as not all are created equal. It is important to consider the connotation of the word because some synonyms can inject a different meaning than the one intended. For example, one synonym of sad is 'gloomy', however, this word carried quite a negative connotation. Depending on the circumstance you can use it, but if you just want to say that someone is 'down' than another synonym such as 'blue' or 'unhappy' would be more applicable.

Word	Synonym	Word	Synonym
Abandon	Desert, leave	Accurate	Exact
Abbreviate	Curtail, abridge	Adversity	Difficult time
Abundance	Plenty	Advantage	Benefit
Abundant	Ample, plentiful	Advancement	Progress
Abduct	Kidnap	Aggression	Attack
Abhor	Hate	Ailing	Having ill health
Abnormal	Irregular, unusual	Auspicious, artful	Joy clever
Abode	Home	Bad	Evil
Abolish	Destroy, remove	Beautify	Adorn, decorate
Abound	Flourish	Baffle	Confuse
Abortive	Fruitless	Beg	Solicit, implore

Contd...

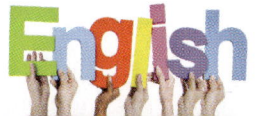

Word	Synonym	Word	Synonym
Addicted	Habitual	Behavior	Conduct
Active	Full of vigour	Big	Huge, large
Ability	Potential, worth	Blame	Reprove
Adopt	Accept	Blessing	Benediction
Adore	Worship, idolise	Brave	Courageous
Alive	Lively, vivacious	Bargain	Agreement
Ally	Colleague, partner	Bright	Clear, brilliant
Alms	Dole, gratuity	Brittle	Frail, fragile
Amend	Improve	Beneficent	Helpful, kind
Anxiety	Misgiving	Behold	Regard
Assent	Consent, agree	Burglar	Bandit, thief
Absolute	Autocratic	Cruelty	Brutality, inhumanity
Busy	Active, alert	Cite	Quote
Beastly	Inhuman	Claim	To ask by virtue
Bliss	Joy	Coarse	Not fine
Bloom	Glow	Cold	Chilly
Blot	Spot	Comfort	Convenience
Beseech	Request	Clutch	Grasp
Blunder	Mistake	Compel	Force
Bluff	Mislead	Collision	Dashing, together
Blunt	Not sharp	Climax	Highest point or degree
Bondage	Slavery	Confirm	Verify
Buy	Purchase	Contagious	Communicable
Binding	Obligatory	Controversy	Dispute
Benevolence	Kindness	Convenient	Well-suited
Candid	Sincere, frank, outspoken	Copy	Imitation of original
Calamity	Misfortune, misery	Create	Produce
Callous	Unfeeling	Cruel	Inhuman
Calm	Quiet	Crude	Refined
Catch	Capture, arrest	Crazy	Unsound
Cause	Reason, purpose	Dangerous	Risky, hazardous
Character	Reputation	Dear	Expensive, costly
Canvass	Solicit	Dead	Lifeless
Capable	Competent	Daunt	Dishearten
Charity	Benevolence	Decrease	Curtail, reduce

Contd...

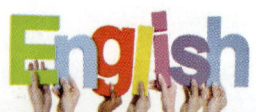

Word	Synonym	Word	Synonym
Choose	Select	Difficult	Hard, unmanageable
Caution	Vigilance	Dazzle	To overpower, glitter
Capacity	Ability, capability	Disaster	Misfortune
Charm	Attraction	Discourse	Lecture, Sermon
Clever	Ingenious	Disease	Sickness, ailment
Clothes	Attire, dress	Eradicate	Eliminate, destroy
Confess	Admit, apologise	Esteem	Love, honour
Constant	Continuous	Eternal	Ceaseless, infinite
Cross	Fretful, ill-tempered	Exaggerate	Magnify, enlarge
Disfigure	Mar, deface	Excess	Surplus, increase
Dishonest	Deceitful	Entreat	Request, beg
Disorder	Confusion, chaos	Ever	Always
Dull	Gloomy, cheerless	Explicit	Clear, expressive
Distant	Remote	Enrage	Irritate, make, angry
Devil	Wicked	External	Exterior
Discourage	Dishearten	Fact	Truth, reality
Dubious	Doubtful	Famous	Renowned, eminent
Differ	Disagree	Fashion	Custom, style
Deep	Profound	Familiar	Known
Dilemma	Perplexing, situation	Fanatic	Extremist
Dwindle	Decline	Feasible	Practicable
Definite	Exact	Fasten	Bind, join
Eager	Keen, enthusiastic	Fatal	Deadly
Earn	Gain, achieve	Fate	Destiny, end
Earthly	Terrestrial	Fault	Error, defect
Ebb	Decline, decay	Fear	Terror
Educate	Train, teach	Fearful	Timid, frightened
Early	Soon	Fight	Battle, struggle
Earnest	Eager, serious	Firm	Durable, lasting
Eject	Expel, emit	Float	Glide, slip
Elevate	Raise, improve	Fond	Affectionate, loving
Elude	Avoid, cheat	Frank	Outspoken, open
Emancipate	Free	Friend	Companion
Embrace	Hug	Frugal	Economical, sparing
Emotion	Feeling, passion	Hinder	Obstruct, impede
Enemy	Foe, opponent	Home	Dwelling

Contd...

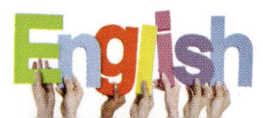

Word	Synonym	Word	Synonym
Enough	Sufficient, adequate	Hollow	Empty, vacant
Enquire	Seek, trace	Hostile	Unfriendly
Entice	Lure, persuade	Hue	Color
Entire	Whole, total	Hush	Silence
Fruitful	Productive	Humble	Modest
Foul	Indecent, bad	Humane	Kind
Foreign	Alien, remote	Humility	Meekness
Flexible	Bending easily	Hazard	Risk, danger
Game	Recreation, sport	Haughty	Proud, arrogant
Gay	Cheerful, lively	Harass	Trouble, worry
Gaze	Stare, espy,	Hard	Difficult
General	Universal, common	Harmony	Peace
Generous	Big-hearted, noble	Terrible	Dreadful
Genuine	Pure, real	Haste	Hurry
Good	True, virtuous	Hypocrisy	Pretention, deceit
Gain	Achieve	Idiot	Foolish
Giddy	Dizzy	Increase	Enlarge, expand
Grievance	Cause to feel pained	Infinite	Endless, everlasting
Guilty	Having, committed a crime	Injure	Hurt, harm
Gradual	Moving little by little	Insolvent	Bankrupt
Great	Large, wonderful	Invasion	Raid, attack
Glory	Fame, brightness	Invoke	Call, summon
Gloomy	Dismal, dusky	Irritate	Tease, provoke
Gaunt	Lean, thin	Import	To bring from foreign country
Gallant	Brave, fine	Impartial	Unprejudiced, fair
Generosity	Nobleness	Illusion	Unreality
Habitual	Customary, custom	Impair	Damage
Habit	Custom, usage	Imposter	Cheat, defrauding
Hateful	Abominable, detestable	Incessant	Uninterrupted
Help	Assist, support	Lack	Deficiency, shortage
High	Tall, lofty, elevated	Liberty	Freedom, independence
Industrious	Hard working	Lasting	Permanent, durable
Include	Comprise, contain	Loathe	Hate, detest

Contd...

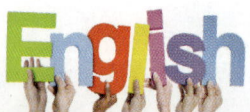

Word	Synonym	Word	Synonym
Indistinct	Unclear	Loyal	Faithful
Ingenuous	Innocent, frank	Luster	Shine, brightness
Ingredient	Component, part	Lad	Boy
Interested	Having interest	Lass	Girl
Innate	Inborn	Labour	Work, toil
Interrogate	Ask, enquire	Lenient	Liberal, mild
Insane	Unsound	Lecherous	Lustful
Jealousy	Envy	Lively	Active
Jeer	Mock, sneer	Lucrative	Profitable
Jest	Joke, taunt	Map	Plan design
Joy	Happiness	Malice	Hate, malevolence
Junk	Rubbish, garbage	Merry	Gay, joyous
Just	Right, fair	Make	Prepare, build
Jovial	Cheerful, merry	Majestic	Grand, significant
Journey	Trip, tour	Major	Important, big
Juvenile	Youthful	Mature	Developed, ready
Justice	Fairness	Mistake	Blunder, error
Jubilant	Rejoicing	Motive	Reason, purpose
Judicious	Wise	Mute	Dumb, silent
Kind	Affectionate, good	Mercy	Pity
Knave	Villain, rogue	Mock	Ridicule
Knowledge	Information, understanding	Morbid	Sickly, ailing
Keen	Sharp, strong	Melancholy	Sad, gloomy
Key	Solution, significant	Magnificent	Superb, great
Knotty	Complicated	Mysterious	Obscure
Lazy	Inactive, idle	Oral	Verbal
Lure	Entice, persuade	Oratory	Eloquence
Lapse	Mistake, slip	Outlaw	Clear
Lead	Guide, direct	Obsolete	Outworn, discarded
Meager	Lean, thin	Obstinate	Stubborn, heady
Menial	Mean	Outstanding	Remarkable, eminent
Mingle	Mix	Oppressive	Cruel, tyrannical
Merit	Worth	Obvious	Clear
Motion	Movement	Optional	Not compulsory
Muscular	Powerful	Ominous	Inauspicious

Contd...

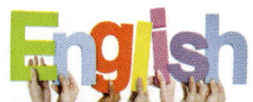

Word	Synonym	Word	Synonym
Mild	Moderate	Omnipotent	Almighty
Myth	Fiction	Optimist	One who looks to bright side of things
Narrate	Say, tell	Orthodox	Firm in religious beliefs
Necessary	Needful, essential	Outward	External
Necessity	Want, need	Odd	Not even, strange
Native	Innate, original	Own	Possess, belonging to oneself
Negligent	Careless	Option	Choice
Nefarious	Unlawful, evil	Outrage	Violence
Niggardly	Miserly	Overt	Public
Non-Plus	Puzzle, perplex	Opulent	Rich, wealthy
Nuptial	Marriage, bridal	Obedient	Meek, respectful, Supporter
Narrow	Not wide, constructed	Pitiful	Sympathetic, merciful
Neutral	Indifferent	Polite	Courteous, civil
Notorious	Infamous	Poor	Needy, destitute
Normal	Usual, regular	Port	Harbour
Nourish	Nurture, support	Proud	Haughty
Nudity	Nakedness	Punctual	Not late, exact
Nervous	Excited	Pursue	Continue
Nullify	Neutralize	Quiet	Calm, still
Obey	Yield, submit	Quote	Cite
Obscene	Indecent	Quest	Search
Oblation	Gift, offering	Queer	Strange, odd
Odious	Hateful	Quell	Suppress, crush
Old	Ancient, antique	Quit	Stop, leave
Omen	Sign	Quarrelsome	Quarrelling, irritable
Poverty	Want	Quick	Prompt
Power	Ability, capacity	Quaint	Old fashioned
Predict	Foretell	Quandary	Difficult situation
Praise	Compliment, applaud	Quite	Completely, fairly
Pretty	Beautiful, lovely	Quiver	Tremble, vibrate
Propagate	Broadcast, advertise	Rash	Careless, tactless
Pain	Suffering, distress	Ready	Prompt, alert

Contd...

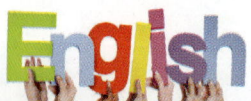

Word	Synonym	Word	Synonym
Pacify	Calm	Real	Genuine
Passion	Emotion	Recruit	Apprentice
Passionate	Intense, excited	Refugee	Outlaw, fugitive
Pale	Sallow	Regent	Viceroy, substitute
Pathetic	Miserable	Riot	Revolt
Prejudice	Bias	Rude	Impolite, abusive
Praise	Chatter, gossip	Rule	Govern, supervise
Precious	Costly, priceless	Rescue	Save
Paradox	Self-contradictory	Rare	Unique, odd
Partial	Incomplete	Reluctant	Unwilling
Part	Portion, share	Remorse	Regret, repentance
Postpone	Delay	Renounce	Give up
Ponder	Reflect	Reliable	Responsible, dependable
Plead	Argue	Rigid	Inflexible, stiff
Pensive	Sad, dejected	Reprove	Condemn, reproach
Persuade	Urge	Ruin	Wreck, destruction
Pardon	Forgive	Suitable	Appropriate, befitting
Pleasant	Delightful	Surrender	Yield, submit
Peevish	Irritable, quarrelsome	Similar	Resembling
Placid	Mild	Simple	Plain, artless
Preserve	Save, protect	Silence	Quiet
Privilege	Rights, special, benefits	Shy	Coy
Profuse	Extravagant, lavish	Shirk	Avoid
Prevent	Hinder	Selfish	One who works for self-interest
Prolong	Extend	Scorn	Hate, dislike
Restrain	Suppress, obstruct	Scold	Reprimand
Reticent	Virtuous, just	Scanty	Small, not much
Religious	Pious	Savage	Uncivilised
Remarkable	Extraordinary	Slender	Lean, thin
Regal	Royal	Sluggish	Inactive
Reduce	Weaken	Soothe	Console, comfort
Radical	Essential	Spiteful	Annoying
Radiant	Shining	Stiff	Hard

Contd...

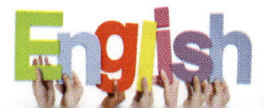

Word	Synonym	Word	Synonym
Regular	Systematic	Suppress	Overpower
Remove	Dismiss, withdraw	Suspicious	Doubtful
Repeal	Revoke	Systematic	Methodical
Resist	Oppose	Synopsis	Abstract, summary
Revenge	Avenge	Steady	Firm, constant
Rogue	Rascal, dishonest	Tame	Control
Risk	Danger	Timid	Cowardly
Rumour	Hearsay	Trust	Rely, believe
Rural	Pertaining village	Try	Attempt
Sad	Sorrowful, mournful	Tedious	Wearisome, monotonous
Sacred	Holy	Transient	Brief, short lived
Sack	Punish, plunder	Temperate	Moderate
Safe	Secure, protected	Temporal	Terrestrial, earthy
Slander	Condemn	Tie	Bind
Scorn	Despise, condemn	Virtue	Excellence
See	View, scan	Vindictive	Revengeful
Silent	Speechless	Vain	Worthless, conceited
Sin	Offence	Valiant	Brave, bold
Sly	Cunning, shrewd	Vehement	Bitter
Small	Tiny, little	Versatile	Changeable
Smell	Scent, odour	Vivid	Clear
Smooth	Level, plain	Voluntary	By free will
Souvenir	Memento, memorial	Vulnerable	Liable to injury
Speech	Eloquence, oratory	Weak	Feeble
Spread	Scatter, disperse	Wreck	Destruction
Stranger	Foreigner, alien	Wicked	Evil, bad
Strong	Powerful, muscular	Wonder	Surprise, amazement
Torture	Physical mental pain	Wretched	Mean, miserable
Torment	Mental pain	Withhold	Restrain, hold back
Tyranny	Injustice	Wholesome	Healthy, salutary
Turmoil	Disturbance	Wax	To grow in size
Triumph	Victory	Want	Deficiency
Tumult	Noise	Waive	Put off
Thrifty	Economical	Woeful	Sad, gloomy
Tragedy	Serious, accident	Wild	Uncivilized, untamed

Contd...

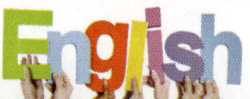

Word	Synonym	Word	Synonym
Tough	Hard, strong	Weary	Tired
Transparent	Through which can be seen	Vax	Irritate, annoy
Typical	Peculiar	Vague	Unclear, indefinite
Urban	Pertaining to city	Venture	Risk, hazard
Ugly	Horrid, hideous	Voracious	Greedy
Utter	Speak, total	Vulgar	Rough, indecent
Unique	Matchless, peerless	Woe	Misfortune, sadness
Urge	Press, exhort	Wrangle	Altercate
Uproar	Commotion, tumult	Yearn	Longer, grieve
Uniform	Regular, constant	Yield	Produce, succumb
Ulterior	Remote, not, immediate	Youth	Young
Universal	General	Yoke	Slavery
Usual	Common	Zenith	Highest
Unfair	Improper	Zone	Area, region
Value	Worth, esteem	Zeal	Enthusiasm, passion
Victory	Triumph, success		

MORE SYNONYMS

Word	Synonym	Word	Synonym
Abase	Degrade, disagree	Chaste	Pure
Abridge	Abbreviate, shorten	Cheat	Defraud
Absurd	Silly, foolish	Colossal	Huge, big
Accessory	Auxiliary, subsidiary	Commerce	Start, begin
Achieve	Gain, attain	Conceal	Cover
Adept	Expert	Conspiracy	Combination
Adequate	Enough, sufficient	Consult	Talk to
Adherent	Follower	Convict	Criminal
Admire	Esteem, praise	Cordial	Friendly
Affliction	Sorrow	Cowardly	Fearful
Amicable	Lovable, amiable	Crafty	Cunning
Anxiety	Worry	Credible	Possible
Astonish	Surprise	Criticism	Stricture, analysis
Audacious	Courageous	Cruel	Savage
Base	Low	Damage	Loss, harm

Contd...

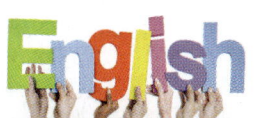

Word	Synonym	Word	Synonym
Behavior	Way	Danger	Risk
Brisk	Fast	Dearth	Lack, want
Brutal	Beastly	Decease	Demise, death
Bystander	Spectator	Deceit	Forgery
Calculate	Count	Decision	Settlement
Cancel	Abandon	Decorum	Gravity, decency
Casual	Uncertain	Defer	Postpone
Category	Group, class	Dejected	Downhearted
Censure	Reprove	Deliberate	Intentional
Demonstrate	Show	Demise	Death, decease
Deny	Refuse	Demolish	Destroy
Desire	Crave, wish	Encounter	Fight
Desolate	Deserted	Endurance	Fortitude, patience
Despondency	Disappointment	Enmity	Hate, hostility
Destruction	Demolition, ruin	Enormous	Gigantic
Devastate	Wrecking	Entertain	Cheer
Dexterity	Cleverness	Enthusiasm	Interest, zeal
Diligence	Care	Enumerate	Number
Diminish	Reduce	Epoch	Era, time
Disapprove	Reject	Erudite	Learned
Disciple	Follower	Ethics	Morality, morals
Disconsolate	Miserable	Evidence	Testimony, proof
Dismay	Discouragement	Extravagant	Stylish
Disgust	Dislike	Fabricate	Invent
Discomfort	Uneasiness	Fabulous	Fictitious, exaggerate
Discredit	Doubt, disgrace	Failure	Collapse
Dispute	Controversy	Fallacy	Mistake
Distinguish	Differentiate	Famine	Dearth
Distribute	Share	Fanatical	Over aspiring
Divine	Heavenly	Fatigue	Weariness
Domicile	Home, residence	Festivity	Merry making
Doctrine	Principle	Fickle	Varying
Dominant	Superior	Filthy	Nasty
Easy	Convenient	Folly	Foolish
Eccentric	Abnormal, odd	Fondle	Caress
Economise	Retrench, save	Forbearance	Refraining

Contd...

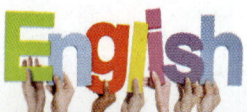

Word	Synonym	Word	Synonym
Effeminate	Weak	Forebode	Denote
Elaborate	Explain, discuss	Formidable	Difficult
Elementary	Primary, introductory	Fragrant	Soothing
Elevated	Upgraded	Fraudulent	Dishonest
Elegant	Graceful	Frivolous	Vain
Eliminate	Discard	Gallantry	Heroism, bravery, courage
Eloquence	Oratory	Genteel	Polite
Elucidate	Illuminate	Ghost	Spirit
Emancipate	Free	Glimpse	Glance
Embarrass	Confuse	Glory	Honour
Embezzle	Cheat	Gluttonous	Greedy
Emphatic	Forceful	Immature	Childish
Grandeur	Glory	Humiliate	Insult
Grateful	Thankful	Humorous	Comical
Handy	Easy	Hypocrisy	Deceit
Hardship	Difficulty	Ideal	Perfect
Heinous	Wicked	Imminent	Close
Heritage	Inheritance	Implicit	Assumed
Hilarious	Joyous	Importance	Value
Hindrance	Obstacle	Inculcate	Generate
Homage	Tribute	Incumbent	Binding
Horizon	Limit	Indicate	Show
Hospitable	Warm	Indolence	Laziness
Humane	Caring	Inevitable	Sure
Identity	Recognition	Infallible	Unfailing
Idolise	Admire		
Ignorant	Ill-informed		

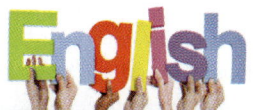

SYNONYMS (MISCELLANEOUS)

Word	Synonym	Word	Synonym
Practical	Realistic	Privilege	Benefit
Brilliant	Shining	Profession	Occupation
Popular	Famous	Prosaic	Dull
Delightful	Happy	Fascinating	Charming
Perfect	Complete	Realize	Understand
Rare	Few	Profile	Side view
Rough	Coarse	Accomplishment	Skill
Charm	Beauty	Bequeath	Give
Patched	Repaired	Ineffectual	Ineffective
Amazing	Wonderful	Consolation	Comfort
Miserable	Wretched	Prudence	Wisdom
Fortune	Luck	Patent	Evident
Attains	Gets	Trance	Dream
Chatter	Speak	Discreet	Tactful
Faint	Fade	Inconsequential	Unimportant
Stroll	Walk	Wit	Wisdom
Probably	Possibly	Dark	Mysterious
Splendid	Marvelous	Ecstatic	Joyful
Magnificent	Exalting	Hysterical	Excited
Growled	Howled	Ardent	Eager
Apology	Pardon	Dandy	Beautiful
Shabby	Dirty	Particular	Special
Blurred	Unclear, hazy	Accidentally	Suddenly
Rapid	Fast	Tempt	Induce, influence
Garment	Cloth, apparel	Glint	Shine
Sparkle	Shine	Explore	Search
Panting	Tired	Jostle	Push
Chilly	Cold	Throng	Push
Anxious	Eager	Inspect	Watch
Generosity	Kindness	Humble	Meek
Terrified	Afraid	Grab	Hold
Nimble	Quick	Wretched	Miserable
Scream	Yell	Composed	Calm
Shell	Covering	Discovered	Found

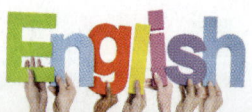

Contd...

Word	Synonym	Word	Synonym
Yearn	Want	Excited	Agitated
Tresses	Hair (tufts)	Blockhead	Stupid
Dusk	Evening	Except	Besides
Precious	Costly	Assistance	Help
Grave	Serious	Embrace	Hug
Frolicsome	Playful	Ails	Troubles
Gravity	Seriousness	Blisters	Swellings
Perplexing	Confusing	Penance	Regret, sorrow
Dispute	Quarrel	Drawn	Pulled
Superintend	Watch	Echoing	Sounding
Ambush	Attack	Tale	Story
Vanish	Disappear	Pray	Request
Ridiculously	Foolishly	Robes	Clothes
Trapper	Hunter	Bow	Stoop
Warily	Cautiously	Radiant	Shining
Collosal	Huge	Holy	Pure, pious
Solicitude	Concern	Reckless	Rash
Crook	Swindler	Intoxicated	Drunk, tipsy
Collect	Gather	Boundless	Free, limitless
Trifle	Unimportant	Spell	Charm
Legacy	Money, bequest	Defile	Pollute
Pelt	Skin, throw	Quench	Put out, satisfy
Knot	Group	Sought	Wanted
Crush	Press, squeeze	Vow	Resolve
Prediction	Prophecy	Exile	Banish
Ague	Unclear	Solemn	Holy
Reveal	Show	Contemplate	Think
Delude	Deceive	Wicked	Bad
Clasp	Hold	Deliverance	Freedom
Doom	End	Infirmity	Weakness
Conform	Comply	Substantial	Enough
Churn	Stir	Accost	Address
Illusion	Fantasy	Mortify	Hurt
Solemnly	Thoughtfully	Exclusive	Reserved
Homage	Respect	Privilege	Advantage
Trample	Crush	Patent	Right

Contd...

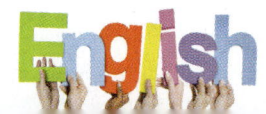

Word	Synonym	Word	Synonym
Momentary	Short	Craft	Cunning
Immense	Great	Single	Unmarried
Quiver	Tremble	Sneer	Contempt
Torment	Torture	Pretend	Show
Writhed	Twisted	Swarm	Crowd
Ferry	Boat	Vicious	Corrupt
Turbulent	Uncontrolled	Pretext	Excuse
Cling	Slick	Advert	Advertisement
Mingle	Mix	Assume	Imagine
Daring	Courageous	Appointed	Fixed
Might	Power	Quiver	Shake
Absolute	Complete	Morose	Unsocial
Scatter	Spread	Brat	Child
Endure	Bear	Snap	Break
Agony	Pain	Makeshift	Temporary
Furious	Angry	Hue	Color
Cords	Threads	Fancy	Imagination
Kindle	Light	Amiable	Pleasant
Weary	Tired	Dainty	Delicate
Glimmer	Shine	Vital	Essential
Bores	Wound	Supplied	Given
Serpent	Snake	Fashion	Vogue
Duel	Fight	Frank	Candid
Casket	Box	Discreet	Tactful
Turmoil	Agitation	Prudently	Tactfully
Attain	Get	Recall	Remember
Slack	Loose	Secretive	Mysterious
Plunge	Jump	Revel	Enjoy
Whisper	Soft talking	Sacred	Holy
Elaborate	Explain	Solemnity	Seriousness
Rhetorical	Impressive	Reverential	Respectful
Delicate	Soft	Thrilled	Excited
Evoke	Summon	Grave	Serious
Solemn	Serious	Sublime	Holy
Exquisite	Excellent	Uplifted	Raised
Amusing	Pleasing	Absurd	Strange
Alien	Stranger		

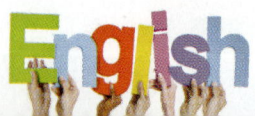

Chapter 16

Building Vocabulary—
One-Word Substitution

WORDS DENOTING NUMBERS

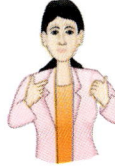

There are words which denote numbers..

A number of sheeps	Flock
A small number of birds, e.g., partridge	Covey
A number of cattle or swine feeding or driven together	Herd
A number of bees, locusts, ants, etc.	Swarm
A colony of seals	Rookery
A number of young pigs, dogs, acts brought forth at one birth	Litter
A number of kittens	Kindle
A collection of fowls, ducks, etc.	Poultry
A number of people listening to a concert or lecture	Audience
A number of people looking on at a football match, etc.	Spectators
A number of people collected together in the street	Crowd
A number of actors	Company
A number of persons, of the same race, character, etc.	Tribe
A number of sailors manning a ship	Crew
A number (more than two) of judges or bishop	Bench
A collection of poems	Anthology
A collection of books	Library
A large collection of trees	Forest
A number of stars grouped together	Constellation
A set of furniture rooms, etc.	Suite
A place where, medicines are compounded	Dispensary
A place for the treatment of sick people	Hospital
A residence for monks or priests	Monastery

Contd...

A residence for nun	Convent
A place where milk is converted into butter and cheese	Dairy
A number of Jurymen engaged on a case	Jury
A collection of slaves	Gang
A number of artists	Troupe
A number of judges	Bench
A number of disorderly people	Mob
A number of beautiful ladies	Bevy
A number of thieves	Gang
A number of directors of a company	Board
A number of people collected for some common purpose	Assembly

MEDICAL TERMS

A vehicle for conveying sick or injured people to the hospital	Ambulance
To cut off a part of a person's body which is infected	Amputate
Low levels of iron in the blood	Anemia
Any medicine which produces insensibility	Anesthetic
A medicine to counteract poison	Antidote
A substance which destroys or weakens germs	Antiseptic
A substance used in surgery to induce unconsciousness	Chloroform
To be able to tell the nature of a disease by its symptoms	Diagnose
A disease confined to a particular district or place	Endemic
A disease affecting many persons at the same place and time	Epidemic
To disinfect by smoke	Fumigate
Free or exempt from infection	Immune
A medicine for relieving, numbing pain	Narcotic
A cure for all diseases	Panacea
The science of diseases of the human body	Pathology
A forecast of the result of a disease or illness	Prognosis
Affecting the lungs	Pulmonary
A disease widely epidemic	Pandemic
A substance used to deaden the gum and nerve	Cocaine
A medicine which gives relief from pain	Anodyne
An instrument used by doctors to listen to someone's heart or breathing	Stethoscope
The mark left after a wound is healed	Scar
A medicine for producing sleep	Narcotic

Contd...

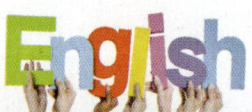

A medicine to cause vomiting	Emetic
One who is recovering from illness	Convalescent
The mosquito which spreads malaria	Anopheles
A substance to keep down evil smells	Deodorant
A device which prevents pregnancy	Contraceptive
A medicine which loosens the bowels	Laxative
Cure of the hands and finger nails	Manicure
A hospital for TB patients	Sanatorium
Suffering for physical or mental weakness because of old age	Senile
A medicine which calms the nerves	Sedative

LITERARY TERMS

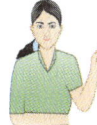

A poem in which the first letters of each line, taken in order, form a name or a sentence	Acrostic
A list of headings of the business to be transacted at a meeting	Agenda
A book with blank pages for putting autographs, pictures, stamps, etc.	Album
A succession of the same initial letters in a passage	Alliteration
A record of one's life written by himself/herself	Autobiography
A handwritten signature	Autograph
A statement which is accepted as true without proof	Axiom
A list of books in a library catalogue, sources used in the preparation of a book	Bibliography
The record of the life of a person written by someone else	Biography
The heading or short description of a newspaper article, chapter of a book, etc.	Caption
A humorous play, having a happy ending	Comedy
The exclusive right of an author or his heirs to publish or sell copies of his writing	Copyright
A principle or standard by which anything is, or can be judged	Criterion
A conversation between two persons	Dialogue
A book in which the events of each day are recorded	Diary
A book containing the words of a language with their definitions, in alphabetical order	Dictionary
A book of names and addresses	Directory
A mournful song (or poem) for the dead	Dirge
A poem of lamentation, especially for the dead	Elegy
A writing or speech in praise of a person, eulogy	Encomium
A book containing information on all branches of knowledge	Encyclopedia
To pronounce words distinctly	Enunciate
A short speech by a player at the end of a play	Epilogue

Contd...

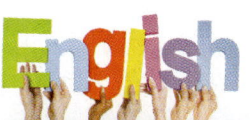

A brief summary of a book, an abstract	Epitome
An error or misprint in printing or writing	Erratum
An extract or selection from a book of writing	Excerpt
To remove the offensive portions of the book	Expurgate
Still in use (of books published long ago)	Extant
Delivered (of a speech) without previous preparation	Extempore
An exact copy of handwriting, printing or of a picture	Facsimile
A picture facing the title of the book	Frontispiece
To make expressive gestures or motions while speaking	Gesticulate
A list of explanations of rare, technical or obsolete words	Glossary
Language that is made commonplace by being used frequently	Hackneyed
A noisy or vehement speech intended to excite passions	Harangue
A list of articles and their descriptions	Inventory
Language which is confused and unintelligible	Jargon
A book of account showing debits and credits	Ledger
Study by night	Lucubration
A declaration of plans and promises put forward for election, a political party or a sovereign	Manifesto
A written account, usually in book form, of the interesting and memorable experiences of one's life	Memoirs
A note to serve as a remainder	Memorandum
The concluding part of a speech	Peroration
Passing off another author's work as one's own	Plagiarism
One who writes play, dramatist	Playwright
Speaking to oneself	Soliloquy
A play with sad or tragic end	Tragedy
The trade mark of the maker seen on paper when it is held up to the light	Watermark
One who pretends to have a great deal of knowledge	Wiseacre
A list of books in a library	Catalogue
A book in which daily events are recorded	Directory
A book in which account are kept	Diary
A play with a happy ending	Comedy
A short speech by a player at the beginning of the play	Prologue
A short speech by a player at the end of the play	Epilogue
A long speech by one character in a play	Monologue
A conversation between two persons	Dialogue
A person's own handwriting	Autography
One who writes plays	Dramatist

Contd...

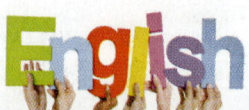

A brief summary of a book	Epitome
A list of explanations of rare or technical words	Glossary
The legal right to be the only producer or seller of a book, play, film, etc.	Copyright
A written declaration made on oath in the presence of a magistrate	Affidavit
A word opposite in meaning to another	Antonym
Words which have similar meanings	Synonyms
Being the only one of its kind	Unique
Concerned with the voice	Vocal

NEGATIVES

That which cannot be taken by assault	Impregnable
That which cannot be injured	Invulnerable
That which cannot be tolerated	Intolerable
That which cannot be resisted	Irresistible
That which cannot be put into practice	Impracticable
That which cannot be digested	Indigestible
That which cannot be destroyed	Indestructible
That which cannot be expressed in words	Inexpressible
That which cannot be touched	Intangible
That which cannot be satisfied	Insatiable
That which cannot be easily understood	Unintelligible
That which will exist for ever	Imperishable
Not endowed with animal life	Inanimate
Without which we cannot do	Indispensable
One who does not favor anyone	Impartial
That which cannot be approached	Inaccessible
That which cannot be calculated	Incalculable
One who cannot pay debts	Insolvent
A step from which there is no going back	Irrevocable
One who does not mix in society	Unsociable
Unable to die	Immortal
That which cannot be moved	Immovable
That which cannot be passed	Impassable
That which cannot be pierced or penetrated	Impenetrable
Enduring for all times	Imperishable
Not admitting the passage or entrance of water, etc.	Impervious

Contd...

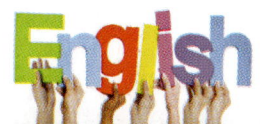

That which cannot be taken by assault	Impregnable
That which cannot be heard	Inaudible
Incapable of being burnt	Incombustible
Incapable from being redeemed from evil, or beyond correction	Incorrigible
That which cannot be erased	Indelible
Incapable of being destroyed	Indestructible
That which cannot be avoided or prevented	Inevitable
That which cannot be made plain or understood	Inexplicable
Incapable of making errors	Infallible
That which cannot be imitated	Inimitable
That which cannot be conquered	Invincible
That which cannot be seen	Invisible
That which cannot be lessened	Irreducible
Not relating to the matter at hand	Irrelevant
That which cannot be repaired or remedied	Irreparable
That which cannot be replaced in case of loss	Irreplaceable

OPPOSITES

Writing that is easy to read	Legible
Writing that is difficult to read	Illegible
One who is unable to read and write	Illiterate
Fit to be eaten	Edible
Not fit to be eaten	Inedible
Fit to be chosen	Eligible
Not fit to be chosen	Ineligible
Loud enough to be heard	Audible
That which cannot be heard	Inaudible
That which can be seen	Visible
That which cannot be seen	Invisible
One who believes in the existence of God	Theist
One who does not believe in the existence of God	Atheist
Born of married parents	Legitimate
Born of unmarried parents	Illegitimate
To move from one country to another	Migrate
One who leaves his country to settle in another	Emigrant
One who comes into a foreign country to settle there	Immigrant

Contd...

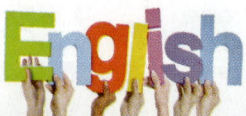

To send back a person to his own country	Repatriate
To banish from one's country	Expatriate
Love of one's country	Patriotism
Goods brought into a country	Import
Goods carried out of a country	Exports
A list of duties payable on exports or imports	Tariff
A list of goods dispatched to the purchaser	Invoice
One to whom goods are dispatched	Consignee

MILITARY WORDS

The killed or wounded in battle	Casualties
A van for carrying patients	Ambulance
The equipment of a soldier	Kit
Something like an umbrella used for jumping from an aircraft	Parachute
Sharp or pointed pieces of a bomb	Splinters
A place where soldiers can have refreshments	Canteen
A soldier recently enlisted for service	Recruit
A foreigner in a belligerent country	Alien
A group of ships travelling together for the sake of safety	Convoy
A promise given by a prisoner to behave well if given temporary release	Parole
To empty a place in order to avoid the destruction of war	Evacuate
To seize for military use	Commandeer
To surround a place in order to capture it	Besiege
To attack the enemy in small groups unexpectedly	Guerrilla warfare
A soldier's holiday	Furlough

SCIENTIFIC INSTRUMENTS

Instrument used for measuring heat or cold	Thermometer
An instrument for taking photographs	Camera
An instrument for measuring gases	Manometer
An instrument for measuring minute distances	Micrometer
An instrument for distinguishing precious stones	Lithoscope
An instrument for seeing distant objects	Telescope
An instrument for measuring electric current	Ammeter
An instrument for detecting earthquakes	Seismograph

Contd...

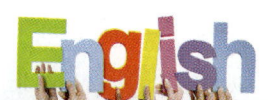

An instrument which when put to both eyes make distant objects look near	Binoculars
An instrument for increasing the volume of the voice	Microphone
An instrument for transmitting the voice to a distance	Telephone
An instrument for measuring the pressure of the air	Barometer
An instrument which makes very small objects appear large	Microscope
An instrument used for arithmetical calculations	Calculator
An instrument for measuring the speed of a motor car	Speedometer

DEATH

The act of killing a human being	Homicide
Death due to being deprived of air	Asphyxia
The dead body of a human being	Corpse
The dead body of an animal	Carcass
A place where dead bodies are temporarily placed	Mortuary
A place where dead bodies are placed for identification	Morgue
A place where dead bodies are cremated	Cemetery
An inscription on a tomb	Epitaph
Which results or ends in death	Fatal

PERTAINING TO MARRIAGE

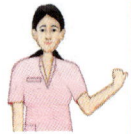

To run away with a lover in order to get married secretly	Elope
A man engaged to be married	Fiancé
A woman engaged to be married	Fiancée
Engaged to be married	Betrothed
A bride's outfit	Trousseau
Practice of marrying one at a time	Monogamy
Legal dissolution of marriage	Divorce
A hater of marriage	Misogamy
One vowed to a single or unmarried life	Celibate
A woman whose husband is dead	Widow
A man whose wife is dead	Widower
Allowance due to a wife from her husband on separation	Alimony
Having two husbands or wives at a time	Bigamist
Man who has more than one wife at a time	Polygynist
Woman who has more than one husband at a time	Polyandrist

Contd...

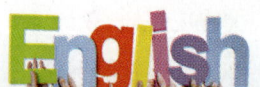

The property which a new wife brings to her husband	Dowry
An unmarried man	Bachelor
An old unmarried woman	Spinster
The state of being married	Matrimony
The state of being unmarried	Celibacy

PERTAINING TO RELIGION

One who has too much religious enthusiasm	Fanatic
One who believes in a single God	Monotheist
One who believes in many Gods	Polytheist
Holding opinions contrary to the true doctrine of religion	Heresy
Showing disrespect to something holy and sacred	Sacrilege
A sacred book of religion	Scripture
Having nothing to do with any religion	Secular
To utter impious language against God and sacred things	Blaspheme
One who is converted from one religion to another	Proselyte
One who believes that nothing can be known about God	Agnostic
One who renounces his religious principles	Apostate
One who breaks religious images and ornaments	Iconoclast
The stand from which a preacher delivers his sermon	Pulpit
The vessel containing for baptism	Font
One who believes in the existence of God	Theist
One who does not believe in the existence of God	Atheist
One who leads a life of self-discipline for religious reasons	Ascetic
To atone one's sins	Expiate
One inspired by God to warn and teach mankind	Prophet
The soul leaving one body and entering another	Transmigration

PERTAINING TO GOVERNMENT

Government of the people, for the people and by the people	Democracy
Government by one man having unlimited powers	Autocracy
Government by the wealthy	Plutocracy
Government by a few	Oligarchy
Government by a military class	Stratocracy
Government by departments of state	Bureaucracy

Contd...

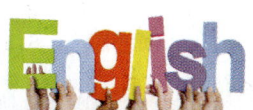

Government by the nobility	Aristocracy
An official numbering of the population	Census
The right of self-government	Autonomy
The science of the government	Politics
The wife or husband of a king or queen	Consort
Facts and figures	Statistics

WORDS DENOTING PLACES

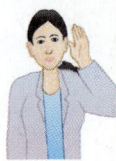

A place where money is coined	Mint
A place where fruit trees are grown	Orchard
A place where orphans are housed	Orphanage
A place where leather is tanned	Tannery
A place for housing cars	Garage
A place for storing grain	Granary
A place where treasures of art are exhibited	Museum
A place for housing aeroplanes	Hangar
A place where milk is converted into butter and cheese	Dairy
A place where clothes are washed and ironed	Laundry
A place where athletic exercises are performed	Gymnasium
A place where scientific experiments are conducted	Laboratory
A place where any manufacture is carried on	Factory
A place where government records are kept	Archives
A place where people may obtain food and refreshment	Restaurant
A place where travellers may obtain lodging and refreshment	Hotel
A place where spirituous liquors are produced	Distillery
A place where animals are slaughtered for the market	Abattoir
A place where bread and cakes are made	Bakery
A place where medicines are compounded	Dispensary
A place where pigs are kept	Sty
A place where rabbits are kept	Hutch
A place where fishes are kept	Aquarium
A place where bees are kept	Apiary
A place where birds are kept	Aviary
A place where women sell their bodies	Brothel
A place where two rivers meet	Confluence
A place of permanent residence	Domicile

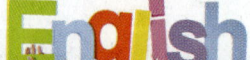

Contd...

A place for criminals in a court	Dock
A place from where we get stone or slate	Quarry
A place where soldiers are quartered	Cantonment
A place for the treatment of sick people	Hospital
A place where water is collected and stored	Reservoir
A place with gambling tables	Casino
A place where ships are built	Dock
A place where ships are loaded and unloaded	Quay
A house or shelter of the eskimo	Igloo
A house or shelter of a gipsy	Caravan
A house or shelter for a dog	Kennel
A house or shelter for a horse	Stable
A house or shelter for a cow	Pen
A house for the residence of students	Hostel
A residence for monks or priests	Monastery
A residence for nuns	Convent
The dwelling place of an animal underground	Burrow
The home of a lion	Den
The home of a squirrel	Dray
A factory for manufacturing beer	Brewery
A building for soldiers to live in	Barracks
A Muslim place of worship	Mosque
The sleeping-rooms in a college or public institution	Dormitory
A receptacle for storing coal	Bunker
A small box in which tea is kept	Caddy
An underground place for storing thing	Cellar
A lady's handbag or workbag	Reticule
A case in which the blade of a sword is kept	Sheath
A variety show performed in the restaurant	Cabaret
A place where books are kept	Library
A place for storing grain	Granary
A place where goods are stored	Depot
A place where fruit trees are grown	Orchard
A place where water is collected and stored	Reservoir
A place frequented for the reason of pleasure or health	Resort
A nursery where children of poor people are cared for while their parents are at work	Creche
A school for infants and young children	Kindergarten

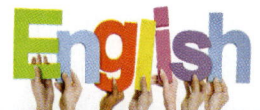

WORDS DENOTING PROFESSIONS

One who deals in writing materials	Stationer
One who writes the shorthand	Stenographer
One who studies the evolution of mankind	Anthropologist
One who gives treatment of diseases of animals	Veterinarian
One who sells sweets and pastries	Confectioner
One who pays out money at a bank	Cashier
One who travels from place to place to sell miscellaneous articles	Hawker
One who makes pots, cups, etc.	Potter
One who mends shoes	Cobbler
One who flies an aeroplane	Pilot
One who studies the stars	Astronomer
One who studies rocks and soils	Geologist
One who studies the past through remains	Archaeologist
One who deals in fruits	Fruiter
The head of a college	Principal
The head of a town council	Mayor
The treasurer of a college or university	Bursar
A person who wants to turn other metals into gold	Alchemist
A woman who sells her body	Prostitute
A person who suddenly rises from a low position to a high position	Upstart
One who attends to the disease of eye	Oculist
One who tests eyesight and sells spectacles	Optician
One who attends to sick people and prescribes medicines	Physician
One who compounds and sells drugs	Druggist/ Pharmacist
One who treats diseases by performing operations	Surgeon
One who attends to the teeth	Dentist
One skilled in the care of hands and feet	Chiropodist
One who drives a motor car	Chauffeur
One who manages or attends to an engine	Engineer
The person in charge of a ship	Captain
One who carves in stone	Sculptor
One who plans and draws the design of the building and superintends their erection	Architect
One who deals in flower	Florist
One who deals in medicinal herbs	Herbalist

Contd...

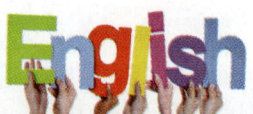

One who deals in fish	Fishmonger
One who deals in lead especially mending water pipes	Plumber
One who deals in clothes and other fabrics	Draper
A professional rider in horse races	Jockey
A woman employed to clean inside buildings	Charwoman
One who sells sweets and pastries	Confectioner
A teacher who travels place to place to give instruction	Peripatetic
One who watches over students taking an examination	Invigilator
The person in charge of a library	Librarian
The head of a college	Principal
The head of a town council or corporation	Mayor
One who writes poetry	Poet
One who writes novel	Novelist
One who writes books	Author
One who sells paper, ink, pens and writing materials	Stationer
One who studies the working of a human mind	Psychologist

PERSONS WITH CERTAIN CHARACTERISTICS

One who dies for a noble cause	Martyr
One who walks in his sleep	Somnambulist
One who talks in his sleep	Somniloquist
One who loves and helps mankind	Philanthropist
One who runs away from justice or law	Fugitive
One who takes refuge in a foreign country	Refugee
A hater of mankind	Misanthrope
One who loves all countries of the world	Cosmopolitan
One who believes things very easily	Credulous
One who pays too much attention to dress	Dundy
One who has strange habits	Eccentric
One who behaves like a woman	Effeminate
One who takes interest in things around him	Extrovert
One who believes in fate	Fatalist
One who talks too much	Garrulous
One who believes in nakedness	Nudist
One who eats everything	Omnivorous
One who is expert in making speeches	Orator
One who tells the future by reading the palm of a person	Palmist

Contd...

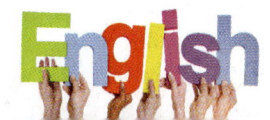

One who is extremely poor and helpless	Pauper
One who signs a document or agreement	Signatory
One who makes a show of superiority	Snob
One who speaks for others	Spokesman
One who accepts pain and pleasure equally	Stoic
One who pays rent for the land, building or house occupied by him	Tenant
One who betrays one's country	Traitor
One having long experience in a field	Veteran
A partner in crime	Accomplice
A hater of marriage	Misogynist
A lover of animals	Zoophiles
A person having extraordinary mental powers	Genius
A person who eats too much	Glutton
A person who has lakhs of rupees	Millionaire
A person with the same name as another	Namesake
A person or thing that causes trouble	Nuisance
A person with magical power	Wizard
A woman with light colored hair	Blonde
A woman with dark hair	Brunette
One who looks in the bright side of things	Optimist
One who looks on the dark side of things	Pessimist
One who delights to speak about himself or thinks only of his own welfare	Egoist
One who devotes his life to the welfare and interests of other people	Altruist
One who runs away from justice or the law	Fugitive
One who offers his service of his own free will	Volunteer
A soldier or a sailor newly enlisted	Recruit
One who eats no animal flesh	Vegetarian
One who feeds on human flesh	Cannibal
One who journeys on foot	Pedestrian
One who journeys to a holy place	Pilgrim
One who goes from place to place begging alms	Beggar
One who loves his country and serves it devotedly	Patriot
One who foretells events	Prophet
One devoted to the pleasures of eating and drinking	Epicure
One who pretends to be what he is not	Hypocrite/Impostor
A messenger sent in great haste	Courier
One who abstains from alcoholic drinks	Teetotaller

Contd...

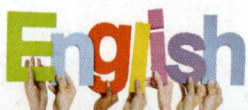

A person who dresses up woman's hair	Hairdresser/Coiffeur
One who shoots with bows and arrows	Archer
One who fishes with a rod	Angler

SCIENCE AND ARTS

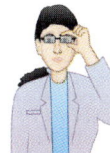

The study of stars	Astronomy
The study of languages	Philology
The study of plants	Botany
The study of human face	Physiognomy
The study of living matter	Biology
The study of birds	Ornithology
The study of rocks and soils	Geology
The study of mountains	Orology
The study of the origin and history of words	Etymology
The study of mankind	Anthropologist
The study of coins	Numismatics
The study of ancient writings	Paleography
The study of heavenly bodies	Astronomy
The study of ancient buildings and ruins	Archaeology
The science of numbers	Mathematics
The science of family descent	Genealogy
The science of triangles	Trigonometry
The science of colors	Chromatics
The science which deals with the varieties of the human race	Ethnology
The science of the structure of the human body	Anatomy
The science which deals with the working of human body	Physiology
The scientific study of industrial arts	Technology
The art of tilling the soil	Agriculture
The art of cultivating and managing gardens	Horticulture
The art of effective speaking	Elocution
The art of telling the future by the study of the stars	Astrology
The art of beautiful handwriting	Calligraphy
The art of making maps and charts	Cartography
The art of metal working	Metallurgy
An institution for education in the arts and sciences	Polytechnic

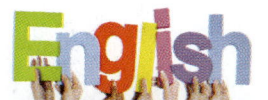

WORDS RELATED TO NATURE STUDY

One who studies plant and animal life	Naturalist
An animal or plant growing on another	Parasite
Animals with backbone	Vertebrates
The animals of a certain region	Fauna
The plants and vegetation of a certain region	Flora
The flesh of sheep	Mutton
The green coloring matter in the leaves of plants	Chlorophyll
A gnawing animal	Rodent
A cud-chewing animal	Ruminant
A preparation for killing insects	Insecticide
Lasting for a single year	Annual
Lasting for two years	Biennial
Lasting for many years	Perennial
The process by which the young plants begin to grow	Germination
The process by which plants manufacture food	Assimilation
The process by which plants take up mineral salts through roots	Absorption
The process by which plants and animals breathe	Respiration
The dead skin cast off by a snake	Slough

MISCELLANEOUS

Loss of memory	Amnesia
A traveller through outer space	Astronaut
Money that remains unpaid	Arrears
Without the name of the writer	Anonymous
A name of celebration coming after a year	Anniversary
That which has got life	Animate
Period of life between childhood and maturity	Adolescence
Fluent in two languages	Bilingual
A song or poem that tells an old story	Ballad
Having no hair on the head	Bald
Which can be easily broken	Brittle
A bird or animal with two legs	Biped
The framework of a car	Chassis
A picture drawn to make people laugh	Caricature
Person held guilty and punished by court	Convict
Two or more things happening together by chance	Coincidence
Bad spelling	Cacography
A person who regards the whole world as his country	Cosmopolitan

Contd...

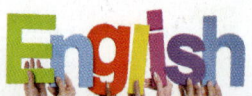

Irresistible craving for alcoholic drinks	Dipsomania
To go from bad to worse	Deteriorate
A song sung by two persons	Duet
A period of ten years	Decade
To lower the worth or value of a thing	Depreciate
Wasteful in spending	Extravagant
To hear something without the knowledge of the speaker	Overhear
Through which light cannot pass	Opaque
Having all power	Omnipotent
Present everywhere	Omnipresent
Believing in old accepted ideas	Orthodox
No longer in use or fashion	Obsolete
Belonging to the earliest times	Primitive
Property inherited from forefathers	Patrimony
Sudden fear which spreads like wild fire	Panic
A line of people waiting for something	Queue
A general knowledge test	Quiz
Once after every three months	Quarterly
A formula to prepare some dish or medicine	Recipe
A report which is not based on truth	Rumour
Recalling of past experiences	Reminiscence
A string of beads for prayer	Rosary
A place appointed for meeting	Rendezvous
The bony framework of the body	Skeleton
Comparison of one thing to another	Simile
Pertaining to sun	Solar
A child who runs away from school	Truant
To pass through another's land without permission	Trespass
Not yet finally decided	Tentative
Communication between minds	Telepathy
A foolish belief that one is God	Theomania
Never done or done before	Unprecedented
With one voice	Unanimous
Able to adapt oneself readily to many situations	Versatile
A sea journey by ship	Voyage
In the nature of farewell	Valedictory
Evening prayers in a church	Vespers
A path which turns right and left	Zig-zag
Love of one's country	Patriotism
Goods brought into a country	Import
Goods carried out of a country	Export
A list of duties payable on export	Tariff
A list of goods dispatch to the purchaser	Invoice
One to whom goods are dispatched	Consigner

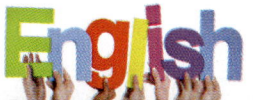

NOTES

Chapter 17

Building Vocabulary—
Idioms and Phrases

Illustrate the meaning of the following English Idioms and Phrases by using them in sentences of your own.

A

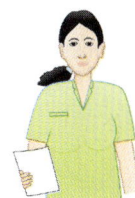

- **The ABC (the most elementary knowledge of a subject):** He does not know even the ABC of India's foreign policy.
- **All and sundry (everyone without exception):** His mother invited all and sundry to the marriage party.
- **Apple pie order (in perfect order):** Everything in his room was lying in an apple pie order
- **Above all (above everything):** The boy is sincere, honest and above all obedient.
- **Apple of one's eye (very dear):** Being the only son, he is an apple of his mother's eye.
- **Apple of discord (cause of quarrel):** A piece of land is an apple of discord between two brothers.
- **Above board (honest and frank):** Everybody raises him because he is above board in his dealings.
- **At an arm's length (to avoid):** He is a bad person; therefore, I keep him at an arm's length.
- **Abide by (act upon, to fulfil):** We must abide by the rules of the game.
- **At daggers drawn with (to be on bad terms, to have enmity):** Both the brothers are at daggers drawn with each other.
- **At a stretch (continuously):** Our mother is so hard working that she can work for ten hours at a stretch.
- **At a stone's throw (very near):** My college from my house is at a stone's throw.
- **Add fuel to the fire (to increase the existing excitement):** The teacher was already very angry but his words added fuel to the fire.
- **At sixes and sevens (in disorder):** His clothes were lying at sixes and sevens in his house.
- **At one's beck and call (to be at one's service):** All the members of the staff are at the beck and call of the Principal.
- **All in all (all powerful):** Our principal is all in all in our college.
- **At a pinch (in a difficulty):** I am thankful to you for your help which you gave me at a pinch.

- **At the eleventh hour (at a late stage):** He dropped the idea of going to Chandigarh at the eleventh hour.
- **Add insult to injury (to give more offence to the already punished):** He added insult to injury by first abusing me and then beating me.
- **At sea (confused):** He found himself at sea when he saw the question paper.
- **At a low ebb (on the decline):** The credibility of political leaders is at a low ebb at this time
- **At the risk of (putting oneself in danger):** The man saved the drowning person at the risk of his own life.
- **At a snail's pace (very slowly):** If you work at a snail's pace, you will not be able to finish your work in time.
- **An eye wash (a pretence or to deceive):** The interview was simply an eye wash because the candidates for the job had already been selected.
- **To feel at home (to feel comfortable):** Try to feel at home at this new place.
- **At large (to be free and not under any control):** The thief is still at large.
- **Aim at (target):** The hunter aimed at the bird.
- **Apple pie order (extreme neatness):** Everything in her house was in apple pie order.
- **Act by (adhere):** I cannot act by these rules.
- **Act on or upon (follow):** Act on (or upon) his advice.
- **Act on (affect):** Wine acts on the brain.
- **Against the grain (against one's bent of mind):** He will not cheat you; cheating is against his grain.
- **An apple of discord (cause of dispute):** Even a small toy becomes an apple of discord between two children.
- **An axe to grind (to serve one's own purpose):** I do not think that he is cooperating with you without having an axe to grind.

B

- **To burn the candle at both ends (to end one resources lavishly):** After his father's death, he started burning his candle at both ends and soon became penniless.
- **A big gun (a person of great importance):** All the big guns of the world were there.
- **To burn the mid-night oil (to work very hard till late at night):** If you want to stand first you will have to burn the mid-night oil.
- **Birds of a feather (persons of the same nature or habits):** Birds of a feather flock together.
- **To be born with a silver spoon in one's mouth (to be born in a rich family):** He was born with a silver spoon in his mouth.
- **To be in the good books of (to be in favor with):** A hard working student is always in the good books of his teacher.
- **To be in the bad books of (to be in disfavor with):** Those students who are not disciplined are in the bad books of their teachers.
- **A broken reed (one who cannot be depended upon):** You should not depend upon your friend because he is a broken reed.
- **A blessing in disguise (a curse that proves to be a blessing in the end):** Poverty proved to be a blessing in disguise in the case of Mahesh.

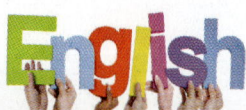

- **To breathe one's last (to die):** His grandfather breathed his last at the age of seventy.
- **To bid a farewell (to give a send-off):** They bade farewell to the officer when he got transferred.
- **Bear in mind (to remember):** You should bear in mind the advice of your teacher.
- **Broad day light (in open day light):** The Advocate was shot dead in the broad day light.
- **Better half (wife):** He went with his better half to see a play.
- **Back up (support):** I shall back up your candidate.
- **Back out (go back on):** He backed out of his promise.
- **Beat off (to repel an attack):** We beat off dogs and ran away.
- **Beat back (to compel to retire):** The enemy was beaten back by our forces.
- **Break loose (to get free):** The dog broke loose from its chain.
- **Break out (spread):** Malaria has broken out in the town.
- **Break down (to open by force):** When they lost the key, they broke open the door.
- **Break off (to stop suddenly):** She broke off in the middle of her speech.
- **Break down (develop a defect):** Our car broke down on the way.
- **Bring forward (to produce):** He brought forward a very good proposal.
- **Bring out (to publish):** He has brought out a new book.
- **Bear away (to win):** He bore away many prizes on the Sports Day.
- **Bear out (to confirm):** He will bear out what I have said.
- **Bear with (to tolerate):** I cannot bear with this insult.
- **Break down (to collapse):** His Health broke down due to overwork.
- **Break into (to enter forcibly):** A thief broke into my house at night.
- **Break open (to open by force):** A thief broke open the box.
- **Bring about (cause):** Gambling brought about his ruin.
- **Bring forth (to bear):** This plant brings forth very beautiful flowers.
- **Bring up (to rear):** Parents bring up their children with love and affection.
- **A bed of roses (comfortable position):** The life of a soldier is not a bed of roses.
- **A bed of thorns (full of sorrows and sufferings):** The job of a principal is often a bed of thorns.
- **A bird's eye view (a general view):** We had a bird's eye view of the town from the high tower.
- **A black sheep (a disgraceful person):** He is a black sheep and cannot be depended upon.
- **Build castles in the air (to make imaginary schemes):** He is always building castles in the air, and can never succeed in his life.
- **By hook or by crook (by fair or foul means):** I must get it done by hook or by crook.
- **Bear a grudge against (to feel hatred for):** He bears a grudge against his former boss.
- **Break out (to spread):** Cholera has broken out in the town.
- **Break off (to stop suddenly):** He broke off while lecturing.
- **Break up (disperse, close):** The meeting broke up.
- **Break forth (to burst out):** He broke forth into shouts.
- **Bring to mind (to recall):** He could not bring to mind where he had seen this man.
- **Bring under (to capture):** The rebels were easily brought under by the army.
- **Beat about the bush (to distress):** Do not beat about the bush, but come to the point.

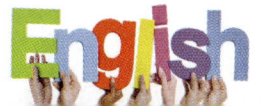

- **Beat down (to crush):** The Indian Army beat down the Pakistan forces.
- **To be done for (to be required):** I am done for because I have lost in business.
- **To bury the hatchet (to end quarrel):** We should bury the hatchet and become friends again.
- **To blow one's own trumpet (to boast):** Do not take his statements at their face value, he often blows his own trumpet.
- **To be on the last legs (about to finish):** The winter is on its last legs.
- **Blessing in disguise (hidden favor):** Failure has proved to be a blessing in disguise; he has become regular in studies.
- **Burning question (hotly debated):** This is the burning question and so everyone is talking about it.
- **To be in one's good books (to be favorite of):** Till you are in the good books of the principal nobody can do any harm to you.
- **To bear in mind (to remember):** I cannot remind you again and again, you will have to bear it in mind yourself.
- **Break into (to enter into a house forcibly):** The dacoits broke into the house at midnight and took away cash.
- **To break the ice (to start speaking in an atmosphere of silence):** There was complete silence in the hall, I broke the ice by requesting him to speak.
- **Bring forth (to produce):** He brought forth many points in favor of this view.
- **A black sheep (one who betrays friends or any other group of persons):** Neither his friends nor his brothers like him because he acts like a black sheep.

C

Schedule your Study

- **To catch a glimpse of (to see):** We caught a glimpse of the Taj while we were travelling by train.
- **A child's play (something very easy):** To pass the PCS examination is not a child's play.
- **To curry favor (to win favor):** He does many odd jobs of his boss to curry favor with him.
- **A cock and bull story (an imaginary story):** He invented a cock and bull story to justify his late coming to college.
- **To catch red-handed (in the act of doing):** The thief was caught red-handed while he was trying to escape through the window.
- **To carry the day (to win victory):** Our college football team carried the day and won the trophy.
- **A cat's paw (to make somebody a tool):** The politicians use poor people as cat's paw to promote their selfish ends.
- **Come to a standstill (to come to a stop):** His business has come to a stand still for want of money.
- **To come off with flying colors (to succeed with credit):** He came off with flying colors in the MBBS examination.
- **A cat and dog life (to lead a life of quarrel):** Both the wife and the husband are leading a cat and dog life these days.

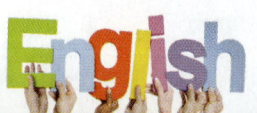

- **Chicken hearted (Cowardly):** A chicken hearted fellow should not think of joining the army or police.
- **To come to light (to be disclosed or to be known):** Many facts have come to light during investigation by the police.
- **To come to terms (to come to an agreement):** Both the partners sank their differences and came to terms with each other.
- **Cut down (to reduce):** The people should cut down their expenses on marriages.
- **To cut one's coat according to one's cloth (to limit one's expenses to the money available):** You will never run into debt if you cut your coat according to your cloth.
- **To count upon (to depend upon):** You can count upon me for help in difficulty.
- **Cut off (kill):** He was cut off in the prime of his life.
- **Cut down (to reduce):** We must cut down our expenses.
- **Call in (call the doctor):** Please call in the doctor.
- **Call off (to withdraw):** The strike has been called off.
- **Call out (say something loudly):** The teacher called out the names of the students.
- **Carry out (obey):** He did not carry out any orders.
- **Carry one's point (gain one point):** In spite of opposition, I carried my point at the meeting.
- **Cast off (to get rid of something):** I have cast off my old shirt.
- **Cast aside (to reject):** His suggestion was cast aside by the members.
- **Come of (belong):** She comes of a noble family.
- **Come up with (to overtake):** India is trying to come up with advanced countries.
- **Come about (to happen):** I do not know when this accident came about.
- **Come at (to come in a threatening way):** Megha came at me with a knife.
- **Come out of (to get clear):** He came out of his difficulty with courage.
- **Cry for (desire):** He is crying for justice.
- **Cry down (to condemn):** His critics cried down his achievements.
- **Call forth (to bring into action):** You will have to call forth all your energy.
- **Carry on (to continue):** It is difficult to carry on our conversation at this noisy place.
- **Carry through (to support):** Having made a promise, you must carry it through.
- **Come down (to reduce):** Prices have come down now.
- **Come off (to happen):** His marriage comes off next Monday.
- **Cut down (to decrease):** You must cut down your expenditure.
- **Call in question (to doubt):** His honesty was called in question.
- **To call names (to abuse):** When he called me names, I abused him.
- **Call you (to call):** I will call you up when I need your help.
- **To carry into effect (to put into practice):** You carry your schemes into effect.
- **To carry away (to be influenced by):** He was carried away by her beauty.
- **To come about (to happen):** How did this come about?
- **To come round (to agree):** After discussion he came round to my views.
- **Come to blows (to fight):** From hot words they came to blows.
- **Come across (to see accidently):** I came across your friend in the street.
- **To come into force (to operate):** This act comes into force.

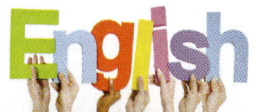

- **To come true (to be fulfilled):** My prediction has come out to be true.
- **Come to light (to be known):** After investigation, the murder came to light.
- **Cut short (to interrupt):** His speech was cut short by protest.
- **To cut a figure (to attract attention):** He always cuts a figure in the public meeting.
- **A cock and bull story (fabricated story):** I cannot believe it because it seems to be a cock and bull story.
- **A cold-blooded murder (murder without any provocation):** The murder of a child is always considered to be a cold-blooded murder.
- **To chew the curd (to ruminate):** You can easily pass time by chewing the curd of old and sweet memories.
- **To crack a joke (to cut a joke):** Do not crack such jokes they do not behove of you.
- **Crocodile tears (hypocritical tears):** I do not think he has any sympathy with you; he is shedding crocodile tears only.
- **A child's play (a simple work):** Passing this exam is not a child's play: work hard.
- **Cry over spilt milk (to repent uselessly):** You cannot do anything about it; do not cry over split milk.
- **Cut a sorry figure (to give a poor show):** He had not prepared well so he had to cut a sorry figure in the examination.
- **To cut teeth (growing teeth):** These days the child is cutting teeth.

D

- **To do away with (to abolish):** Let us take a pledge to do away with dowry system.
- **To die in harness (to die while working):** Pt. Nehru died in harness in 1964.
- **A dead language (a language which is no longer in use):** Urdu has become a dead language in Punjab.
- **A dead letter (a document of no value):** The Shimla Agreement between India and Pakistan has become a dead letter now.
- **A dark horse (a person of unknown capabilities):** Archana turned out to be a dark horse when she stood first in the competition.
- **Double dealing (not to be sincere):** I do not like those people who indulge in double dealing.
- **To draw the line (to fix the limit):** She invited one after the other to her birthday party and did not know where to draw the line.
- **Do away with (to abolish):** Corruption must be done away with.
- **Do over (do again):** This sum is wrong, do it over.
- **Draw in (to involve someone):** I do not want to be drawn in any controversy.
- **Draw up (arrive):** The taxi drew up at the gate.
- **Drop in (to come unexpectedly):** Guests drop in when they like.
- **Drop off (to begin to sleep):** Just when I was dropping off somebody knocked at the door.
- **Do away with (to abolish):** The dowry system should be done away with.
- **To do a good turn (to be kind):** He did me a good turn when I needed him.
- **To do without (to dispense with):** I cannot do without a servant.
- **To do one's best (to try utmost):** He did his best to win her over but failed.

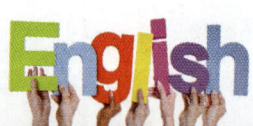

- **Drawn game (game in which neither party wins):** They had to play again because the first was a drawn game.
- **Drop in (appear suddenly):** When we were discussing something confidential, he dropped in.

E

- **An eye wash (deception):** The interview of the candidates was only an eye wash.
- **An eye opener (something that brings one to sense):** His failure in the examination proved to be an eye opener for him.
- **Eye to eye (to agree):** I do not see eye to eye with you at least on this point.

F

- **To fly in the face of (to oppose openly):** No student can dare fly in the face of the new science teacher because he is very strict.
- **From hand to mouth (a miserable condition):** Most of the people in India live from hand to mouth.
- **To follow suit (to do what the person before you have done):** When a boy left the class the others followed suit.
- **To feather one's nest (care for one's selfish interest):** The politicians in India are feathering their own nest in the name of public service.
- **To follow in the footsteps of (to follow somebody's example):** We should follow in the footsteps of good people in order to become good.
- **A fair-weather friend (a selfish friend):** When our purse is full, many fair weather friends gather around us.
- **Fair and square (just, honest):** We should be fair and square in our dealings with others.
- **To feel at home (to feel comfortable):** He does not feel at home in the new atmosphere.
- **A fish out of water (to feel uneasy):** In the absence of my parents, I feel like a fish out of water.
- **A fool's paradise (a state of joy based on false hopes):** He is living in a fool's paradise if he thinks that Ginni will marry him.
- **To fish in troubled waters (to take advantage of the trouble of others):** The English fished in troubled waters during their stay in India.
- **To find fault with (to find shortcomings):** I am not in the habit of finding fault with what others do.
- **Fall off (to decline):** The number of passengers in night trains has fallen off.
- **Fall short (to be deficient):** The result fell short of our expectations.
- **To fall through (to fall):** The scheme fell through for lack of planning.
- **To fall to (to start eating):** The hungry man just fell to dish.
- **To fall flat (to be unsuccessful):** My advice fell flat on him.
- **To fall out (to quarrel):** The two friends fall out property.
- **To find fault with (to pick holes):** Do not find fault with every one, it is a bad habit.
- **From pillar to post (from one place to another):** He had to run from pillar to post for getting a job.

G

- **To give a good account (to acquit oneself well):** He gave a good account of himself in the interview.
- **A get together (meeting):** The tea party given by him was only a get together of old friends.
- **To go to the dogs (to be ruined):** If you do not mend your ways, you will surely go to the dogs.
- **To give a piece of one's mind (to rebuke):** The teacher gave the boys a piece of his mind for coming late in the class.
- **To go without saying (to be clear):** It goes without saying that corruption is in full swing in India.
- **To give a cold shoulder (to treat in a cold manner):** I went to one of my relative to borrow money but he gave a cold shoulder.
- **To get on one's nerves (to be a cause of worry):** Do not get on my nerves because I am already tired of life.
- **To get into hot water (to get into trouble):** He got into hot water when he was found cheating.
- **To go up in flames (to be destroyed):** All his plans went up in flames when his parents refused to give him financial help.
- **To go against the grain (against one's liking):** To admire a worthless fellow whom I dislike goes very much against the grain.
- **Give and take (the making of mutual concession):** The policy of give and take has undermined the moral values of life.
- **Get over (to overcome):** Finally, he succeeded in getting over his difficulties.
- **Get through (to pass):** He got through his examination in first division.
- **Give out (to announce):** It was given out that the minister was dead.
- **Give rise to (to cause):** Your absence from house has given rise to suspicion.
- **Give away (to distribute):** The Chief Minister gave away the prizes.
- **Go astray (to be misled):** His son has gone astray in life.
- **Go on (continue):** The children went on making a noise.
- **Get over (to overcome):** You will get over your difficulties if you have enough courage.
- **Get rid of (to be free from):** You should try to get rid of these selfish friends.
- **Get up (to rise):** What time do you get up?
- **Give in (to yield):** The enemy had to give in at last.
- **Give up (to stop):** You should give up your bad habits.
- **Go through (to enquire):** I have not gone through the accounts yet.
- **To get off (to escape):** When the thief saw the policeman, he managed to get off.
- **To get hold of (to seize):** He has got hold of house.
- **To go off (to pass):** I am sure everything will go off smoothly.
- **To go hard with (to be in real danger):** It goes hard with him as he is unemployed.
- **To grope in the dark (to search in vain):** He does not know anything about this course; he is still groping in the dark.
- **To go to dogs (to be ruined):** He went to dogs only because of bad planning.
- **To give way (to fall):** Under heavy traffic the bridge gave way.

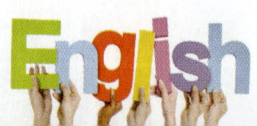

- **Gave away (to distribute):** The Prime Minister gave away the prizes.
- **To give ear (to listen):** Please give ear to what I say.
- **To give out (to abandon):** I have given out the project because of pressure.
- **To go back on (to fall back):** I shall not go back on my word.
- **Go astray (to wonder from the course):** Check him he is going astray.
- **To grind one's teeth (to have a feeling of disappointment or rage):** The captain ground his teeth when he missed to score an easy goal against the rival team.

H

- **Horns of a dilemma (to be in a fix):** He was on the horns of a dilemma and did not know what to do next.
- **A hard nut to crack (a problem difficult to solve):** The Kashmir issue has proved to be a hard nut to crack.
- **To hang heavy (difficult to pass):** Time hangs heavy on my head when I have no work to do.
- **To have a finger in the pie (to interfere):** You will get into trouble if you unnecessarily have a finger in the pie.
- **Hall mark (main quality):** Honesty is the hall mark of his character.
- **To lend a hand (to help):** She always lends a hand to her mother in the kitchen.
- **To hit below the belt (to use unfair means):** A true sportsman never hits below the belt.
- **Hard and fast (strict):** Hard and fast rules have to be followed.
- **Hue and cry (a loud noise):** The students raised much hue and cry when they found the question paper difficult.
- **Hen-pecked husband (a husband under the control of his wife):** He is a hen-pecked husband and has no voice in the family.
- **A haunted house (a house where ghosts live):** I shall not stay here any longer because it is a haunted house.
- **To hope against hope (to hope even when there is no hope):** He has not done his papers well, and yet he hopes against hope he will pass.
- **Head and shoulders (very superior):** Rabindranath Tagore stand head and shoulders above other Indian poets.
- **To hit the nail on the head (to touch the exact point):** The speaker hit the nail on the head when he said that all politicians were corrupt.
- **To hold one's tongue (to keep silent):** Please hold your tongue otherwise you will have to repent in the end.
- **Hold back (to hide):** Why are you holding back the facts?
- **Hold out (to offer):** The doctors hold out little hope of his recovery.
- **Hold over (to postpone):** The matter was held over until the next meeting.
- **To hold water (to be well-grounded):** Your argument does not hold water.
- **To hold back (to delay):** The train was held back due to rain.
- **Hold to (to stick to):** She still holds to her old views.

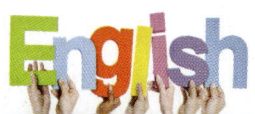

- **From hand to mouth (earning very little):** He does not have spare money, he lives from hand to mouth.
- **To hit below the belt (to use unfair means):** Criticise openly; do not hit below the belt.
- **To have no stone unturned (to do one's utmost):** He will leave no stone unturned for getting this job.

I

- **In cold blood (cruelly):** The murder was committed in cold blood.
- **In black and white (in writing):** He gave his statement in black and white in the court of law.
- **In lieu of (in place of):** In lieu of translation you can write a paragraph on any topic.
- **In hot water (in difficulty):** The clerk used to accept hush money and now he is in hot water.
- **In a nut shell (in brief):** He told us the story in a nut shell.
- **In the twinkling of an eye (in no time):** The pick-pocket disappeared from the sight in the twinkling of an eye.
- **In full swing (in great progress):** The fair was in full swing when we reached there.
- **In the nick of time (just in time):** We reached the station in the nick of time and caught the train.
- **Ins and outs (full details):** The head clerk knows the ins and outs of the office work.
- **An irony of fate (happening of events contrary to natural expectation):** He expected to win the assembly election, but by the irony of fate he lost even his security deposit.
- **In one's heart of hearts (from the depth of one's heart):** Everyman in his heart of hearts wish to become wealthy overnight.
- **The irony of fate (stroke of ill luck):** By the strange irony of fate he lost his job.

J

- **To jump to the conclusion (to arrive at a conclusion):** They jumped to the conclusion that Rajan was at the root of this trouble.
- **Jack of all trades (a person who has knowledge of everything but is a master of none):** A person who is Jack of all trades but master of none hardly ever progresses in life.

K

Keep going you are doing good

- **To keep an eye (to watch):** Parents must keep an eye on the activities of their children.
- **To knock down (to defeat):** Our hockey team knocked down the rival team by a big margin of goals.
- **To keep away (to keep aloof):** Always keep away from bad company.
- **To keep an eye on (to attend to):** Keep an eye on him because he is not good.
- **To keep aloof (to avoid):** You should keep aloof from bad company.
- **To keep at arm's length (to keep at a distance):** He is a dangerous man, keep him at an arm's length.
- **To keep one's word (to keep one's promise):** You should keep your word otherwise people will lose faith in you.

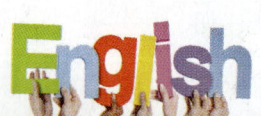

L

- **Laughing stock (an object of ridicule):** His foolish behavior made him the laughing stock of all the boys.
- **To leave in the lurch (to leave in difficulty):** When he fell on bad days, his friends left him in the lurch.
- **Loaves and fishes (material comforts):** He is prepared to sacrifice all the principles of life for the sake of loaves and fishes.
- **To lead a dog's life (a miserable life):** Both the husband and wife are leading a dog's life.
- **Lame excuse (false excuse):** He invented a lame excuse to justify his absence from the hospital.
- **To leave no stone unturned (to make all possible efforts):** He left no stone unturned to secure the top position in the university examination.
- **A left-handed compliment (a false praise):** When he admitted my ability to work, I knew that it was only a left-handed compliment.
- **To lead a cat and dog life (to lead a life of quarrel):** The husband and the wife are leading a cat and dog life these days.
- **Leap in the dark (a careless action):** By marrying a foreign girl he has taken a leap in the dark.
- **To lead astray (to mislead):** I am afraid your friend will be led astray in their company.
- **To let the grass grow under one's feet (to remain inactive):** Those who let the grass grow under their feet do not succeed in life.
- **A lump in the throat (feeling of grief):** He felt a lump in the throat when he narrated the story of his parent's death.
- **Look after (to take care of):** Parents look after their children with love and affection.
- **Look for (search):** He is looking for a job.
- **Look out for (to be on the watch):** You go to the station and look out for your brother?
- **To lay hand on (to seize):** I will read all I could lay my hands on.
- **To lay waste (to destroy):** America laid waste to Vietnam in the name of saving it.
- **To look down upon (to treat with contempt):** Do not look down upon the poor.
- **To look forward to (to wait anxiously):** I am looking forward to the day when India is prosperous.
- **To look up (rise in price):** The prices are looking up.
- **Look up to (to regard with respect):** We look up to God for help.
- **Look through (to understand thoroughly):** The magistrate will look through the case.
- **Look sharp (to lose no time):** Please look sharp we are getting late.
- **To lay by (to save for future):** We must lay by something for our evil days.
- **To lay down (to prescribe):** He is prepared to lay down his life for the sake of reputation.
- **A leap in the dark (An adventure which is not properly reasoned out):** His decision to resign is a leap in the dark as he has no other source of income.

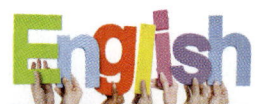

M

- **To make the most of (to take the full advantage):** You should work hard in order to make the most of this opportunity.
- **Maiden speech (the first speech made by a person):** He had to cut a sorry figure in his maiden speech.
- **To make a mark (to distinguish):** He is a hard-working person and is sure to make a mark in his field.
- **A man of letter (a scholar):** Shakespeare was not only a writer but also a man of letters.
- **To make the both ends meet (to live within one's means):** The prices are rising so high that it has become difficult for poor people to make the both ends meet.
- **To mind one's own business (to confine to oneself):** You should mind your own business and not interfere in others' work.
- **To make amends for (to compensate for an injury):** You will not be allowed to leave this place unless you make amends for the loss.
- **To mind one's P's and Q's (to be careful in one's behavior):** A cultured person always minds his P's and Q's while talking to others.
- **Make for (to go in the direction of):** The bull made for me and I had to run.
- **Make out (to understand):** I cannot make out what you want to say.
- **Make up one's mind (to decide):** I have made up my mind to leave this place.
- **To make it up with (to settle one's differences):** Till they make it up with each other, their business will not prosper.
- **To make the most of (to get the best advantage):** Try to make the most of the bad bargain.
- **To make up for (to compensate):** I will make up for this wrong which I have done to you.
- **To make away with (to kill):** A dacoit made away with a money lender.
- **Make out (to prove):** You make your case, then I will support you.

N

- **Nook and corner (everywhere):** He looked for his missing shoe in every nook and corner of the house.
- **A narrow escape (to be saved with difficulty):** He had a narrow escape in a car accident.
- **To nip in the bud (to destroy in the beginning):** All evils should be nipped in the bud.
- **A nine days wonder (something short lived):** Beauty is a nine days wonder.
- **Null and void (invalid):** His election as Mayor was declared null and void.

O

- **Out of date (out of fashion):** Tight dress is out of date today.
- **On the spur of the moment (at once):** He answered all my questions on the spur of the moment.
- **Order of the day (something common):** Corruption is order of the day in every office.
- **On the horns of a dilemma (in a fix):** I am on the horns of a dilemma and do not know what to do next.
- **Odds and ends (big and small things):** He left all odd and ends behind him when he was transferred to Delhi.

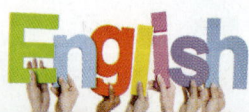

- **Open secret (a secret which everybody knows):** It is an open secret that Mukesh and his wife are leading a cat and dog life.
- **Out of question (impossible):** He is so careless that his success in the examination is out of question.
- **Off hand (without previous preparation):** He spoke off hand at the meeting but his speech was greatly admired.
- **On the alert (to be watchful):** India should be on the alert against the evil designs of Pakistan.
- **Open question (debatable):** It is an open question whether right to property should be scrapped.
- **Of one's own accord (of one's free will):** He donated his property to a charitable trust of his own accord.
- **Over head and ears (completely):** He has been taking loans and is now over head and ears in debt.
- **At one's beck and call (ready to serve):** You have a sincere person in him; he is always at your beck and call.
- **An oily tongue (flatterer):** In the present-day world only an oily tongue can get promotion in the organisation.
- **On the spur of the moment (without getting time to think):** He cannot speak on the spur of the moment; it was his prepared speech.

P

- **To put in cold storage (to neglect):** Many schemes have been put in cold storage for want of funds.
- **To play with fire (to do something dangerous):** Those who try to create differences between Indians are playing with fire.
- **To pick a quarrel (to begin a quarrel):** It is not good to pick a quarrel always.
- **To put heads together (to hold consultation):** Let us put heads together and find out some solution to the problem.
- **To poison one's ears (to prejudice):** My friend Mina poisoned the ears of my teacher against me.
- **To pay in the same coin (tit for tat):** We should return good for evil and not pay in the same coin.
- **Part and parcel (an essential part):** Games are a part and parcel of education.
- **To play false (to deceive):** Never play false with your friends.
- **To pour oil over troubled waters (to pacify an angry person):** When the boys of our locality were about to fight, it was I who poured oil over troubled waters.
- **To pull one's leg (to make a fool of):** In his family if one is about to march ahead, the others begin to pull his leg.
- **To pocket the insult (To bear insult):** No human being can pocket this insult.
- **Pillar to post (from place to place):** He is running from pillar to post in search of some good job.

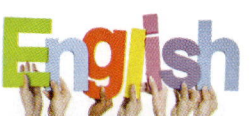

- **To play one's trump card (to use unexpected means):** They played their trump card towards the end and won the case.
- **A pleasant surprise (a surprise that pleases):** It was a pleasant surprise for the parents when their son was selected in the I.P.S.
- **Pull over (to stop the vehicle):** The Policeman signalled him to pull over.
- **Push ahead (to continue with a plan):** Finally, we decided to pull ahead with the deal.
- **Push aside (to try to forget):** You should push aside the bitter memories of hostel life.
- **Put down (to crush):** The rebellion was put down.
- **Put off (to postpone):** Do not put off till tomorrow what you can do today.
- **Put on (to wear):** Put on your clothes now.
- **To pull through (to recover):** Her illness is serious but I think she will pull through it.
- **To pull down (to demolish):** Many old houses were pulled down.
- **To pull up (to rebuke):** The boy was pulled up for his bad conduct.
- **Put forth (to exert):** I put forth his power to defeat me.
- **Put up with (to tolerate):** I cannot put up with this insult.
- **To play ducks and drakes (lavish with money):** His father is lenient so he is playing ducks and drakes with money.
- **To play truant (to miss classes without permission):** He is punished for playing truant.

Q

- **A queer fish (a strange person):** Nobody likes to have any relations with him because he is a queer fish.

R

- **To run short of (to be exhausted):** It became a problem for us when we ran short of money during our journey to Mumbai.
- **To rest on one's laurels (to be satisfied with one's success):** We should not rest on our laurels but work for more and more success.
- **To rain cats and dogs (to rain heavily):** It has been raining cats and dogs since yesterday.
- **A rolling stone (one who never sticks to one place):** A rolling stone gathers no moss
- **To rub shoulders with (to come into contact):** We rub shoulders with all types of people in our life.
- **Run into (to be involved):** He has run into debt.
- **Run across (to meet suddenly):** I ran across an old friend last week.
- **Run through (to waste):** He has run through his property.
- **Run after (to pursue):** Everybody is running after wealth these days.
- **Run short of (to be exhausted):** I ran short of money and had to come back.
- **To run down (to criticise, to become weak):** He is always running down leaders. His health has run down.
- **Run into (to be involved):** You will run into debt if you do not live within your income.
- **Run through (to waste):** He ran through his fortune and became bankrupt.
- **Run out (to expire):** The time has run out.
- **A red-letter day (auspicious day):** August 15, 1947 is a red letter day in the history of our country.

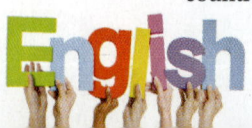

S

Read carefully

- **To see eye to eye with (to agree):** I do not see eye to eye to with you in this matter.
- **A sharp tongue (a bitter langue):** Since she has a sharp tongue, nobody likes to talk to her.
- **To smell a rat (to suspect):** The police smelled a rat and found drugs in his bag.
- **A snake in the grass (a hidden enemy):** You regard him as your true friend but I think that he is a snake in the grass.
- **A standing joke (an object of laughter):** His multi-colored clothes are a standing joke for his class fellows.
- **Shoulder to shoulder (in cooperation):** Let us all work shoulder to shoulder for the progress of our country.
- **To sail in the same boat (equally exposed to risk):** I told my friend that he alone was not unlucky but many others were also sailing in the same boat.
- **A stiff-necked person (on obstinate person):** Karan is a stiff necked fellow, therefore, nobody likes his company.
- **Set in (start):** Rainy season has set in.
- **Set aside (to reject):** The judge set aside his petition for mercy.
- **Set apart (to keep aside):** He has set apart fifty thousand rupees for the marriage of his daughter.
- **Set apart (to reverse):** I have set apart some money for my daughter.
- **Set off (to start):** They have set off on their journey.
- **Set on (to incite):** The poor beggar was set on by the street dogs.
- **Set aside (to reject):** The judge has set aside the judgment of the lower court.
- **Set up (to stand business):** He has set up a new shop.
- **Set about (to begin happily):** He set about his work happily.
- **To smell a rat (to suspect correctly):** The police smelt the rat and arrested him; he was a terrorist.
- **A stumbling block (an obstacle):** Their nature is a stumbling block in the way of their progress.
- **A slip of tongue (a mistake in talk):** A slip of tongue is never excusable.
- **To stand on one's legs (to become independent):** Do not think of getting married unless you stand on your own legs.
- **To stand in the way (to obstruct):** We wanted to start a joint business but my friend's father stood in the way.
- **To start from a scratch (to start afresh):** After loss in business we had to start our business from a scratch.
- **A sleeping partner (a partner in a business who is not active but shares its profit):** I am only a sleeping partner in my new business.
- **To step into another's shoes (to take the charge):** When our Principal retired, the Vice principal stepped into his shoes.
- **Small talk (gossip):** The ladies generally indulge in small talk when they meet at marriages.
- **A square peg in a round hole (misfit):** After retirement from service when he started business, he found himself as a square peg an a round hole.

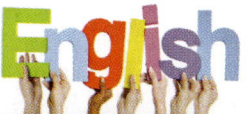

- **To serve one right (to treat as one deserves):** You have served him right by not inviting him to your house for his rude behavior.
- **At snail's pace (very slowly):** If you work at a snail's pace, you will not be able to finish it in time.

T

- **To take a heart (to feel):** You should not take your failure to heart but try again.
- **To turn a deaf ear (refuse to listen):** He turned a deaf ear to my advice and continued to smoke secretly.
- **To take the cue (to take the hint):** When they started discussing something personal, I took the cue and left the place.
- **Take after (to resemble):** She takes after her mother.
- **Take off (to remove):** Please take off your shoes.
- **Takeover (to take charge):** He has taken over the charge of the office.
- **To be taken aback (to be surprised):** I was taken aback by the news.
- **Take up the cause (support):** We should take up the cause of the poor.
- **Throw away (to get rid of):** You should not have thrown away the receipt.
- **Turn up (to come):** Nobody turned up for the meeting.
- **Turn against (go against):** The people have turned against the government.
- **Turn down (reject):** The Principal turned down his request.
- **Turn aside (to deviate):** I shall not turn aside from the path of virtue.
- **Take after (resemble):** She takes after her mother.
- **Take off (remove):** I took of my clothes and jumped into the river.
- **Turn up (to appear):** He promised to come, but has not turned up yet.
- **Turn off (to dismiss):** Turn off this fellow as he is rude.
- **Taken down (to record):** The steno took down the dictation.
- **Take to (to adopt the profession):** He has taken to medicine.
- **To take the bull by the horns (to face danger bravely):** He is success in life because he takes the bull by the horns.
- **To throw out of gear (disturb):** Owing to riots normal life has been thrown out of gear.
- **Tooth and nail (violently):** If we are attacked, we will fight tooth and nail.
- **To take ill (to feel offended):** He took my words ill and did not speak to me.
- **To turn turtle (capsize):** The car turned turtle, as it collided against the pole.
- **To turn one's head (to fill with pride):** Wealth has turned his head.

U

- **Ups and downs (rise and fall):** Her life is full of ups and downs.
- **Under lock and key (under safety):** He keeps his wife's ornaments under lock and key.
- **Underdog (the poor and needy):** The government should take steps to improve the lot of the underdog.
- **Up to the mark (up to a standard):** Your answer is not up to the mark, therefore you should write it again.

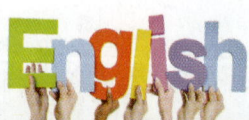

V

- **To vie with (to compete with):** Women vie with each other to steal the limelight.
- **Via media (middle course):** Some via media will have to be found to solve the problem.

W

- **A white elephant (costly to maintain):** SUV is a white elephant for a middle class family.
- **A wild goose chase (a foolish pursuit):** To find real happiness in the world is only a wild goose chase.
- **To wet blanket (one who spoils joy):** Whenever we plan to go on a trip Gurdeep proves to be a wet blanket.
- **To win laurels (to win glory):** By standing first in the university examination she has won laurels for her college.
- **A wolf in a sheep's clothing (a hypocrite):** Do not depend on him, he is a wolf in a sheep's clothing.
- **With one accord (with one voice):** All the students went to the principal and requested him with one accord to let them go on a trip.
- **Wear and tear (damage caused by use):** The company made him payment for the wear and tear of his car.
- **Worth one's weight in gold (of great value):** A glass of water is worth its weight in gold in a desert.
- **Wear one's heart on one's sleeve (to show one's emotion publicly):** He is a very sensitive person and wears his heart on his sleeve.
- **Work out (to solve):** I cannot work out these algebraic problems.
- **Work up (to excite):** He worked himself up into a bad temper.
- **To win laurels (win honour):** By his adventurous actions he has won laurels.
- **A wolf in sheep's clothing (hypocrite):** This man seems to be innocent but he is a wolf in sheep's clothing.
- **Work wonders (to bring about good results):** This medicine has worked wonders.

Y

- **Yeoman's service (very good service):** As a social worker he has rendered yeoman's service to reform the society.
- **Yearn for (long far):** Every student yearns for holidays.

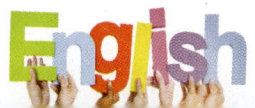

NOTES

Chapter 18

Confused Words

Mistakes in the use of words frequently occur while reading or using words which have some similarity with other words. This is particularly so when some words are similar, though not necessarily identical, in appearance, spelling and sound, but which have different meanings. The following is the a list of words which are similar in appearance, spellings or sound but different in meanings.

1. **Abject** (wretched; as low as possible): The whole family is living in abject poverty.
   Object (an article; to take exception): They saw a suspicious object lying on the road.

2. **Aboard** (on/into a ship, aircraft, train, etc.): All aboard the ship were drowned during the storm.
   Abroad (in another country): Her family decided to settle abroad.

3. **Accede** (grant; accept): He acceded to her request to appear only in final exams.
   Exceed (be more than required; be much more): His punishment far exceeded his crime.

4. **Accept** (receive): Mohit accepted the gift from his uncle.
   Except (save [as a preposition; exclude [as a verb]): All except Rahul were present in the class.

5. **Access** (approach): This poor man has no access to any high officer.
   Excess (more than usual or required): He admired her beauty to excess.

6. **Accomplice** (a person who helps another in a crime): The thief's accomplice ran away.
   Accomplish (achieve something with effort): The minister's visit accomplished nothing

7. **Adapt** (make suitable for new needs or situation): Romesh adapted himself to the new situation.
   Adept (skilled, proficient): The new typist is adept in his job.
   Adopt (take someone, especially a child): The issueless couple adopted an orphaned baby.

8. **Affect** (Verb: have a bad effect on; feel; pretend): Your actions will affect your reputation.
   Effect (Noun: influence; Verb: bring about): The new principal has effected many changes.

9. **Affection** (strong feeling; love): Reena's mom has a great affection for me.
   Affectation (artificiality in manners, etc.): Her English accent reveals a clear affectation.

10. **All ready** (entirely ready): He is all ready to do anything for me.
    Already (by this time; before): Rajan has already left for Shimla.

11. **All together** (taken collectively): All together we were twenty persons in the party.
    Altogether (completely): You are altogether right in your choice.

12. **Allusion** (indirect reference): Her speech contained an allusion to the treatment given to him.
    Illusion (false impression; mirage): The heat in the desert produces an illusion of water.

13. **Altar** (place of offering inside the church): The couple offered prayers at the altar of the goddess.
    Alter (change; modify): The secretary altered the time of my appointment with the minister.

14. **Alternate** (leaving a gap of one): The doctor visited the college on alternate days.
    Alternative (choice between two things): We had to come back from the alternative road.

15. **Angel** (a heavenly creature with wings): Fools rush in where angels fear to tread.
    Angle (the space between two lines that meet each other at a point): A triangle has three angles.

16. **Anyone** (anybody, any person): Does anyone know Renu's address?
    Any one (any one of the given three or more): You can answer any one of these three questions.

17. **Apposite** (exactly suitable): It was an apposite comment on her style of acting.
    Opposite (contrary; as different as possible): They have started moving in opposite directions.

18. **Ascent** (act of going/moving up/climbing): They made a successful ascent of the mountain.
    Assent (formal agreement): As soon as we get his assent, we will start the work on this project.

19. **Ensure** (make certain): Your timely help has ensured the success of our project.
    Insure (protect against loss of money, life, etc.): Raman's shop is insured for a crore of rupees.

20. **Attention** (serious care): You must pay attention to what I am going to say.
    Intention (inclination): He shows no intention of appearing in the examination.

21. **Bail** (money or guarantee given to a court to set a prisoner free): Anil was released on bail.
    Bale (bundle): How many bales of cotton are lying in the store?

22. **Bare (**Uncovered): His head was bare. Children ran about bare-footed on the road.
    Bear (accept; suifer): No mother can bear to see her child in pain.

23. **Berth** (a seat in a railway compartment): He booked a berth for himself in the Frontier Mail.
    Birth (being born; coming into the world): Freedom is our birth right.

24. **Beside** (by the side of): He was sitting beside her in the theatre.
    Besides (in addition to): Besides his house in Delhi, he has a flat in Mumbai.

25. **Born** (came into the world; took birth): Mahatma Gandhi was born on October 2, 1869
    Borne (carried; suffered): He has borne so much suffering and yet he can smile at his fate.

26. **Brake** (apparatus for checking a vehicle's motion): He applied the brake and the car stopped.
    Break (make discontinuous or fragmentary): Why did you break that window pane?

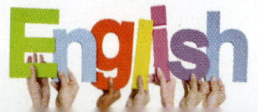

27. **Bridal** (pertaining to a bride): How much did she pay for her bridal make-up?
    Bridle (headgear of the harness of a horse): The horse ran away with the bridle.

28. **Canvas** (strong, rough cloth used for tents, sails, etc.): He bought a pair of canvas shoes.
    Canvass (ask for political support or votes): He is now busy canvassing support for his friend.

29. **Career** (job or profession for which one is trained): His career as a novelist came to a sudden end.
    Carrier (one or something that carries something): In the past there used to be carrier pigeons.

30. **Cast** (throw; give): Many people refused to cast their votes.
    Caste (social class based on one's birth): There are reservations for people of backward castes.
    Cost (involve expenditure on buying): How much did this house cost you?

31. **Cattle** (animals, usually pet, such as cows): Many herds of cattle perished during the famine.
    Kettle (a pot or vessel): The kettle cannot call the pot black.

32. **Cell** (a small room in a prison): The prisoner-lived in his solitary cell.
    Sell (give in retum for money): He has decided not to sell his ancestral house.

33. **Censor** (cut out, considered suitable): Some scenes of the movie have been censored.
    Censure (criticize unfavorably): The assembly censured the remarks of the minister.

34. **Cereal** (grains for food): Oats and barley are cereals with a rich food value.
    Serial (coming in a series): The new television serial is enjoying great popularity.

35. **Choir** (band of singers in church service): John is a member of the parish choir.
    Coir (coconut fiber): This is a coir mattress.

36. **Cite** (quote from a book or article): He cited many authors in support of his critic theory.
    Site (place/ground for a building, school, etc.): This site is reserved for a public school.

37. **Coarse** (rough): School bags are usually made of coarse cloth.
    Course (path): He had to chart out his own course in life.

38. **Coma** (a state of unconsciousness): The patient is still in coma.
    Comma (a punctuation mark): Take proper care of your commas and colons.

39. **Comprehensible** (which can be understood): His Latin was scarcely comprehensible.
    Comprehensive (thorough): He gave a comprehensive description of the nuclear blasts.

40. **Conscious** (aware; fully seized of something): I am conscious of my duty towards my wife.
    Conscience (moral sense of right and wrong): He had the conscience to betray his old friend.

41. **Council** (assembly; official body): He is member of the state legislative council.
    Counsel (advice; also a lawyer): His good counsel was ignored and the result is there before you.

42. **Cue** (hint about one's part in a drama or in general): I followed his cue and left the hall.
    Queue (file of persons waiting for their turn): Much of our life is spent in standing in the queue.

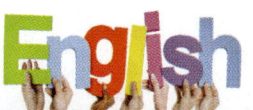

43. **Deceased** (dead): He inherited the estate and property of his deceased grandfather.
     Diseased (showing signs of disease): This plant has become diseased and will wither soon.

44. **Descent** (downward journey through a hill): Barb found the descent hike quite pleasant.
     Decent (nice): She has a nice bearing and decent manners.
     Dissent (disagreement): My dissent may please be put on record.

45. **Desert** (abandon; give up): Avinash deserted his post and hid himself in the fields.
     Dessert (course of fruit, sweet dish at the end of a dinner): What was served in the dessert?

46. **Dose** (quantity of medicine given at a time): You must stick to the dose prescribed for you.
     Doze (sleep): Soon he dozed off into sleep in the sofa where he had been sitting.

47. **Draft** (rough form of a piece of writing): You must first write a rough draft of the precis.
     Draught (liquid for drinking at one time): She took a draught of water and went to sleep.
     Drought (a long period of dry, rainless weather): The drought led to a famine in the area.

48. **Elicit** (draw forth what is latent): All my questions failed to elicit any response from her.
     Illicit (illegal): His father is involved in illicit trade.

49. **Eligible** (fit to be chosen): You are not eligible to join a course in engineering,
     Illegible (which cannot be read): Your handwriting is almost illegible; you must improve it.

50. **Emigrate** (move from one's country to settle in another): Ajitabh emigrated from India to Peru.
     Immigrate (move into a country with a view to settling there): Amit immigrated to the USA.

51. **Fair** (periodical gathering for sale of goods; beautiful): We visited the book fair held in Delhi.
     Fare (cost of a passenger's conveyance): Both bus and train fares have been increased.

52. **Farm** (piece of land on which crops are grown): Michael worked on his own farm.
     Form (shape; kind): How many forms does a verb have?

53. **Farmer** (a person who grows crops or raises animals on a farm): Her husband is a cotton farmer.
     Former (first of the two in subsequent references): Her former boy-friend is now married.

54. **Farther** (refers to distance): They traveled much farther than they had initially planned.
     Further (refers to direction; quality): They made no further progress in their studies.

55. **Fate** (destiny): We should work hard and leave nothing to fate.
     Fete (festival): The college fete was attended by a large number of people.

56. **Fiance** (betrothed man; a man engaged to be married): Her fiance is a mechanical engineer.
     Fiancee (a girl engaged to be married): Sumit's fiancee is very beautiful.

57. **Foul** (dirty; wicked): You Should not hope for a fair result by adopting foul means.
     Fowl (a farmyard bird, such as the hen): Many fowls have perished due to a strange fowl disease.

58. **Gait** (manner of walking): Her gait has a peculiar charm about it.
     Gate (main door at the premises of a building): You must lock the gate before 10 o'clock.

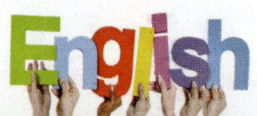

59. **Ghastly** (extremely bad or unpleasant): It was a ghastly holiday that we spent.
   Ghostly (like a ghost): I saw a ghostly light ahead of me in the darkness.

60. **Hair** (fine thread-like growth on the skin): His hair has turned grey.
   Heir (successor; inheritor): The king died without announcing his heir.

61. **Heal** (cure; treat): The wound will take quite long to heal.
   Heel (back part of the foot or the shoe): Women's high heels are almost out of fashion.

62. **Heard** (received [sound] through the ears): Have you heard the latest news from the USA?
   Herd (group of cattle): We saw a herd of cattle grazing in the valley.

63. **Historical** (belonging to history): This building is of historical importance.
   Hysterical (disturbed emotionally): She cried hysterically at the sight of the robbers.

64. **Impassable** (which cannot be passed through): This road becomes impassable during winter.
   Impossible (not possible): Nothing seems impossible when one is young and healthy.

65. **Knotty** (difficult; complicated): The problem turned out too knotty for a simple solution.
   Naughty (mischievous): Now don't be naughty and concentrate on your homework.

66. **Later** (after a particular time): He said that he could come later in the afternoon.
   Latter (the second of the two earlier mentioned): Ajit told Sham that the latter need not wait.

67. **Lessen** (reduce; decrease): Take this tablet; it will lessen your pain.
   Lesson (instruction in a subject): We must draw the right lesson from our past experience.

68. **Loose** (the opposite of tight): He was dressed in a loose gown.
   Lose (suffer a loss): How much money did he lose in this bargain?

69. **Medal** (piece of metal awarded as distinction): He won a gold medal in athletics.
   Meddle (interfere): He does not like anyone meddling in his private affairs.

70. **Miner** (a person who works in a mine): Miners are demanding increase in their wages.
   Minor (underage): She is still a minor.

71. **Moral** (relating to morality or ethics): Science is not concerned with moral issue.
   Morale (spiritg; confidence): The morale of our team is very high at the moment.

72. **Necessaries** (things needed): All the necessaries have been packed.
   Necessities (basic needs): Many people do not have even the basic necessities of life.

73. **Patrol** (go regularly to see there is no trouble): The police are patrolling the trouble Street.
   Petrol (refined mineral oil used as fuel in cars, etc.): This car uses less petrol then your old car.

74. **Peace** (lack of war/conflict): Peace has her own victories more renowned than those of war.
   Piece (fragment): Remove these pieces of glass carefully.

75. **Plain** (frank; straightforward): She pretends to like plain speaking..
   Plane (an instrument used for levelling wood): The carpenter was sharpening his plane.

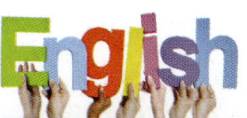

76. **Pole** (a long stick of a pillar): Many electricity poles fell down due to the storm.
    Poll (cast vote in election): Are you going to poll your vote?

77. **Pray** (offer prayers): She used to pray in the morning as well as evening.
    Prey (victim): The knight became the latest prey of the lady without mercy.

78. **Principal** (head of a school or college): His mother was the principal of a college.
    Principle (rule or code): I cannot give up my principles for petty gains.

79. **Profit** (gain): How much profit did you make in this business?
    Prophet (revealer of God's will to the people): Prophets show us the right path.

80. **Quiet** (calm): Rajat is a quiet child.
    Quite (completely): I could not quite make out what he was saying.

81. **Right** (just, morally good): You must do only that which your conscience calls right.
    Rite (solemn religious ceremony; procedure): The marriage rites took several hours.

82. **Root** (part of the plant inside the soil): The plant has now taken a firm root in the soil.
    Rout (defeat) The enemy was badly routed.
    Route (way): They opted to go by the shortest route.

83. **Sail** (launch in a boat of ship): They sailed toward the island in a motor-boat.
    Sale (process of selling): His house is for sale.

84. **Soar** (go up in the sky): Prices are soaring day by day.
    Sore (tender aggrieved): He has a sore throat today.

85. **Stationary** (unmoving, fixed): The sun is stationary but the earth revolves round the sun.
    Stationery (pens, pencils, paper, etc.): His father deals in stationery goods.

86. **Suit** (set of clothes): You need a new suit of clothes for yourself.
    Suite (a set of rooms in a hotel): The actress was found dead in her suite.

87. **Vain** (useless): He did his best but all his efforts were in vain.
    Vein (a tube carrying blood to the heart): Our veins carry blood to our heart. Wane (decrease): The moon begins to wane after the full moon night.

88. **Waist** (part of the body below ribs and above hips): How much does your waist measure?
    Waste (spend recklessly): Don't waste your parents hard earned money.

89. **Whether** (either this or that): It does not matter to me whether you go or stay here.
    Weather (atmosphere around at a particular time): The weather is pleasant today.

90. **Zest** (feeling of being excited and eager): He does everything with a rare zest.
    Jest (joke): The clown was trying to entertain us with his stale jests.

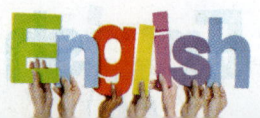

WORDS WITH SHADES OF MEANING

Words very similar in appearance but differing slightly in meaning, usage can be very confusing. If interchanged, these words can completely change the meaning of a sentence or an answer.

Amiable	He has amiable manners.
Amicable	The parties came to an amicable settlement.
Abstain	I abstained from food for two days.
Refrain	He will not refrain from gambling.
Accident	There was a motor accident on the Mall.
Incident	A strange incident took place last night.
Admit	He admitted that he had cheated.
Admit	He was admitted into the class.
Acknowledge	Please acknowledge the receipt of this parcel.
Confess	He confessed his crime.
Artist	A painter is an artist.
Artisan	A carpenter is an artisan.
Alter	He asked the tailor to alter the length of his trousers.
Change	I change my clothes everyday.
Assent	The Governor gave his assent to the new bill.
Consent	My father has consented to my going to England.
Ascent	The ascent to the top of the hill is very hard.
Battle	The first Battle of Panipat was fought.
War	A war may see many battles won and lost.
Character	He was a man of noble character.
Conduct	His conduct was praiseworthy.
Custom	The custom of early marriage used to be popular.
Habit	Drinking is a bad habit.
Cheat	He cheated me of two rupees.
Deceive	Do not try to deceive your teacher by telling lies.
Childish	He has childish habits.
Childlike	His childlike ways are appealing.
Conscious	I am conscious of my shortcomings.

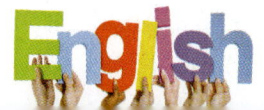

Conscientious	He is a conscientious worker.
Clean	He is neat and clean in his dress.
Clear	There is a spring of clear water nearby.
Continuous	It rained continuously for two hours.
Continual	He is continually coming late.
Cold	After the fall of snow it has been very cold here.
Cool	A cool breeze is blowing today, bringing relief to many.
Contagious	Small-pox is a contagious disease.
Infectious	Her laughter was very infectious.
Contented	He leads a contented life.
Satisfied	He was satisfied with what we gave him.
Cloth	Cloth is manufactured at Ahmedabad.
Clothes	He always wears fashionable clothes.
Corporal	Corporal punishment is forbidden in schools.
Corporeal	Angels are not corporeal beings.
Deadly	It was a deadly wound.
Deathly	She became deathly pale during her illness.
Deny	He denied having told a lie.
Refuse	He refused to lend me money.
Devoted	He is devoted to village service.
Addicted	He is addicted to drinking.
Discover	Columbus discovered America.
Invent	Edison invented a gramophone.
Explore	David Livingstone explored Africa.
Drown	The ship sank and all the sailors were drowned.
Sink	Wood cannot sink in water.
Doubt	I doubt his honesty.
Suspect	I suspect that my servant has stolen my purse.
Delightful	We had a delightful trip to the hills.
Delicious	He served us a very delicious dinner.

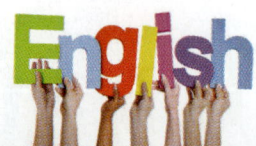

Freedom	Freedom is our birthright.
Liberty	India is fighting for liberty.
Famous	Browning was a famous poet.
Notorious	He is a notorious dacoit.
Farther	The train moved farther and farther away from the station.
Further	Do you have anything further to say on this matter?
Fetch	Please fetch me a glass of water.
Bring	Bring your camera when you come.
Graceful	He is a man of graceful bearing.
Gracious	God is gracious and merciful to all.
Hear	We heard a noise outside.
Listen	Listen to what I say.
Hope	He hopes to get through the examination every year.
Expect	We expect him this evening.
House	He has built a house of his own.
Home	There is no place like home.
Ice	There are many ice factories.
Snow	The high mountains are always full of snow.
Idle	I have been idle for the last two months waiting for work.
Lazy	My dog is too lazy to come the first time I call him.
Ill	He is ill with fever.
Sick	Florence Nightingale looked after the sick and injured.
Sickly	He is a sickly child.
Imaginary	His fears were imaginary.
Imaginative	He is an imaginative poet.
Industrious	He is a very industrious boy.
Industrial	Industrial education is the crying need of India.
Judicial	He intends joining the judicial service.
Judicious	He has made a judicious selection of books.

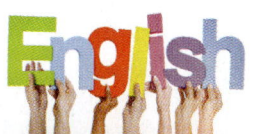

Kind	It is very kind of you to help me now.
Kindly	Kindly refer to the paragraph on page three.
Luxurious	The prince led a luxurious life.
Luxuriant	The Himalayas are covered with luxuriant forests.
Lovely	The rose is a lovely flower.
Loving	This is a letter from my loving sister.
Lovable	He is a man of lovable nature.
Momentary	The joys of this world are momentary.
Momentous	Many momentous problems were discussed at the conference.
Neglect	He was fined for neglect of duty.
Negligence	You must suffer for your negligence.
Part	He divided his property into three equal parts.
Portion	She received a good portion out of her father's property.
Physics	Nowadays we are studying physics in class.
Physique	He is a young man of sound physique.
Remember	I do not remember your name.
Recollect	I cannot recollect what you told me last month.
Respectable	He belongs to a respectable family.
Respectful	We must be respectful to our elders.
Respective	Now go to your respective classes to meet new friends.
Rob	The traveller was robbed at gunpoint of what be had.
Steal	The thieves stole everything in the house during the night.
Sensible	He is a sensible young man.
Sensitive	My eyes are sensitive to light.
Social	We must observe social customs.
Sociable	He is a sociable man.
Stop	The train has stopped.
Stay	Will you stay with me tonight?
Strict	Our teacher is a strict disciplinarian.
Severe	He was suffering from severe pain.

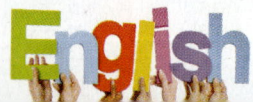

Union	The trade union was able to unite the workers.
Unity	Our Premier is trying to bring about Hindu-Muslim unity.

Walk	We went out for a, walk.
March	The soldiers marched to the battle.
Weather	After the rain, there was fine weather.
Climate	I do not like the Bengal climate.

SOME MORE IMPORTANT WORDS THAT ARE OFTEN CONFUSED

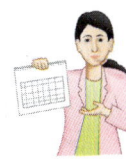

Reply-Answer

A reply is an answer in which an opinion is expressed. An answer is given to a question and contains only the information required.

1. The counsel for the defendant replied that the arguments used against his client were false.
2. The witness answered that he was present at the time of the crime.

Haste-Hurry

Haste denotes quickness or urgency of action. Hurry denotes confusion and want of collected thought.

1. I made haste to reach the station on time.
2. In my hurry to catch the train, I forgot my purse.

Robber-Thief

A robber comes and openly plunders, or takes away our property by brute force. A thief secretly does his job and takes away things by stealth.

1. The traveller was stopped on the road-side by the robbers.
2. The thieves broke into our house in our absence.

Sin-Crime-Vice

Offence against the commands of God is sin. Offence against law is crime, and a habitual offence against morality is vice.

1. To tell a lie is a sin.
2. Murder is a crime.
3. Gambling is a vice.

Big-Large-Great

Strictly speaking, big means of large size, bulk or extent. Large means of great breadth or comprehensiveness, and great means of importance, eminence or distinction.

1. The rat was too big to be swallowed by the snake.
2. A large house was given to guests. Or a large army was sent against the rebels.
3. Rabindranath Tagore was a great poet.

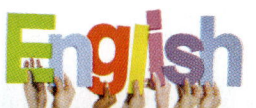

High-Tall-Lofty

High is opposed to 'low' and means extending upward tall is opposed to 'short' and means high as compared with others of kind. Lofty means of great or of imposing altitude.

1. Our country is bounded on the north by high hills.
2. She is the taller of the two sisters. Or What a tall person.
3. The Qutub Minar is a lofty building.

Reason-Cause

Reasons are logical; causes are natural. We give reason for actions; and causes for things.

1. There is reason in what you say.
2. The cause of the accident is not known.

Impracticable-Impossible

Impracticable means that which cannot be put into practice or accomplished by human skill. What is contrary to the laws of nature or to common sense is impossible.

1. We abandoned the plan, as it was found to be impracticable.
2. It is impossible that two and two should make anything but four.

Vacant-Empty

Vacant is that which requires something in it. Empty is that which has nothing in it.

1. The front seats were left vacant for the distinguished guests.
2. Empty vessels make much noise.

Servant-Slave

The servants serve their masters for wages according to some but slaves are servants deprived of all liberty or choice. Slaves can be bought and sold.

1. She was a maid servant at a hotel.
2. There were many slaves in the West Indies.

To forgive-To pardon

Small offences are forgiven between those of the same condition in life. Pardon are granted for serious offences by those in authority to their inferiors.

1. We forgave each other after the quarrel.
2. The king pardoned the rebels.

To see-To look

To see is to use the eyes. To look is to see a particular object.

1. We must see if our eyes are open, but we must make up our mind to look at a thing.
2. On looking at the picture, I saw that the paint was still wet.

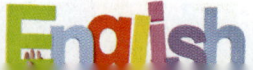

A fault-A mistake

A fault usually has in it something morally wrong; a mistake is simply an error due to carelessness or ignorance.

1. It is a great fault to allow children to have their own way all the time.
2. It is a mistake to trust a stranger.

To avenge-To revenge

We avenge others; we take revenge for ourselves

1. I will avenge the insult of my brother.
2. I will take my revenge on him.

Cost-Price-Value

Cost is money paid by the purchaser for a thing, price is demanded by the seller. Value is what the article is considered to be worth.

1. This book cost me two hundred and fifty rupees.
2. The bookseller demanded a higher price.
3. Its price is two hundred and fifty rupees, but the value of the book is much less.

Boots-Shoes

A boot is a covering for the foot and the lower part.
A shoe is a covering for the foot only.

1. Boots are a part of a soldier's uniform.
2. I have always worn shoes.

Pin-Needle

A pin has a head, it is used for stitching paper; a needle, has an eye, and it is used for sewing clothes.

1. I fastened the pieces of paper with a pin.
2. Will you thread this needle for me?

Bush-Hedge

A bush is a shrub thick with branches. A hedge is a fence or boundary made of bushes.

1. Bushes planted in a line will make a hedge.

Coat-Blazer

A coat is an outer garment for the upper part of the body. A blazer is a light jacket, usually of wool, of silk and of a bright color, for tennis, cricket or other sports.

1. The Old man took off his coat and sat in the sun.
2. Our Cricket Eleven looked smart in their blue blazers.

Bench-Stool

A bench is a long seat and differs from a stool in its length.

1. The spectators in the third class had benches to sit on.
2. Every student is given a stool to sit on in the drawing classroom.

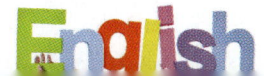

Desk-Table

A table is a simpler article of furniture than a desk. Both have a top for reading or writing; but a desk may have a seat or compartments.

1. I placed books on the table.
2. The children were sitting at their desks.

Telegram-Telephone

Telegram is a message sent by telegraph, an apparatus which communicates at a distance by means of signals. To telephone is to actually speak from a distance. In a telephone, the actual words of the speakers are carried from one end to the other.

1. I received a telegram to the effect that I had passed the examination.
2. I had a talk on the telephone with my friend.

Smile-Laugh

When we laugh, we produce a sound and show a muscular movement of the face. When we smile, there is no sound and very little, if any, muscular movement of the face.

1. The clown was so funny that we could not help laughing.
2. He caught my eye and smiled.

Incident-Accident

Anything that falls or takes place is an incident. All events and occurrences are therefore, incidents. But only unforeseen occurrences of an unfortunate character, where damage is done are accidents.

1. It was the strangest incident of my life.
2. My brother broke his left arm in a motorcycle accident.

Friend-Acquaintance

A friend is an intimate associate; acquaintance is a person who is not very well known to you.

1. I have many acquaintances, but very few friends.

Shade-Shadow

Shade is opposite to light. It means a place sheltered from the sun. Shadow means a figure.

1. This tree gives cool shade.
2. The dog saw his shadow in the water.

Rent-Hire

Rent is a tenant's payment for the use of land or house. Hire is payment for the use of a thing.

1. The rent for this house is two thousand rupees a month.
2. We hired a tonga for one hour.

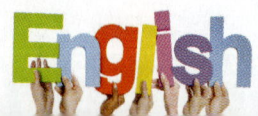

Chapter 19

Phonetics

INTRODUCTION

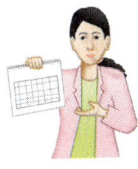

Language has a very important social purpose, because it is mainly used for linguistic communication. Communication is quite possible without the use of language. For example, a dog barks and informs its master of the approach of a stranger. A child cries and informs his/her mother that he/she is hungry, thirsty or uncomfortable. In both the examples we have cited above, communication does take place, but no language is used. Here we will deal with linguistic communication.

A language can be used in two ways for the purposes of communication. It can be *spoken* or *written*. In other words, we can communicate, using the same language, using the spoken *medium* or the written *medium*.

The medium of speech is more important than the medium of writing. This is because speech comes **first** in the history of any language community in fact it came centuries before writing was introduced in the history of any language community. **Secondly**, speech comes first in the history of any individual. We started speaking long before we started writing. **Thirdly**, speech as a medium of communication is used much more than the medium of writing. **Fourthly**, written language is only an attempt to represent the sounds used in spoken language, using marks on paper.

Phonetics is a branch of linguistics and it is the branch dealing with the medium of speech. It deals with the production, transmission and reception of the sounds of human speech.

PHONETICS

Speech is an important medium of communication. The spoken language consists of a succession of varying sounds whereas the written language consists of a succession of marks arranged systematically on a surface of paper or a board. There are specific muscular activities performed in specific medium of communication like we use our lungs, larynx, tongue, teeth, lips and some other organs in the spoken medium of communication and this medium is addressed to the listener's ears. When we use the written medium of communication we use our arm and fingers and the medium is addressed to the reader's eyes. The spoken medium is the aural medium, whereas the written medium is the visual medium of communication. We also communicate with others by use of other mediums of communication, like the medium of touch.

English as spoken by educated people in India does not have much difference from that spoken by the Britishers and the Americans in grammar and vocabulary. But, however, in pronunciation it is different from British English and American English. Phonetics studies are concerned with the spoken medium of communication. In phonetics, we study how production, transmission and reception of the sounds of a particular human language take place. Language learning involves the process of learning to reproduce the sounds and patterns used by other human beings. Each language has its own system. Therefore while learning a language we have to resist the pull of our mother tongue. The learning of the spoken medium is very important because it is used more than the written language. The written language is based on representing the sounds with the help of signs or symbols. There is a relationship between the sounds and symbols representing these letters. This relationship is not consistent in English. Modern technological developments, like telephone, tape recorder, radio, compact disc system, etc. have also contributed to the importance of the spoken medium of language.

SPEECH MECHANISM

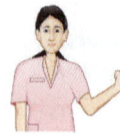

A speech event involves a number of consecutive operations. First a concept is formulated in the brain of a speaker, and then the nerves transmit the linguistic codification of it to the speech organs. The speech organs are set in motion and the movements setup disturbances in the air and the listener receives these sound waves. His or her nervous system then carries the message to the brain where it is interpreted in linguistic terms and the communication takes place.

To speak, we use a special mechanism to produce sound with the help of an **energiser, avibrator and resonators (Fig. 1)**. The energiser is the exhaled breath, the vocal cords act as the vibrator and the resonators are the passages of the throat, mouth and nose. The airstream when passes from lungs through windpipe to the mouth or the nose it produces sound. When the airstream passes through the mouth or the oral passage, oral sounds are produced. When it passes through the nose or the nasal passage, the nasal sounds are produced.

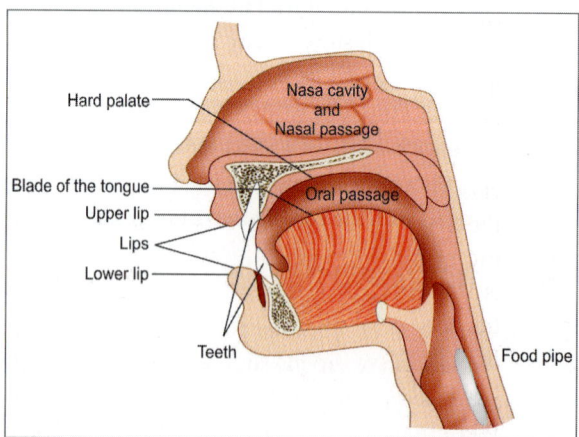

Fig. 1: Speech organs

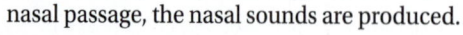
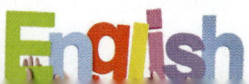

Organs of Speech

The organs of speech can be divided into three groups:

1. The respiratory system which consists of the lungs, the muscles of the chest and the wind pipe.
2. The phonatory system which consists of the pharynx and the larynx.
3. The articulatory system which consists of the nose, mouth, the tongue, the teeth, the root of the mouth and the lips, etc.

The Pharynx

It is a tube which begins just above the larynx. At its top it is divided into two parts, one part being the back of the mouth and the other being the beginning of the way through the nasal cavity.

The Larynx

These are two vocal cords which are like a pair of lips, placed horizontally from front to back. The larynx is at the top of the wind pipe through which the air stream comes after it is released by the lungs. They are joined in the front but separated at the back. The opening between them is called *glottis*.

The vocal cords are held loosely together. The pressure of the air stream coming from the lungs makes them vibrate. The vibration of vocal cards produces sound. The frequency of vibration is the number of times the vocal cords open and close. The frequency of vibration determines the pitch of the voice.

The Soft Palate

The roof of the mouth can be divided into three parts: the teeth ridge, the hard palate and the soft palate. The part which is just behind the teeth is called the teeth ridge or the alveolar ridge. It is a hard convex surface behind the upper front teeth. The hard concave surface that follows the teeth ridge is called the hard palate. The back part of the root is called the soft palate or the vellum. The end of the soft palate is called the uvula.

The soft palate can be lowered to open the nasal passage, or it can be moved up or raised to close the nasal passage. When the nasal passage is closed, the sounds that are produced with the air stream escaping through the oral passage, are called the oral sounds. All English sounds except the sounds—m, n and k as in me, not and king are oral sounds. When the nasal passage is open and if simultaneously the oral passage is blocked closing the lips or by some part of the tongue making a firm contact with some part of the roof of the mouth, the air stream coming from lungs passes through the nasal passage. Such types of sounds are called nasal sounds. If both of the passages are open for air stream to escape from both the passages, the sounds thus produced are called *nasalized sounds*.

The Tongue

The surface of the tongue is divided into four parts: the tip or the extreme end of the tongue, the blade or the part that lies opposite the teeth ridge, the front or the part which lies opposite

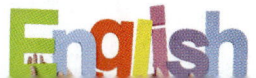

to the hard palate and the back or the part which lies opposite to the soft palate. The tongue can take up different positions to articulate different vowel and consonantal sounds in the production sounds. For example, to produce vowel sounds, we generally keep the tongue low, whereas some other part of the tongue is raised towards the roof of the mouth.

The Lips

The lips play an important role in the articulation of some of the consonantal sounds. The lips can be tightly shut or loosely brought together or kept with a narrow gap in between or drawn apart. The lips also assume different positions for articulating different vowel sounds. They can be spread, neutral, open or rounded. It is convenient to use the phonetic symbols suggested by the International. Phonetic Association to represent the sounds of speech.

CLASSIFICATION OF SOUNDS

Vowel Sounds

Vowels	Pure vowels of short vowels or weak vowels	Monophthongs short, strong vowels with single sound	Diphthongs combination of strong and weak vowel glides closing diphthongs
			/fu/
			/ai/
Front	/i/	/ i: /	/ei/
Vowels	/e/		/au/
	/ae/		/fi/
Central	/f/	/3: /	Central Diphlongs
			/if /
Vowels	/A/		/ef/
Back	/u/	/u:/	/uf/
Vowels	/f/	/a:/	

There are twenty distinct vowel sounds in British Received Pronunciation (RP). Received pronunciation implies a form of English, i.e., Educated Southern British English is socially well received in all over the world. There are twelve pure vowels or monophthongs. They are pure vowels because in their production the point of articulation does not change.

The diphthongs are so called because in their production the tongue glides from one point of articulation to another.

The Figure 2 depicts the mouth. The positions closed, half-closed, half-open and open are the positions of the mouth during the articulation of the vowel sounds. They also are the pointers to the position of the tongue at the time of articulation of these sounds. The pure vowels are shown in figure as the points denoting the exact places from where the sounds are produced.

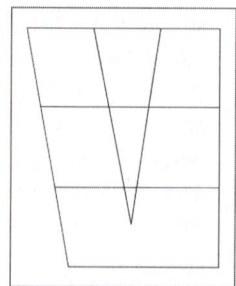

Fig. 2: Positions of month during articulation of vowel sound

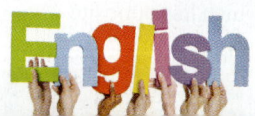

In the articulation of the vowels any part of the tongue can be raised towards the root of the mouth. There are different degrees of the raising of the tongue for the articulation of different vowels. The vowels for which the front part of the tongue is used are called the **front vowels**, for which it is the central part they are called the **central vowels** and for which if the back part of the tongue is used these are called **back vowels**. According to the degree of Figure 3.

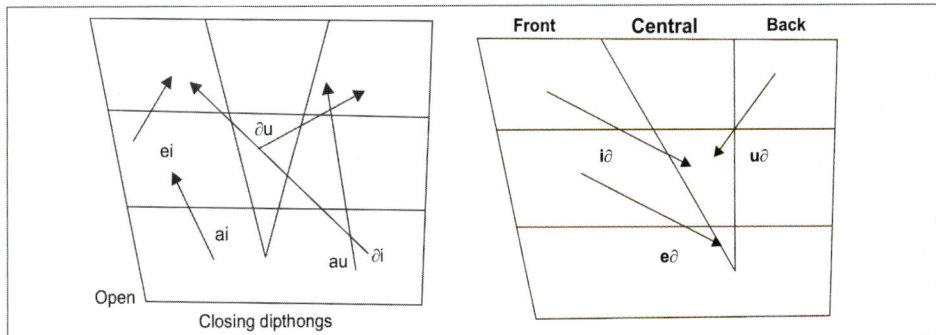

Fig. 3: Articulation of pure vowels (left) articulation of front, central back vowels (right)

In the production of vowels, the air stream from the lungs comes out continuously through the mouth. During their articulation the vocal cords vibrate. In articulating vowel sounds there is no closure of the air passage. Nor is there any narrowing of the passage which would cause friction. The notes produced by the larynx are modified by the resonating cavities of the pharynx, the mouth and the nose. They are further dependent on the positions of the soft palate, the tongue and the lips. The vowels get nasalized in the environment of nasal sounds.

Consonantal Sounds

In the production of consonantal sounds there is an audible friction due to the narrowing of the air passage and there are modifications too due to the different positions of soft palate, tongue, lips, etc. The consonantal sounds are also **voiced** and **voiceless** depending upon position of vocal cords. If they are drawn closer they vibrate. If they are drawn apart they do not vibrate when aggressive (coming out) lung air passes through them. In the articulation of consonantal sounds stricture has also an important role apart from the place of articulation and the manner of articulation. The stricture involves different ways in which the air passage is restricted. In the stricture of complete closure, the active and passive articulators make a firm contact with each other ([p], [b]). The passive articulators are 'the upper lip, the upper teeth, the root of the mouth' (the teeth ridge, hard palate, soft palate) and the back wall of the throat or pharynx. The active articulators are the lower lip and the tongue. The closure is also done when the soft palate is raised and air cannot pass through the nasal passage either. Sometimes the tongue makes a firm contact with the part of the root of the mouth just behind the teeth ridge ([t], [d]). The stricture of complete closure also takes place when the back of the tongue makes a firm contact against the soft palate ([k],[K]). The stricture may be of complete oral closure ([y]). There can be intermittent closure between the passive and active articulators, causing vibration of the active articulators ([r]). For some consonants the active articulator strikes the passive articulator just

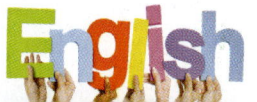

once (r in English phonetics, *very*). The stricture can be of **close approximation** in which the articulators are brought very close leaving a narrow space between them causing the air stream pass with an audible friction. The stricture can be of the **contact of articulators** at the centre of the vocal tract causing air stream to pass through sides called lateral passage ([l]): The stricture can be of **open approximation** in which although two articulators are brought to each other, there is a wide gap between the two ([i], [w]). Consonants are classified on the basis of the place of articulation and the manner of articulation.

Place of Articulation

Bilabial – Articulation by two lips

Labiodental – Articulation by the lower lip against the upper teeth

Dental – Articulation by the tip of the tongue against the upper teeth

Alveolar – Articulation by the tip or the blade of tongue against the back of the teeth ridge

Post alveolar – Articulation by the tip of the tongue against the back of the teeth ridge

In several languages there is no 'one-to-one' correspondence between the letters of the alphabet and the sounds they represent and English being a notorious example. A child who learns that the letters 'ch' in the word *chin* have to be pronounced in a certain way will get into trouble if he pronounces the *same two letters 'ch' in the word machine* the same way as he was taught to pronounce the *ch* in *chin*. His concentration will grow worse if later on he is introduced to a word like *character* in which the same two letters *ch* represent a sound totally different from the *ch* in *chin* and the *ch* in *machine*.

The letter '*c*' represents a certain sound in the word *scale* and the same letter represents a different sound in *cease*. The letter '*g*' is pronounced differently in *give* and *gin*. The letter '*j*' is pronounced like the letter g in *gin*. The letters '*gh*' are pronounced differently in *ghost* and *cough*. The same two letters '*gh*' aren't pronounced at all in a word like *bough*, '*gh*' in *cough*, '*f*' in *fun*, if in *coffee* and '*ph*' in *physics* are pronounced exactly alike! The letter '*l*' in film is pronounced whereas it is not pronounced at all in *palm and calm*. The letters '*ee*' in *see*, '*ea*' in *sea*, '*i*' in *machine* and *police* are pronounced alike. *Key* and *quay* are pronounced alike. How many unnecessary letters are there in the English word *queue*!

In English, therefore, one letter of the alphabet stands for more than one sound and conversely, the same sound is represented by different letters of the alphabet. This problem of non-existence of a one-to-one relationship between spelling and pronunciation is not something that is peculiar to English. In French, for example, the final letter '*p*' is not pronounced in the word like *drap* or 'cloth' nor is the final letter '*e*' pronounced in a word like *dame*, i.e., 'lady'. In Hindi, the letter (ओ) is pronounced like the *ow* in the English word *cow* when it is pronounced in isolation (during alphabet recitation, for example) but the same letter (ओ) is not pronounced like the *ow* in *cow* in a word like (और).

While analysing speech, we will have to consider units higher than individual speech sounds. A word is made up of one or more syllables. It is perhaps fairly easy to point out with a fair amount of accuracy how many syllables a given word has. What is more difficult is to

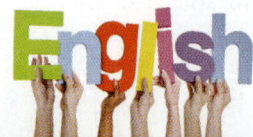

delimit the syllable, i.e., to say precisely where one syllable ends and the next begins in a given word which has several syllables. Words like *girl, bay, shirt, came, go, ant, up, cut, bus* and *bill* have one syllable each. They are also called monosyllabic words. Hindi words like, (एक) 'one' (सब) 'all', (बस) 'enough', (कुछ) 'a little' and (काम) 'work' are also monosyllabic. Words like *teacher* and *doctor* have two syllables each; *remember* has three syllables; *population* has four and *examination* has five.

Usually syllable division is marked with a hyphen thus; *tai-lor*; *cu-cum-ber*; *pen-cil*; *re-mark*; *be-com-ing*; *po-pu-la-tion*; *pho-ne-tics* and so on. It should be pointed out here that it is not always possible to mark syllable-division in the orthographic representation (spelling form) of English words for example, *example* is an *English* word which has three syllables. The letter in this word represents two sounds, [g] and [z]. In the pronunciation of several English speakers, the [g] is part of the first syllable and the [z] part of the second syllable. How can we mark syllable-division then? It is therefore better to write a phonetic transcription of words and mark syllable-division in the transcribed versions of words. Some examples are given below:

Mispronounce	mis-prə-nauns
Cigarette	si-gə-ret
Possibility	po-sə-bi-li-ti
Captain	kæp-tin
Relationship	ri-lei-ʃn-ʃip
Computation	kɔm-pju-tei-ʃn

We said earlier on that it is not always easy to point out where one syllable ends and where the next one begins. For example, the word *cigarette* is to be divided as:/si-gə-ret/or/sig- ə-ret/? Is *teacher* to be divided/ti: tʃə/or/ti:tʃ -ə/? There are no hard and fast rules regarding the way in which a word is divided into syllables as long as our syllable-division does not violate any rules of the phonology of the language in question. The word *examination*, for example, cannot be divided as /i/gzæ/mi/nei/ʃn / because in such a division, the consonants '/g/' and '/z/' occur together initially in the second syllable and English does not permit these two consonants to begin a syllable.

THE ENGLISH VOWELS

Given below are the phonetic symbols used to transcribe the vowels of English. It should be pointed out that the vowels listed below are those that occur in one type of British English. We shall discuss this and one other type of English.

The second point to note is that several systems of transcriptions are available for English.

While transcribing English words of more than one syllable, the syllable that is pronounced more prominently than the other syllables in the same word (the syllable which receives the accent) has to be marked. We shall discuss the concept of word-accent also. Here let us learn how to mark the accented syllable. A phonetic transcription is incomplete without marking word-accent. There is no need of marking this in monosyllabic words.

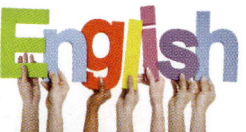

The word is a linguistic entity composed of one or more phonemes. The words '*I*,' '*oh*', consist of one phoneme each. The diphthong '/ai/' and '/əu/' respectively. The words *bee* and *saw* have two phoneme each /b/ and /i:/ and /s/ and /ɔ:/ respectively. The words *cat* and *big* have three phonemes each '/k/, æ/ and /t/' and 'b/, /i/ and /g/' respectively. The words *crack* and *train* have four phonemes each '/k/, /r/, /æ/' and '/k/ and /t/, /r/', /ei/ and /n/, respectively. The words blast and friend have five phonemes each—/b/, /1/, /a:/ /s/' and /t/ and /f/, /r/ /e/, /n/ and /d/ Though the words cited above have different number of phonemes each. All of them have one syllable each and all of them are monosyllabic words.

There are a number of words in every language which have more than one syllable. The English words *tailor* and *teacher* have two syllables each. The second syllable in these words have the vowel /ə/.

	Symbol	Key Word with the Letters
Pure Vowels	i:	Bead
	i	Bid
	e	Bed
	æ	Bad
	a:	Bard
	ɔ	Cot
	ɔ:	Caught
	u	Book
	u:	Boot
	ʌ	Cup
	ə:	Heard
	ə	About
Diphthons	ei	Play
	ai	Ply
	ɔ i	Boy
	əu	Go
	au	Now
	iə	Near
	uə	Poor
	ɛə	Hair

WHAT IS WORD STRESS?

Stress within a word and in a sentence is an important aspect of English speech. A world can be divided into segments which are called syllables. Each syllable usually has a vowel. A word can be monosyllabic or polysyllabic. The syllable which is used with greater breath force gains more prominence and has the accent, which is indicated by a vertical mark above the syllable.

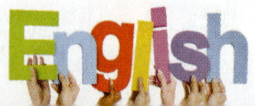

Mono Syllabic Words

[1]Time

[1]burst

be [1]gun (2)

ill .[1]ness (2)

[1]tea.cher (2)

[1]fam.i.ly (3)

be.[1]gi.nning (3)

[1]con.sci.ous (3)

[1]ab.so.lute.ly (4)

The English stress pattern is fixed and can fall on any syllable of the word. For example.

[1]Melancholy	(Stress on the 1st syllable)
Re[1]markable	(Stress on the 2nd syllable)
Diplo[1]matic	(Stress on the 3rd syllable)
Impossi[1]bility	(Stress on the 4th syllable)
Personifi[1]cation	(Stress on the 5th syllable)
[1]advertise	(Primary accent on the *first* syllable)
Ad[1]vertisement	(Primary accent on the *second* syllable)
ex[1]amine	(Primary accent on the *second* syllable)
exami[1]nee	(Primary accent on the *third* syllable)
exami[1]nation	(Primary accent on the *fourth* syllable)
in[1]ferior	(Primary accent on the *second* syllable)
inferi[1]ority	(Primary accent on the *fourth* syllable)
[1]photograph	(Primary accent on the *first* syllable)
pho[1]tographer	(Primary accent on the *second* syllable)
photo[1]graphic	(Primary accent the *third* syllable)
[1]politics	(Primary accent the *first* syllable)
po[1]litical	(Primary accent on the *second* syllable)
poli[1]tician	(Primary accent on the *third* syllable)
res[1]ponsible	(Primary accent on the *second* syllable)
responsi[1]bility	(Primary accent on the fourth syllable)

Pronouncing every word correctly leads to poor pronunciation. Good pronunciation comes from stressing the right words. This is because English is a time stressed language. The non-stressed words and syllables are often 'swallowed' in English. Always focus on pronouncing stressed words well, non-stressed words can be glided over. We need not focus on pronouncing

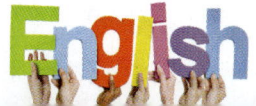

each word. Focus on the stressed words in each sentence. Understanding word stress, helps to understand syllables. Each word is made from syllables. Each word has one, two, three or more syllables.

Word		No. of Syllables
Dog	Dog	1
Green	Green	1
Quite	Quite	1
Quiet	Qui-et	2
Orange	Or-ange	2
Table	Ta-ble	2
Expensive	Ex-pen-sive	3
Interesting	In-ter-est-ing	4
Realistic	Re-al-is-tic	4
Unexceptional	Un-ex-cep-tion-al	5

It is difficult to learn the stress pattern through theoretical rules but repeated listening to the language would give a general idea. When a word has two or more syllables, one of them has the main stress. In these examples the main stress follows the symbol:

'¹acent, pre'fer, edu¹ cation, ¹necessary, Ja'pan and Japa'nese'. If you put the stress on the wrong syllable it may be difficult for listeners to understand what you are saying. There are many words in English where a letter is not pronounced like fasten, plumber, calm, knee, wrong and comb. There are also many words' where we almost 'eat' one of the syllables and as a result a vowel sound almost disappears and a word, for example, with three written syllables may be two or two and a half in spoken English.

FAculty	FANtasy	FElony
Filament	FORmula	FREquency
GARrison	GEnesis	Government
GOvernor	HARbinger	HARmony`
HOroscope	HOSpital	hyPOcrisy
HyPOthesis	IGnorance	INcident
INdustry	INfluence	INstrument
INterval	INterview	JUpiter
KErosence	LAByrinth	LEprosy
LuKEmia	LIBerty	LITera
LUnacy	MAINtenance	MAjesty
MAnager	MERcury	MESsenger
MInister	MInistry	NIGHtingale
Nitrogen	NOvelty	Orient

Contd...

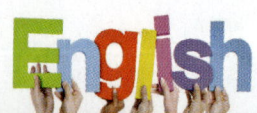

ORnament	Origin	ORthodox
PAnama	PANcreas	PAradise
PAradox	PAragraph	PArallel
paRAlysis	PArasite	PArody
PARticle	PASsenger	PEnalty
PRophecy	PROtestant	PYramid
REgiment	Register	REmedy
REvenue	RHEtoric	ROYalty
SAbotage	SAcrifice	SCHOlarship
secreTAriat	SEMinar	SIGnature
SYLlable	SYLlabus	SYMpathy
SYMphony	SYNthesis	TElephone
TEMperature	TYranny	Uniform
uRAnium	Uterus	VAcancy
VAlency	verNAcular	Video

NOUNS (WITH MAIN STRESS ON THE PENULTIMATE SYLLABLE)

ABsence	Adult	ADVerb	DUplex	Echo	ecoNOmics
ADvent	aGENda	Agent	emPLOYment	enCLOsure	ENtrance
AlBIno	Any	appaRAtus	ENzyme	Ethos	Evening
ARchives	aROma	asBEStos	eXAMple	exPOsure	fiANce
atTORney	baNANa	BENzene	fiASco	FORmat	forMIca
BENzine	BIceps	Bishop	FRIgate	FURlong	GADget
CArol	caTHEdral	CAthode	HARvest (n,v)	HAzard	haemoGLObin
CERtain	CLImate	COMfort	HONey	hoRIzon	HUman
CObalt	comMITtee	COMpass	HUNdred	Husband	HYgiene
COMplex	comPUter	conDUCtor	iDEa	Image	INcome
COLleague	COLlege	comPARTment	INdex	INsect	INset
CONsort	conSULtant	CONvent	InsPECtor	insurance	INterest
CONvoy	corresPONdence	CREdence	InTEStine	ISland	JUDGEment
CREScent	CREole	CYclone	KNOWledge	LAdy	LIbel
CYMbal	deCOrum	dePARture	LIcence	LINGuist	LUGgage
DePENdant	dePOsit	deTERgent	lieuTEnant	MAGnet	MERchant
diagNOsis	DIAlect	DIAlogue	MOment	moMENtum	MOney
DIFference	dipLOma	diRECtor	MORtar	MOUNtain	MUsic

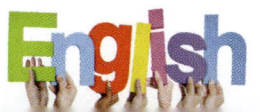

MUStard	MUTton	NECtar
neuROsis	N Itrate	NOmad
NONsense	NOthing	NOtice
noVEMber	NUIsance	NYlon
oAsis	obSERver	ORphan
paGOda	paPAya	PArent
PEAcock	PEnance	PEon
PERfurme	PETrol	PHYsics
PILLar	PIvot	PORtrait
poTAto	PREfect	PREference
PRElude	PREview	PROduct
proFESsor	proPRIEtor	PROverb
PROvince	RAdar	SAlad
SAtire	SCHEdule	SEnate

SERgeant	SERvant	SIlence
soCIEty	SOMEthing	sucCESsor
SYMbol	TARmac	THUN der
TOFfee	toMAto	TOpaz
triBUnal	TRI bute	TRIbune
TRIumph	TYphoid	TYrant
Ulcer	ultiMAtum	umBRELla
Umpire	uRAnus	Urine
Usage	uTENsil	VACcine
vaNILla	VIcar	VILlage
VINtage	Visa	Visit
volCAno	VOlume	VORtex
VOYage	WARrant	WINdow
PROtein		

NOUNS (WITH MAIN STRESS ON THE FINAL SYLLABLE)

aBUSE(n,v)	acCOUNT	afterNOON
asCENT	asSAULT	asSENT
atTACK (n,v)	atTEMPT (n,v)	balLoon
baTIK	baBOON	baZAAR
berLIN	braZIL	beLIEF
briGADE	caNAL	chimpanZEE
conCEIT	conCERN (n,v)	conTROL (n,v)
deCEIT	deFENCE	deGREE
deLAY (n,v)	deLIGHT (n,v)	desCENT
deSIGN	desSERT	deTENTE
deVICE	disGRACE	disGUISE (n,v)
disGUST (n,v)	disPUTE(n,v)	disSENT (n,v)
exCUSE (n,v)	faTIGUE	guiTAR
jaPAN	kangaROO	laGOON
laMENT (n,v)	maNURE	maDRID
misTAKE (n,v)	noBEL	ofFENCE
oK	poLICE	ratioNALE
reCEIPT	reCLUSE	reCOURSE
reCRUIT (n,v)	reGRET (n,v)	ReQUEST (n,v)
reTURN (n,v)	reVOLT (n,v)	routine
saLOON	susPENSE	taBOO

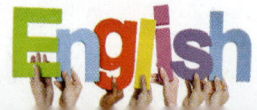

VERBS (WITH MAIN STRESS ON THE PENULTIMATE SYLLABLE)

aBOlish	adMOnish	apPEar
asSEMble	astonish	BELow
conSIder	conTInue	deLIver_
dePOsit (n,v)	deTERmine	deVElop
diMInish	disCOver	disTEMper
disTINguish	disTRIbute	Edit
eLIcit	emBArrass	enCIRcle
enDANger	Enter	esTABlish
exAmine	exHIbit (n,v)	Exile (n,v)
exTINguish	FInance (n,v)	FInish
FLOUrish	FOREcast (n,v)	GOvern
HARvest (n,v)	HIjack (n,v)	iMAgine
inHAbit	inHErit	inHIbit
INjure	inTERpret	LIcense (n,v)
OFfer	ORder	PErish
PROfit	proHIbit	PROmise
PROSper	PUBlish	PUnish
PURchase	reMEMb¢r	reOpen
rePLEnish	REvel	SIlence (n,v)
surRENder	SWALlow (n,v)	TRESpass (n,v)
TRIumph (n,v)	VIsit (n,v)	

VERBS (WITH MAIN STRESS ON THE FINAL SYLLABUS)

aBIDE	absorb	abSTAIN	creATE	creMATE	deCAY
accept	acQUIT	adJUST	deCIDE	deCLARE	deCLINE (v,a)
adMIRE	adMIT	afFECT	deCREE (n,v)	deFER	deFINE
AGREE	appreHEND	arRANGE	deLAY	deLETE	deMAND (n,v)
arREST	asSESS	atTEST	deNY	deNOTE	deRIVE
augMENT	beGET	beGIN	deTEST	dicTATE	disARM
beHAVE	capSIZE	caREER	disCERN	disCUSS	disRUPT
caRESS	colLAPSE	com MIT	disSECT	disSOLVE	diVERGE
conCEAL	conCEDE	conCEIVE	diVORCE	diVULGE	eLECT
conCLUDE	conCUR	conDENSE	emBRACE	eMERGE	eMIT
conDOLE	conFER	conFESS	emPLOY	enCLOSE	enJOY
conFIDE	conFINE	conFIRM	enLARGE	eQUIP	esCAPE (n,v)
conFORM	conFOUND	conFRONT	exACT (v,a)	exCHANGE (n,v)	eXHAUST (n,v)
conFU SE	conNECT	conSIST	exIST	exPEL	exPLAIN
conSTRAIN	conTEST	contraDICT	eXPLODE	exPLOIT	exPLORE
conVENE	conVERT	conVEY	exPRESS (v,a)	exTRACT	foMENT
ConVINCE	CorRECT (v,a)	corRUPT (v,a)	forBID	forGET	forGIVE

Contd...

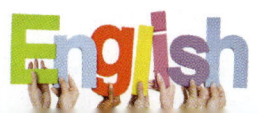

forSAKE	igNORE	imBIBE	proVOKE	purSUE	reBUKE (n,v)
imPAIR	imPRESS	imPRINT	reCALL (n,v)	reCEIVE	recomMEND
imPROVE	inCLINE	inCLUDE	recolLECT	reCUR	reDRESS
InDENT	inDI CT	inDUCE	reFER	reFLECT	reGRET (n,v)
inDUCT	inFECT	inFER	reLENT	reLEASE	reLIEVE
inFEST	inFLICT	inFORM	reLIVE	reLY	reMAIN
insPECT	insPIRE	insTALL	reMARK (n,v)	eMIT	reMOVE
inTEND	interCEPT	interSECT	reNEW	rePAY	rePEAT
introDUCE	inVENT	inVEST	rePORT (n,v)	reSIST	resPECT (n,v)
inVITE	laMENT (n,v)	mainTAIN	reSULT (n,v)	reVENGE (n,v)	reVIEW (n,v)
misbeHAVE,	misGUIDE	misLEAD	reVOLT (n,v)	reWARD (n,v)	saLUTE (n,v)
misRULE (n,v)	misUSE (n,v)	obLIGE	seDUCE	seLECT (v,a)	subMIT
obSERVE	obTAIN	ocCUR	sugGEST	subVERT	supPLY (n,v)
ofFEND	opPOSE	paTROL	supPRESS	surPASS	surPRISE (n,v)
perCEIVE	porTRAY	posSESS	susPEND	susTAIN	transCEND
preDICT	preFER	preSERVE	transACT	transCRIBE	transFORM
preSUME	pretend	preVENT	transLATE	transMIT	transPLANT
preVAIL	proCLAIM	proCURE	underSTAND	underTAKE	disMISS
proMOTE	proNOUNCE	proVIDE	oMIT	inCUR	

ADJECTIVES (WITH MAIN STRESS ON THE PENULTIMATE SYLLABLE)

aBUNdant	aDEPT	adJAcent	imPAtient	imPORtant	indePENdent
aDULT	aNOther	Any	inSIpid	INStant (a,n)	LAtent
BACKward	BANKrupt	BLAtant	Modern	MOdest	NARrow
BUOyant	CAnine	CERtain	NONsense	PAtient (a,n)	POtent
clanDEStine	CLEment	conVERsant	PUNgent	RAMpant	reDUNdant
CURrent (a,n)	conSIStent	DEcent	reMITtent	SAline	SAvage
deFlant	DIStant	diVERgent	SEcond (n,a,v)	SEnile	SERvile
DORmant	EARnest	FEmale	seVEre	Silent	sinCEre
FERvent	FERtile	FRAgrant	transPArent	URgent	VAcant
HANDsome	HOStile	HUman	VAgrant		

ADJECTIVES (WITH MAIN STRESS ON THE FINALE SYLLABLE)

abRUPT	abSURD	aFRAID	eNOUGH	exPRESS (a,v)	OBESE
asTUTE	comPLETE (a,v)	corRECT (a,v)	obsCURE	obLIQUE	obSCENE
corRUPT (a,v)	deLUXE	deVOUT	poL1TE	preCISE	roMANCE (a,n)
diRECT (a,v)	disTANT	diVINE	seCURE	seRENE	subLIME
			SUPREME		

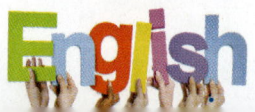

STRESS ON WORDS ENDING IN –al, able,- ible - ous, etc.

aBOminable	aboRIginal	amBItious
ADmirable	adMISsible	AFfable
auTOnomous	aNOmalous	aMEnable
auDAcious	conSIderable	asSIduous
aTROcious	ausPIcious	aVAIlable
CONtinuous	COvetous	CREditable
CULtivable	CUrable	desPIcable
juDIcial	HOnourable	hosPItable
ilLUStrious	imPRESsionable	imPRObable
inAlienable	inaPplicable	inAUdible
gramMAtical	inCALculable	inCApable
inCOMparable	incomPAtible	indisPUtable
inDUStrial	INtegral	INterval
IRresistible	juDIcious	LAmentable
LAUghable	LOVable	MArriageable
mediEval	MIserable	muNIcipal
obJECtionable	PALpable	PAStoral
PItiable	PRACticable	preSENtable
auTHOratative	colLECtive	comMUnicative
comPArative	comPEtitive	compreHENsive
comPULsive	conSERvative	conSEcutive
consTRUCtive	conSULtative	coOperative
coRECTive	corROsive	deCEPtive
deClsive	DEcorative	deFENsive
deFInitive	deMONStrative	deRIsive

deRIvative	desCRIptive	deTECtive
diGEStive	diMInutive	diRECtive
disTINctive	disTRIbutive	eLECtive
eLUsive	eVAsive	exCLUsive
eXEcutive	exPENsive	exTENsive
FiGUrative	ILlustrative/ illUStrative	iMAginative
imperative	imPRESsive	inDIcative
inDUCtive	iNItiative	inSENsitive
intensive	inVECtive	LAXative
LEgislative	locoMOtive	LUcrative
NARrative	NOminative	obJECtive
obsTRUCtive	ofFENsive	OPtative
persPECtive	POsitive	NEgative
preDIcative	preROgative	presCRIptive
preSERvative	preSUMptive	preVENtive
PRImitive	proDUCtive	proGRESsive
proHIbitive	prosPEctive	proTECtive
proVOcative	PUnitive	PURgative
PUtative	RElative	rePEtitive
represENtative	rePULsive	resPECtive
resPONsive	resTOrative	SEdative
reTRIbutive	SEcretive	SPEculative
subMISsive	SUBstantive	sucCESsive
sugGEStive	TENtative	vinDICtive
VOcative		

VOWEL SOUNDS

Observe these sentences:

- ❑ **He is big.**
- ❑ **Please peel the pill.**
- ❑ **Did you deal?**

Vowel sounds can be long or short. Some words carry long sounds and need to be stretched:

- ❑ he
- ❑ please
- ❑ peel
- ❑ deal

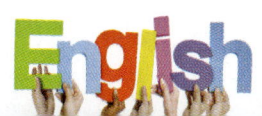

Some words carry short sounds and need to be clipped:
- big
- is
- pill
- did

ih-pronounced 'ih' as in 'hit'	ee - pronounced 'ee' as in 'see'
big	beat
pig	peep
did	deal
tip	teeth
gill	gee
kill	keep
sip	see
zip	zeal
ship	sheet
Gin	jeep
chip	cheek
hit	heat

Vowel sounds can be either open or closed.
- For certain words you need to open your mouth wide, e.g., matter and these are known as open vowels.
- For certain words your mouth remains relatively closed, e.g., medicine and these are known as closed vowels.

eh-pronounced 'eh' as in 'let'	æ - pronounced 'æ' as in 'cat'
bet	bat
Pet	pat
death	dad
tell	tap
get	gap
kept	cat
set	sat
zeppelin	zap
shelf	shaft
jell	jack
chess	chat
help	hat

Practice with these words:

Set	sat
bet	bat
led	lad
bed	bad

ten	tan
lend	land
medal	matter
better	batter

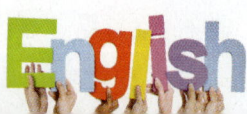

Other Vowel Sounds

'long ah' as in 'heart'	'short ah' as in 'got'
bar	bought
par	paw
dark	dot
tar	taught
Garth	got
carpet	caught
sergeant	saw
Zagreb	Zola
sharp	shawl
John	Jot
charred	chocolate
Heart	hop

'long uh' as in 'put'	'short uh' as in 'up'	'oo' as in 'shoe'
butcher	but	boot
put	pup	proof!
(none)	duck	do
Tokay	tough	tooth
good	gulp	Google
cook	cup	cool
soot	supper	suit
(none)	(none)	zoom
shook	shut	shoot
(none)	jump	June
churn	Chuck	choose
Hook	hup!	who

TRANSCRIPTION

Vowels and Diphthongs

Symbol	Word	Pronunciation
iː	seat	siːt
ɪ	sit	sɪt
e	set	set
æ	sat	sæt
ɑː	card	kɑːd
ɔː	born	bɔːn
ɒ	box	bɒks
ʊ	book	bʊk
uː	boon	bʊːn
ʌ	bus	bʌs

Symbol	Word	Pronunciation
ɜː	bird	bɜːd
ə	bigger	bigə
eɪ	play	pleɪ
ɑɪ	buy	baɪ
ɔɪ	boy	bɔɪ
au	out	aʊt
əu	go	gəʊ
ɪə	here	hɪə
eə	there	ðeə
uə	poor	pʊə

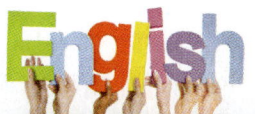

Consonants

1. p	pin	pin	13. s	soon	su:n
2. b	bin	bin	14. z	zoo	zu:
3. t	tin	tin	15. ʃ	shine	ʃain
4. d	din	din	16. ʒ	please	pleʒə
5. k	kin	kin	17. h	help	help
6. g	gun	gʌn	18. m	man	mæn
7. tʃ	church	tʃɜ:tʃ	19. n	neat	ni:t
8. dʒ	jug	dʒʌg	20. ḥ	sing	siŋ
9. θ	thin	θin	21. l	live	liv
10. ∂	that	ðæt	22. w	win	win
11. f	fine	fain	23. r	run	rʌn
12. v	van	væn	24. j	young	jʌŋ

Examples

1. Caps	kæps	26. Go	gəu	51. Texts	teksts
2. Cats	kæts	27. Paper	peipə	52. Kettle	ketl
3. Cooks	kuks	28. Potato	pəteitəu	53. Cattle	kætl
4. Laugh	la:fs	29. Remember	rimembə	54. Little	litl
5. Bulbs	bʌlbz	30. Matter	mætə	55. Subtle	sʌtl
6. Rods	rɔdz	31. Come	kʌm	56. Cotton	kɔtn
7. Bags	bægz	32. Some	sʌm	57. Mutton	mʌtn
8. Loves	lʌvz	33. Gone	gɔn	58. Sudden	sʌdn
9. Pulls	pulʒ	34. Boat	bəut	59. Ridden	ridn
10. Names	neimz	35. State	sleit	60. Have	hæv
11. Keys	ki:z	36. State	steit	61. Does	dʌz
12. Saws	sɔ:z	37. Spin	spin	62. Could	kud
13. Goes	gəuz	38. Stun	stʌn	63. Do	du:
14. Cigarette	sigəret	39. School	sku:l	64. Has	hæs
15. Captain	kæptin	40. Praise	praiz	65. Would	wud
16. Eye	əi	41. Scream	skri:m	66. His	hiz
17. Am	æm	42. Spleen	spli:n	67. Us	ʌs
18. All	ɔ:l	43. Stream	stri:m	68. Who	Hu:
19. Up	ʌp	44. Screen-	skr:n	69. Were	wə
20. Engage	ingeidz	45. Box	bɔks	70. I	əi
21. Ambition	æmbiʃn	46. Fox	fɔks	71. oh!	əu
22. Under	ʌn-də	47. Bond	bɔnd	72. ah!	a:
23. Be	bi:	48. Bold	bəuld	73. ass	æs
24. She	ʃi:	49. Tents	tents	
25. So	səu	50. Bands	bændz	

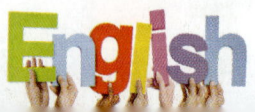

WORDS

74.	Absent	/ 'æbsent /	111.	Right	raɪt	
75.	Concert	/ 'kɔnsət /	112.	Street	striːt	
76.	Conduct	/ 'kɔn,dʌkt /	113.	City	sɪtɪ	
77.	Contact	/ 'kɔn,tækt/	114.	Clean	kliːn	
78.	Contract	/ 'kɔn,trækt/	115.	Have	hæv	
79.	Contrast	/ 'kɔn,traːst/	116.	Leave	liːv	
80.	Convict	/ 'kɔnvikt/	117.	Like	laɪk	
81.	Desert	/'dezət/	118.	Miss	mɪs	
82.	Digest	/ 'daidʒest/	119.	Never	nevə	
83.	Export	/ 'ekspɔːt/	120.	Play	Pleɪ.	
84.	Import	/ 'impɔːt/	121.	Rise	raɪz	
85.	Object	/ 'ɔbdʒikt/	122.	Speak	spɪːk	
86.	Perfect	/ 'pəːfikt/	123.	Start	staːt	
87.	Permit	/ 'Pəmit/	124.	Ride	raɪd	
88.	Present	/ preznt/	125.	Fruit	fruːt	
89.	Produce	/ 'prɔ,duːs/	126.	Eat	iːt	
90.	Categorical	/,kætigorikl/	127.	Tennis	tenis	
91.	Comprehensible	/,kɔmpri'hensəbl/	128.	Baby	beɪbi	
92.	Conventionality	/kɔn,venʃə'næliti/	129.	Cry	kraɪ	
93.	Deposition	/,depə'ziʃn/	130.	Cut	kʌt	
94.	Examination	/ig,zæmi'neiʃn/	131.	Die	daɪ	
95.	International	/,intə'næʃnl/	132.	Lie	laɪ	
96.	Interpolation	/in,tə:pə'leiʃn/	133.	Move	muːv	
97.	Notification	/,nəutifi'keiʃn/	134.	Rain	reɪn	
98.	Passes	/paːsiz/	135.	Read	riːd	
99.	Roses	/rəuziz/	136.	Sit	sɪt	
100.	Edges	/edʒiʒ/	137.	Stay	steɪ	
101.	Bushes	/buʃiz/	138.	Tie	taɪ	
102.	Bag	bæg	139.	White	raɪt	
103.	Bike	baɪk	140.	Fly	flaɪ	
104.	Cold	kauld	141.	Busy	bɪzi	
105.	Dentist	dentɪst	142.	Cost	kest	
106.	Easy	iːzi	143.	Ghost	gaust	
107.	Family	fæmli	144.	Hair	heə	
108.	Happy	hæpɪ	145.	Beer	bɪə	
109.	House	haus	146.	Every	evri	
110.	Ill	ɪl	147.	Hard	haːd	

Contd...

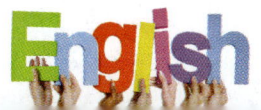

148.	Hate	heɪt
149.	Call	Kɔ:l
150.	Marry	mærɪ
151.	Party	Pa :ti
152.	Letter	letə
153.	Shoe	ʃu:
154.	Bring	brɪŋ
155.	Feel	fɪ:l
156.	Meat	mɪ:t
157.	Stand	stænd
158.	Cake	keɪk
159.	Fast	fa:st
160.	Hat	hæt
161.	Money	mʌnɪ
162.	Find	faɪnd
163.	Stand Up	stænd ʌp
164.	Break	breɪk
165.	Drive	draɪv
166.	Past	Pa:st
167.	Wave	weɪv
168.	Pepper	pepə
169.	Room	ru:m
170.	Sleep	sli:p
171.	Traffic Jam	træfɪk dzæm
172.	Meal	mɪ:l
173.	Bang	bæg
174.	Battery	bætri
175.	Empty	empti
176.	Push	pʊʃ
177.	Engineer	endziniə
178.	Matter	mætə
179.	Steal	sti:l
180.	Biscuit	bɪskɪt
181.	Clap	klæp
182.	Bear	beə
183.	Collar	kelə
184.	Peace	pi:s
185.	Round	raʊnd

186.	Boat	bɔut
187.	Glove	glʌv
188.	Wild	waɪld
189.	Addup	æd ʌp
190.	Ant	ænt
191.	Factory	fæktri
192.	Fried	fraɪd
193.	Doubt	daʊt
194.	Carry	kærɪ
195.	Boot	bu:t
196.	Blood	blʌd
197.	Weight	weɪt
198.	Sister	sistə
199.	Son	sʌn
200.	Wife	waɪf
201.	Baker	beɪkə
202.	Tailor	teɪlə
203.	Cooker	kʊkə
204.	Mirror	mɪrə
205.	Course	Kɔ:S
206.	Fork	Fɔ:K
207.	Suck	sʌk
208.	Knife	naɪf
209.	Leaf	lɪ:f
210.	Life	laɪf
211.	Sheep	ʃi:p
212.	Dry	draɪ
213.	Friendly	frendli
214.	Paper	peɪpə
215.	Rice	raɪs
216.	Stamp	stæmp
217.	Wood	wʊd
218.	Brush	brʌʃ
219.	Seat	sɪ:t
220.	Lucky	lʌki
221.	Push	pʊʃ
222.	Matter	mætə
223.	Steal	sti:l

Contd...

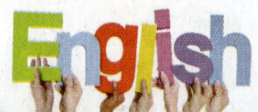

224.	Biscuit	bɪskɪt		263.	Stair	steə
225.	Clap	klæp		264.	Storm	stɔ:m
226.	Bear	beə		265.	Cook	kuk
227.	Handle	hændle		266.	Married	mærid
228.	Race	reɪs		267.	Plan	plæn
229.	Sound	saʊnd		268.	Back	bæk
230.	Tasty	teɪstɪ		269.	Later	leɪtə
231.	Wheel	wi:l		270.	Mine	main
232.	Puppy	pʌpɪ		271.	Dark	da:k
233.	Carpet	ka:pɪt		272.	Free	fri :
234.	Funny	fʌnɪ		273.	Moon	mu:n
235.	Form	fa:m		274.	Soon	su:n
236.	Couple	kʌpl		275.	Heavy	hevi
237.	Cross	kres		276.	Fact	fækt
238.	Desert	dezet		277.	Safe	seɪf
239.	Fancy	fænsi		278.	Kidnap	kidnæp
240.	Blood	blʌd		279.	Mask	ma:sk
241.	Weight	weɪt		280.	Fun	fʌn
242.	Sister	sistə		281.	Might	naɪt
243.	Son	sʌn		282.	Park	pa:k
244.	Wife	waɪf		283.	Sude	ru:d
245.	Baker	beɪkə		284.	Stamp	stæmp
246.	Captain	kæptɪn		285.	Gum	gʌn
247.	Glasses	gla:sɪz		286.	Waste	weɪst
248.	Short	ʃɔ:t		287.	Cool	Ku:l
249.	Team	ti:m		288.	Fat	fæt
250.	Train	treɪn		289.	SIck	sɪk
251.	Lose	lu:z		290.	Sky	skaɪ
252.	Travel	trævl		291.	Food	fu:d
253.	Key	ki:		292.	Milk	mɪlk
254.	Ticket	Tɪkɪt		293.	Pay	peɪ
255.	Centre	Sentə		294.	Laugh	la:f
256.	Foot	fʊt		295.	Bread	bred
257.	Bite	baɪt		296.	Fun	fʌn
258.	Ever	evə		297.	Smile	smaɪl
259.	Since	sɪns		298.	Fizzy	fɪzɪ
260.	Town	taun		299.	Shout	ʃaʊt
261.	Light	lait		300.	Sweet	swi:t
262.	Room	ru:m		301.	Fire	faɪə

Contd...

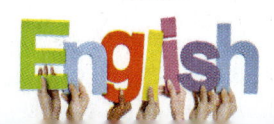

302.	Light	laɪt
303.	Luck	lʌk
304.	Plane	pleɪn
305.	Suit	suːt
306.	Tie	taɪ
307.	Dish	dɪʃ
308.	Feed	fiːd
309.	Tray	treɪ
310.	Bark	baːk
311.	Hook	hʊk
312.	Hunt	hʌnt
313.	Lizard	Lizəd
314.	Traffic Light	traefik lait
315.	Cloudy	klaʊdi
316.	Windy	windi
317.	Crash	kræʃ
318.	Dizzy	dizɪ
319.	Bush	bʊʃ
320.	Fence	fens
321.	Field	fiːld
322.	Guess	ges
323.	Pool	puːl
324.	Chemist	kemist
325.	Track	træk
326.	Rise	raɪz
327.	Dark	daːk
328.	Bride	braid
329.	Friendly	frendlɪ
330.	Groom	gruːm
331.	Sick	sik
332.	Silly	sili
333.	Strike	strɪːk
334.	Thin	θin
335.	Tired	taɪəd
336.	Believe	bɪliːv
337.	Boss	bes
338.	Brave	breɪv
339.	Comfort	kʌmfət
340.	Deep	diːp

341.	Health	helθ
342.	Long	leŋ
343.	Marry	mæri
344.	Vain	veɪn
345.	Ache	eɪk
346.	Briefly	brːfli
347.	Call	Kɔːl
348.	Calmly	kaːmli
349.	Clear	klɪːə
350.	Court	Kɔːt
351.	Deadly	dedli
352.	Elder	eldə
353.	Disease	dɪziːz
354.	Fight	faɪt
355.	Flat	flaet
356.	Hard	haːd
357.	Neat	niːt
358.	Shuttle	ʃʌtl
359.	Survive	səvaɪv
360.	Breath	breθ
361.	Caught	kɔːt
362.	Mad	mæd
363.	Pass	paːs
364.	Spare	speə
365.	Wide	waɪd
366.	Clip	klɪp
367.	Keeper	kiːpə
368.	Lean	liːn
369.	Stick	stɪk
370.	Cash	kæʃ
371.	Credit	kredɪt
372.	Debt	det
373.	Fence	fens
374.	Roof	ruːf
375.	Cry	kraɪ
376.	Death	deθ
377.	Glad	glæd
378.	Great	grːt
379.	Cap	kæp

Contd...

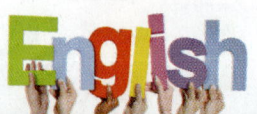

380.	Bust	bʌst
381.	Sleve	sli:v
382.	Wrist	rist
383.	Blood	blʌd
384.	Palm	pa :m
385.	Wear	weə
386.	Crack	kræk
387.	Flu	flu:
388.	Spark	spa:k
389.	Seat	si:t
390.	Cast	ka:st
391.	Knock	nek
392.	Castle	ka:sl
393.	Beef	bi:f
394.	Butter	bʌtə
395.	Grape	greɪp
396.	Lamb	læm
397.	Mix	miks
398.	Peel	pi:l
399.	Plum	plʌm
400.	Slice	slaɪs
401.	Care	keə
402.	Mark	ma:k
403.	Bee	bi:
404.	Blast	bla:st

405.	Crab	kræb
406.	Duck	dʌk
407.	Snake	sneɪk
408.	Gun	gʌn
409.	Nail	neɪl
410.	Pump	pʌmp
411.	Broom	bru:m
412.	Hook	hʊk
413.	Pin	pɪn
414.	Crab	kræb
415.	Damp	dæmp
416.	Puppy	pʌpi
417.	Root	ru:t
418.	Screw	skru:
419.	Zipper	zɪpə
420.	Ruler	ru:lə
421.	Sign	saɪn
422.	Miser	maɪzə
423.	Fool	fu:l
424.	Stamp	stæmp
425.	Staff	sta:f
426.	Weed	wi:d
427.	Snake	sneɪk
428.	Cast	ka:st

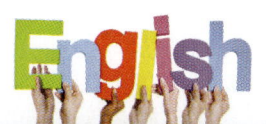

NOTES

Chapter 20

Public Speaking

WHAT IS DEBATING?

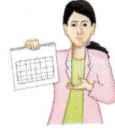

We live in a world where we communicate with others all the time. Debating is a more formal way of communicating. It builds confidence and self-esteem in people.

If we can speak publicly and convey our ideas and thoughts coherently and passionately, we have a valuable tool that can aid us in our public, private and future lives.

Rules

A debate has two teams an Affirmative and a Negative. Each side consists of three speakers. The First Affirmative speaker begins the debate, and is then followed by the First Negative speaker. This pattern is maintained for the second and third speakers of each team. Each speaker speaks for a set time, with a warning bell, to give them a little time to sum up and finish, then a final bell.

Each speaker has certain 'duties' to attend to as they speak (see 'Duties of Speakers').

All debaters must begin with "Madam/Mr Chairman, Ladies and Gentlemen".

A debater may have an interesting opening which she may use just before "Madam Chairman, etc..." which is fine.

Speakers don't have to say "thank you" when they finish, but may if they wish.

Room Layout

A debate is set up as shown in the following diagram:

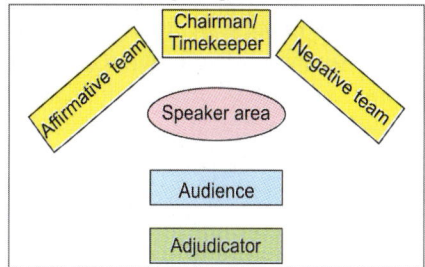

DEBATING CONTENT

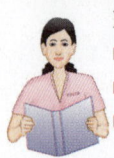

Each speaker is awarded a score out of 100 which is divided as follows:

❑   Argument 50
❑   Presentation 30
❑   Structure 20

Argument is the argument, evidence and proof of the team's case and its disproof of the other side's case. It also includes the definition and interpretation of the topic.

Presentation is how the speaker presents his/her arguments physically. It's a speaker's style, and includes things like eye contact, gestures, stance, deportment and voice.

Structure is the individual form (i.e., structure) of a speakers speech and how that speech links into speeches of the rest of that speaker's team.

Definition and Interpretation

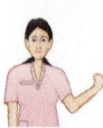

The definition of the topic consists in the first instance of defining individual or key words of the topic. The interpretation is the establishment or explanation of the meaning or significance of the topic as a whole.

The definition and interpretation of the topic should be outlined by the First Affirmative speaker. The Negative team must either agree or disagree with the Affirmative team's definition and interpretation.

How to Define the Topic

1.   Select the key words from the topic and look up their meanings in a range of dictionaries, choosing the most appropriate definition for each word.
2.   Interpret the topic.
3.   Formulate a sentence which explains the topic using the dictionary definitions (in the case of a literal interpretation), or the context of the topic (in the case of a figurative interpretation).

Topic Interpretation

Occasionally, the two teams may have a different interpretation of the topic. No one side has a right to the definition, and as long as a side can support its interpretation and attack the opposition's interpretation and argument with rebuttal of the form "even if we agreed to the topic which we don't, the opposition arguments are wrong because..." the team's interpretation and rebuttal is valid.

The exception to this is where a team has' defined' a topic in such a way as to render it senseless as in the case of sayings. For instance, "A chip off the old block" when interpreted as individual words from a dictionary does not maintain the integrity of the meaning. A much better interpretation would be to explain the meaning of the phase in its entire context.

A team which adopts a quirky interpretation often has a hard time finding evidence to support its case. However, there are occasions when both teams have a viable and valid interpretation of the topic and good arguments for each case. In such a case the debate will be awarded based on whose interpretation and argument was most convincing.

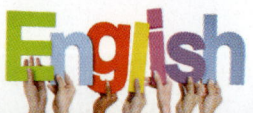

If one side has a reasonable interpretation but poor arguments to support its case, low marks in the Argument section would reflect that.

PREPARING YOUR ARGUMENTS

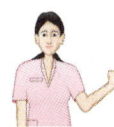

As a debater it's important that you make points that are clear, relevant and easy to understand. The use of a verbal illustration or an analogy may help you to clarify complicated terms.

However, you should remember that examples are not proof of a point.

An effective way of constructing your argument is to arrange it with the least important point first to most important point last. People generally remember what has been said last.

In presenting and developing your argument remember to explain what you mean to prove, what the scope and implication will be, and why it is true with facts and evidence (not just assertions) to support your case.

Planning

There are a number of things that you can do in preparation for a debate. Below are some suggestions:

- ❐ Keep up with newspapers magazines and books
- ❐ Record material, ideas and keep notes
- ❐ Observe and assess other speakers including public figures
- ❐ Evaluate your material
- ❐ Talk to other people, ask their opinions

Open a file and keep articles quotes or humorous cartoons.

Learn to express your thoughts in a more word enriched way-develop word pictures use a dictionary or thesaurus to improve your vocabulary.

Your Argument

You will feel a lot happier approaching a debate if your preparation has been thorough. Explore your topic, discuss it with friends, look through books, etc. to help support your argument. If you believe in what you are saying you will convince your audience as well. Have the strength of your convictions (sometimes after research we can truly see both sides of the coin!).

Notes

Keep notes short and succinct on small cards, but in big writing. Number each card so that if they fall you can sort them easily. Notes are a little reminder of what you want to say. You rule them, not they.

Timing

Before your debate, you need to run through roughly what you are to say so that you can be confident of your timing. If your speech is too short, expand on some of your material, give examples, or analogies.

If your speech is too long, is some information irrelevant, is there too much padding?

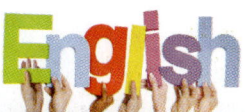

What You Say

Keep a dictionary or thesaurus handy to improve your vocabulary. You don't have to be pretentious or use 26 syllable words, but an extended vocabulary makes what you say more interesting. Humour can go a long way in getting a message across. Keep a file of jokes and cartoons which may come in handy. Quotes of famous people also help to substantiate your point of view.

Two important things to remember:

1. Think of your opening—exactly what you are going to say—it has to grab everyone's attention.
2. End on a positive note firmly expounding your view (possibly with a quote).

A strong opening and a strong finish will give you confidence.

PRESENTATION

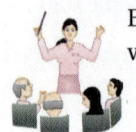

Everyone has his/her own personality and style when it comes to debating. Some very convincing debaters have very subdued but forceful styles.

You don't have to be outgoing, in fact, too dramatic is off-putting.

It's helpful to keep the following in mind:

1. Develop eye contact with the audience.
2. Use your hands and body naturally to emphasise points.
3. Speak clearly.
4. Vary your voice pitch and modulation.
5. Don't speak too quickly.

Hints

1. Don't write your debate in full-make headings and notes on your cue cards.
2. Number each card.
3. Avoid slang -use good conversational English.
4. Open and close your speech with a device such as a joke, illustration, or quote.

How to Speak

Speaking and talking are different things. When we talk we are often interrupted, but when we debate, we are able to speak uninterrupted.

This can be difficult. We may feel uncomfortable at being the centre of attention and so our anxiety becomes heightened. As a result, we may:

1. Speak too quickly
2. Speak too softly
3. Have poor diction (too nervous, lockjaw sets in)
4. Monotonous

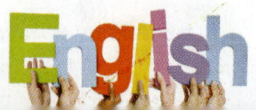

All of the above plus others can be overcome. Firstly, take pleasure in the fact that you now have a chance to air your views, uninterrupted for a few minutes. The audience is there because they want to hear what you have to say. Don't disappoint them. Secondly, remember that you can discard the negative inside messages and develop a balanced view about yourself and your self worth and self-esteem.

Types of Speakers

Those who speak from the mouth have given little thought or preparation to their work—they like the sound of their own voice.

Those who speak from the head have lots of facts and figures but are very boring and dry.

Those who speak from the heart are very emotional. Some of the great orators spoke from the heart.

What we need to do in debating is find a balance between the three. Which one are you? How do you need to balance your presentation?

Speaking

A number of things make up how we sound to other people when we speak. These are some of those elements that make up our speech:

- ❑ Tone
- ❑ Volume
- ❑ Rhythm and cadence
- ❑ Pitch
- ❑ Modulation

When debating you need to slightly exaggerate these, more so 'than if you were just speaking to a friend'. Record your voice so that you can hear how it sounds and the adjustments you need to make.

Points to Remember

Speak clearly and slowly, give time for your words to sink in, especially after a question. Pauses can be very effective.

Modulate your voice so that it has an up and down sound about it.

Feel confident about what you are saying and you'll avoid 'ums', 'errs' and the like.

Use verbal emphasis, e.g., "No" can be said in a number of ways, loud or soft, to catch people's attention.

Body Language

How you stand and move your head, eyes and hands, will help to convey your message in a very powerful way. Stand tall shoulders back, You'll look good and feel confident. When you pause, look at the audience. Maintain good eye contact by looking at individuals within the audience (this also gives you feedback—are they going to sleep? Do you need to speak with more emotion? They look puzzled. Are you speaking too quickly or softly?)

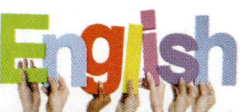

Large hand gestures are good. Think of yourself as larger than life. There may be some distance between yourself and the audience, small gestures may be lost.

Here are some things to avoid:

1. Shifting your weight from foot to foot repeatedly. It's a nervous reaction which is then conveyed to the audience.
2. Keep reading your notes. When your head is bowed it's hard to hear, and you lose eye contact with the audience.
3. Shuffling your notes. This may make you look nervous and is distracting.
4. Personal Peccadilloes (e.g., twirling hair, pulling on ear). This is very distracting.

STRUCTURE

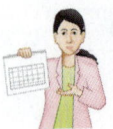

Structure is comprised of the following two things:

1. Individual speaker form: How the speech was constructed. Was it easy to follow? Was it in a logical sequence, and ordered? Did it follow an organised plan with a good introduction and conclusion?
2. Team plan: Did the speaker (as in the case of the First Affirmative and Negative) introduce the remaining speakers and what they were going to do? Did she refer to the team outline and plan, e.g., "as our first speaker said...."

    Points may be deducted if a speaker does not perform the tasks expected of him/her.

    Debates are not three individual speeches.

    Each team has a case, an outline and a theme.

All speakers need to link into their own speakers, and not contradict each other. They must vigorously defend the case, and rebut (except the first Affirmative speaker) the other side.

EXTEMPORE SPEAKING : WHAT IS IT?

Extempore speaking is the term used for a non-formally prepared speech. Explaining to your parents why you arrived home later than your curfew is a form of extempore speaking. When you watch a beauty pageant on television and the contestants have to draw a question and answer it for the judges, they are extempore speaking.

Every time you speak you are preparing for extempore speaking. You probably prepare without even knowing it. You have to read to learn new things for this type of speaking. When doing extempore speaking, you need to use the knowledge that you have and use a strong delivery.

Extemporaneous Speaking Contests

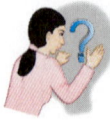

For this contest, you are given forty-five minutes to prepare an original speech indicating your knowledge of current events about an assigned topic. The purpose of an extemporaneous speaking contest is to encourage you to gain a broad knowledge of current events and to prepare, in a short period of time, a meaningful speech that can be delivered skillfully.

Topics usually concern events that have been of state, national, or international importance at any time from the beginning of the current 4-H or school year to the date of the contest. They are worded in the form of questions, which do not require only a yes or no answer.

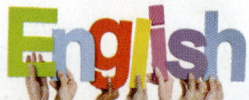

How it Works

You will draw three topics and, in one minute, choose the one that you want to speak about. The other two topics will be returned to the packet.

Each contestant has a maximum of 45 minutes of preparation. You may not talk to anyone or leave the room without permission. You may use an annotated bibliography and consult books, magazines, newspapers, and summary notes. You must provide your own preparatory materials. You may not use a typewriter. You can use the notes you organize during the preparation period.

The maximum time limit for your speech is six minutes. You will not be penalized if you speak for less than six minutes. The information you use should be accurate, pertinent, and demonstrate a thorough knowledge of the topic. You should not deviate from the topic. You should progress with your topic and demonstrate a reasonable analysis. The introduction should gain attention and preview the main points, which are clear and in a logical order. The conclusion should be convincing.

Sense Fair Score Card	Very Good	Needs Improvement Some	Much
Appearance			
Confidence			
Audience Appeal			
Voice Quality and Grammar			
Introduction			
Knowledge of Topic			
Pertinent Information			
Reasonable Analysis			
Conclusion			

State Fair time requirement: 4–6 minutes

Extempore is the art of speaking without any preparation on a given topic. Most often, the term is used in the context of speech and stage acting.

Why do we need it?

Appropriately put, Why do we need extempore. The answer to this may be that many a time, decisions have to be taken on the spot by the man-in charge (reed 'Manager'). At the same time, proper justification has to be given by the manager to his juniors to allay the frayed tempers of the people around him (if at all the tempers rise).

Accordingly, the manager has to be equipped with the skill in order to give an instant 360 degree turn to attitudes. The collateral impact that this makes is that it builds an instant rapport with the people around him. At the same time, this also brings out the leadership quality and the risk-taking ability of the individual, both at the policy and execution levels.

The body language and confidence level that the manager exudes coupled with the ability to express his thoughts articulately and fluently in English are few other abilities tested through this skill.

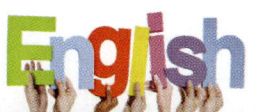

COMMON PROBLEMS FACED WHILE BUILDING THIS SKILL

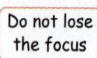

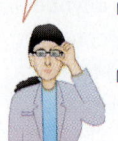

- A sound knowledge base: How much knowledge is required for the individual to tactfully handle a contemporary, as well as, an abstract topic is the biggest question.
- Getting intimated by the knowledgeable people giving you an in-your-face expression is one common problem encountered while building this skill.
- Constructing sentences properly, without disturbing the logical flow of the sentence is worth the consideration. From where we start to where we finally end, within that stipulated time, is yet another concern. Most often cross-questioning by people, coupled with numerous facial expressions from the panel leads to nervousness with the result than one often digresses from the topic.
- Most often, the extempore round is followed by an interview round. At times, if one feels that the extempore was not up to the mark then the apprehension wins and affects the interview as well, especially if the panel for the interview happens to be the same.

How to build the skill

- Now, let's talk about the solutions to the problems mentioned above. Needless to say, the solution lies in building the skill against all odds.
- Start building your knowledge brick by brick. Develop your reading habit. Start subscribing to a magazine, which has a mix of all topics, The knowledge thus gained will give you confidence to tackle any topic that comes your way. The editorial section in the newspapers has to be given. utmost importance. You may work through them by taking a stand on a particular topic and thinking about points to corroborate your position.
- Start speaking loudly on a topic, either in front of a mirror or even without one. The idea is that you should be able to speak, with a fair degree of fluency for about a minute on any topic you get. Practicing by speaking aloud, will ensure that you are able to control your nervousness. Watch your body language while speaking on a topic. There should not be any sign of nervousness, Also, speak in two postures- sitting as well as standing. Try to speak non-stop for five minutes and keep an alarm clock to keep track of time.
- Watch your body language. Too much of hand movements can be taken as a sign of nervousness. The objective is to appear calm and composed, and so you should not use your hands excessively.
- Do not start speaking as soon as the topic is given to you. Think for a few seconds before you start. It has also been observed that those who start off immediately; run out of ideas and don't know what to say. Thus, they end up finishing their speech in hardly 35–40 seconds, or even lesser, in some cases.
- Structure your speech properly. Try and give it an introduction, a body and a conclusion. Define the topic adequately. Try giving examples to drive home your point of view. if the topic provides scope for narrating personal experiences, use the opportunity to do so.
- Time yourself well. If the panel has given you two minutes to speak, try to speak within that time frame. It may not be a good idea to stop in the middle of one of your sentences.
- You should be clear with your career graph. Moreover, your character traits should be visible in your extempore. This will create a positive impact in the interview, which may immediately follow the extempore. There is a high probability that like panel judging you

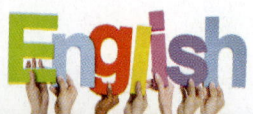

in the extempore and the interview will nearly be the same with a functional expert joining in the interview.

Common topics that are asked range from the Abstract (summers have come, black is beautiful, etc.) to 'Concrete' issues such as those related to Finance (disinvestment, black money, etc.) and those of national importance (Lokpal Bill, overdose of fasts, corruption, etc). Most importantly, maintain your poise during the extempore. This will send the right signal to the panel judging you.

DECLAMATION

Debate and Oratory

A declamation speech is the term used to describe the *re-giving* of an important or famous speech. It could be a political, graduation or commencement speech, a eulogy, or a sermon. The speaker re-interprets the original, reproducing its power afresh.

Often this exercise will be set as part of studying public speaking skills. The purpose is to have the student directly experience the power of masterfully crafted language. Through their interpretation the techniques and skills of the original orator are learned.

The action or art of declaiming; The repeating or uttering of a speech, etc. with studied intonation and gesture.

1. A public speech or address of rhetorical character; a set speech in rhetorical elocution.
2. Declaiming or speaking in an impassioned oratorical manner; fervid denunciation with appeals to the audience.
3. A speech of a rhetorical kind expressing strong feeling and addressed to the passions of the hearers; a declamatory speech, a harangue.
4. Renunciation, repudiation, disclaimer.

Declamation or declamatio (Latin for "declaration") was a genre of ancient rhetoric and a mainstay of the Roman higher education system. It was separated into two component subgenres, the controversia, speeches of defense or prosecution in fictitious court cases, and the suasoria, in which the speaker advised a historical or legendary figure as to a course of action. Roman declamations survive in four corpora: the compilations of Seneca the Elder and Calpurnius Flaccus, as well as two sets of controversiae, the Major Declamations and Minor Declamations spuriously attributed to Quintilian.

Declamation had its origin in the form of preliminary exercises for Greek students of rhetoric: works from the Greek declamatory tradition survive in works such as the collections of Sopater and Choricius of Gaza. Of the remaining Roman declamations the vast majority are controversiae only one book of suasoriae survive, that being in Seneca the Elder's collection.

As a critical part of rhetorical education, declamation's influence was widespread in Roman elite culture.

This method of teaching was used in ancient Greece where public speaking was considered a necessary art for anybody embarking on a career in public service. A declamation was a practice piece set by a teacher for exactly the same reason they are set now: to have a student learn the skills of combining eloquent language- with equally eloquent delivery.

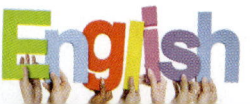

Choosing a Declamation Speech

What you choose is critical. Firstly, you must like it. There's no good to be gained from choosing something because you think it will please or impress your teacher and likewise, judges. You're going to work on this piece to make it your own. Therefore it needs to genuinely reflect you in theme and message.

And secondly, it needs a combination of the qualities listed in the following areas:

- ❑ **Style of language:** Elevated, inspirational, elegant, poetic, masterful—the speech should be an example of 'beautiful' language and construction.
- ❑ **Structure:** Look for unity of purpose. The piece needs to be structurally coherent—have a beginning, development and close. It is not a loose ramble or collection of impressions without form.
- ❑ **Theme:** The message or theme running through it should be worthy of its oratorical treatment, i.e., the style of language specified above. It must be important and applicable beyond the time it was first delivered. For example, Martin Luther King's *I Had a Dream* speech has carried its theme down the years without any loss of potency or relevance. (But be warned—choose carefully. A famous speech such as King's will have been heard and heard again. You need something of similar impact but with considerably less profile.)
- ❑ **Impact:** The speech must have reached and grabbed the hearts and minds of its listeners. It will, persuasively challenged and changed the way people thought and acted, uniting and inspiring them towards a common goal or course of action.

If you're choosing for a competition before you make your choice be sure to *review the guidelines* and do take note of the allocated time. Be prepared to cut your selection to fit.

WHAT IS GROUP DISCUSSION?

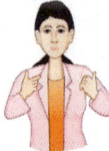

Group Discussion is a methodology or in a simple language, you may call it an interview process or a group activity. It is used as one of the best tools to select the prospective candidates in a comparative perspective. GD may be used by an interviewer at an organization, colleges or even at different types of management competitions.

A GD is a methodology used by an organization to gauge whether the candidate has certain personality traits and/or skills that it desires in its members. In this methodology, the group of candidates is given a topic or a situation. Given a few minutes to think about the same, and then asked to discuss the topic among themselves for 15–20 minutes. Freshersworld.com brings you an elaborate section for GD as you had ever seen anywhere else. It is a very useful tool to screen the candidate's potential as well as their skills.

GD evaluation is done by the subject experts based on the discussions. A report will be prepared on analyzing the facts at the end of the discussion.

Some of the personality traits the GD is trying to gauge may include:

- ❑ Communication skills
- ❑ Interpersonal skills
- ❑ Leadership skills
- ❑ Motivational skills

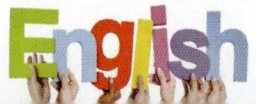

- ❏ Team building skills
- ❏ Analytical/Logical skills
- ❏ Reasoning ability
- ❏ Different thinking
- ❏ Initiative
- ❏ Assertiveness
- ❏ Flexibility
- ❏ Creativity
- ❏ Ability to think on ones feet

Why GDs are Implemented Commonly?

The reason why institutes put you through a Group discussion and an interview, after testing your technical and conceptual skills in an exam, is to get to know you as a person and gauge how well you will fit in their institute. GD evaluates how you can function as a part of a team. As a manager or as a member of an organization you will always be working in teams. Therefore how you interact in a team becomes an important criterion for your selection. Managers have to work in a team and get best results out of teamwork. That is the reason why management institutes include GD as a component of the selection procedure.

Company's Perspective

Companies conduct group discussion after the written test to know more about your:

- ❏ Interactive skills (*how good you are at communication with other people*)
- ❏ Behavior (*how open-minded are you in accepting views contrary to your own*)
- ❏ Participation (*how good an active speaker you are & your attention to the discussion*)
- ❏ Contribution (*how much importance do you give to the group objective as well as your own*)

Aspects which make up a group discussion are:

- ❏ Verbal communication
- ❏ Non-verbal behavior
- ❏ Confirmation to norms
- ❏ Decision making ability
- ❏ Cooperation

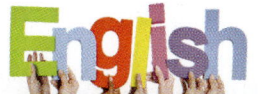

NOTES

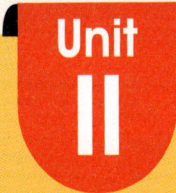

Reading

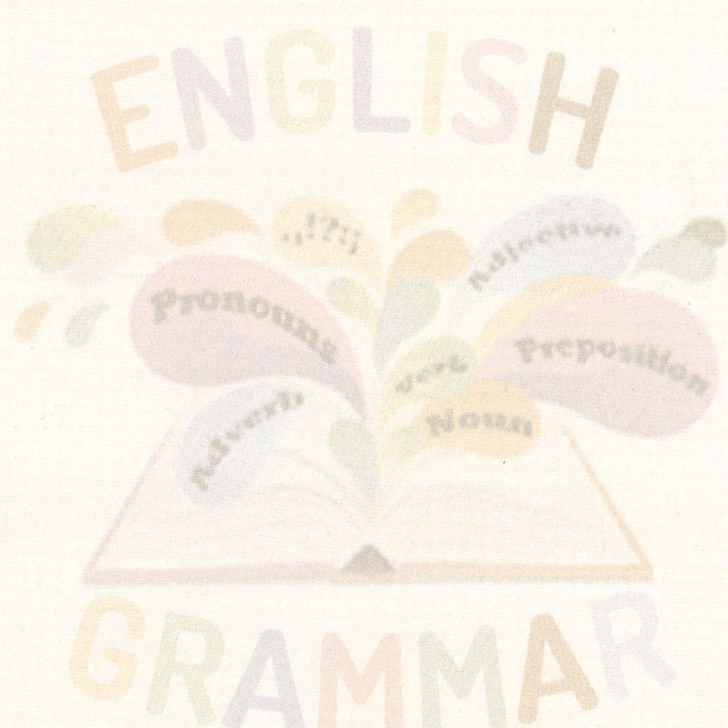

Chapter 21

Reading Comprehension

INTRODUCTION

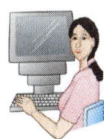

Comprehension of a passage means understanding the gist of the given text thoroughly. It forms a very good exercise for intelligent reading, judicious selection and correct expression. It is meant to test the intelligence of the student to express his/her thoughts independently in a simple, clear, direct, correct and precise manner. This form of exercise eliminates memorising and forms the stepping stone to precis-writing.

HOW TO PROCEED WITH THE PASSAGE

1. Before trying to answer the questions given at the end you should read the passage two or three times till you understand it fully. After that, the questions at the end are to be read and the passage should be read once again paying particular attention to the questions asked.

2. Then you should find out the central idea or the main idea or thought of the passage. This forms the title of the passage. The title or the heading should not be in the form of a sentence. It should either be a word or a phrase or a proverb or an expression which gives the theme of the passage. Generally, the title or the heading is found in the beginning or the end of the passage. All the important words of the title or the heading should be written with a capital letter.

3. The questions should be read and answered carefully. The language of the passage should not be copied as far as possible. Answers must be simple, brief, grammatically correct and direct.

4. Each answer should be given separately. It should be clearly numbered and its number should correspond to that of the question. Several answers should never be put together in one paragraph.

5. Sometimes you may be asked to replace italicised words or phrases in the passage. For this the knowledge of 'Synonyms', and 'One Word Substitution' is necessary.

6. Finally, we must read the questions one by one and compare them with our answers to see whether they confirm with the spirit and requirement of the question.

Passage-1

Read the following passage and answer the questions that follow:

❑ If we look back at India's long history we find that our forefathers made wonderful progress whenever they looked out on the world with clear and fearless eyes and kept the windows of their minds open to give and receive. And, in later periods, when they grew narrow in out look and shrank from outside influences, India suffered a set back politically and culturally. What a magnificent inheritance we have, though we have abused it often enough. India has been and is a vital nation, in spite of all the misery and suffering that she has experienced, That vitality in the realms of constructive and creative effort has spread to many parts of Asian World and elsewhere and brought splendid conquest in its, train. Those, conquests were not so much of the sword, but of the mind and heart which bring and which endure when the men of the sword and their work are forgotten. But that very vitality if not rightly and creatively directed, may turn inward and destroy and degrade.

❑ Even during the brief span of our lives we have seen these two forces at play in India and the world at large—the forces of constructive and creative effort and the forces of destruction. Which will triumph in the end? And on which side do we stand? That is a vital question for each one of us, and more especially for those from whom the leaders nation will be drawn, and on whom the burden of tomorrow will fall. We dare not sit on the fence and refuse to face the issue. We dare not allow our minds to be befuddled by passion and hatred when clear thought and effective action are necessary.

❑ What kind of India are we looking for and what kind of world? Are hatred and violence and fear and communalism and narrow provincialism to mould our future? Surely not, if there has been any truth in us and in our professions. Here in this city of Allahabad, dear to me not only because of my close association with it but also, because of India's history. My boyhood and youth were spent in dreaming dreams seeing vision of India's future. Was there any real substance in those dreams or were they merely the fancies of fevered brain? Some small part of those dreams has come true but not in the manner I had imagined, and so much still remains. Instead of feeling of triumph at achievement, there is an emptiness and distress at the sorrow that surrounds us and we have to wipe the tears from a million eyes.

❑ Vast responsibility, therefore rests on our educational institutions and those who guide their destinies. They have to keep their lights burning and must not stray from the right path even when passion convulses the multitude and blinds many amongst those whose duty it is to set an example to others. We are going to reach our goal through crookedness or flirting with evil in the hope that it may lead to good. The right end can never be fully achieved through wrong means.

❑ Let us be clear about our national objective. We aim at the democratic India where every citizen has an equal place and full opportunity of growth and service, where present day inequalities in wealth and status have ceased to be, where our vital impulses are directed to creative and cooperative endeavor. In such an India communalism, separatism, isolation, untouchability bigotry and exploitation of man by man have no place and while religion is free it is not allowed to interfere with the political and economic aspects of a nations life.

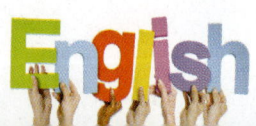

If that is so then all this business of Hindu and Muslim and Christian and Sikh must cease in so far as our political life is concerned and we must build a united but composite nation where both individual and national freedom are secure.

❑ We have passed through grievous trials. We have surprised them but at a terrible cost and the legacy they have left in our tortured minds and stunted souls will pursue us for a long time. Our trials are not over. Let us prepare ourselves for them in the spirit of free and disciplined men and women stout of heart and purpose, who will not stray from the right path and forget our ideals and objectives. We have to start this work of healing and we have to build and create. The wounded body and spirit of India call upon all of us to dedicate ourselves to this great task. May we be worthy of the task and of India!

Questions

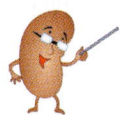

1. **Answer the following questions as briefly as possible:**
   a. How according to Nehru, can India's vitality prove destructive?
   c. How does Nehru describe India's national objectives?
   b. What is the special responsibility of our educational institutions?
   d. What is meant by 'this business of Hindu and Muslim and Christian and Sikh?
   e. How have we faced our trials?

2. **Find from the passage words which mean the same as the following:**
   a. Legacy (para 1)
   b. Period (para 2)
   c. Dishonesty (para 4)

Passage-2

When Algu Chaudhari's name was proposed in the chaupal as a person to act as the Chief Judge, the aunt agreed to accept him. Jumman was overjoyed but he hid his feelings. Algu said, 'Aunty, you know Jumman and I are close friends, She replied, 'Son, nobody sells his conscience for friendship.' Algu said, 'We have been old friends but at this moment I cannot favor anyone. Please state your case before Panchayat.' Jumman was so confident of his victory that he imagined the talk of Algu was mere show. He had to face questions from his friend that were too difficult for him to answer. He was much amazed. Finally Algu gave the judgment. 'Jumman Sheikh, the elders think that the property of your aunt yields enough profits for monthly expenses to be paid to her. If you do not agree, the property should be returned to her.' Hearing this the audience cheered the village judges noisily.

Questions

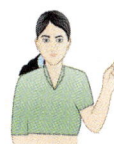

1. What feelings did Jumman hide and why?
2. Why did the aunt have full faith in Algu?
3. How did Jumman feel when Algu said he couldn't favor any one?
4. What amazed Jumman?
5. What was Jumman asked to do in case he did not agree to pay the aunt her monthly expenses?
6. Give a suitable heading to this passage.

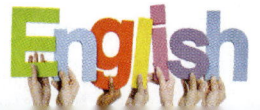

Passage-3

When Mr Jones went to a restaurant one day, he left his coat near the door. There was nothing in the pockets of the coat when he left it. So he was very surprised when he took his coat after his meal and found the pockets full of jewelry.

There was a waiter near the door. Mr Jones said to him, 'Somebody has made a mistake. He has put some jewelry in my coat. Take it, and when he comes back, give it to him.' The waiter took it and went away. Suddenly another man came in with a coat just like Mr Jones. 'I am sorry,' said this man. 'I made mistake. I took your coat and you have got mine. Please give me my coat and jewelry.' Mr Jones answered, 'I gave the jewelry to the waiter. He will give it to you.'

Mr Jones called the manager of the restaurant; but he said, 'We have no waiters here. We have only waitresses.' 'You gave the jewelry to a thief!' shouted the other man, 'I shall send for the police!' Mr Jones was frightened and paid the man a lot of money for the jewelry.

Questions

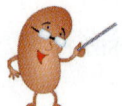

1. What did Jones think about the jewelry in the pockets of his coat?
2. What mistake did Mr Jones make?
3. What mistake had the owner of the jewelry made?
4. When did Jones come to know of his mistake?
5. What had Jones to do in order to save himself from trouble?
6. Give a suitable heading to the passage.

Passage-4

Gandhiji's mother was a very sweet, kind and religious woman. She visited the temple daily, often taking her little son with her. She fasted frequently, too. Once she made a vow to eat only one meal a day for four months, and not to take even that one meal unless she had first seen sunshine. As she had made this vow in the rainy season, it was often difficult to see sunshine at all. Her children, who could not bear to think of their dear mother going without food all the 24 hours, would stand staring up at the sky, waiting to catch the first gleams of the sun. As soon as a ray appeared, they would dash into the house and call their mother to come and see for herself. By the time she came out, the sun had often gone behind the clouds again. 'It does not matter,' she would say cheerfully. 'God does not want me to eat today,' and back she would go to her household, tasks. In this way Gandhiji learnt from his good mother how to do penance cheerfully for love of God.

Questions

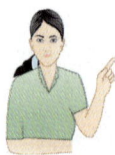

1. What vow did Gandhiji's mother make?
2. What could the children not bear?
3. What did the children do if they saw some sunlight in the sky?
4. What did Gandhiji learn from his mother?
5. What did she do daily?
6. Why was it often difficult to see the sunshine?
7. Give a suitable heading to the passage.

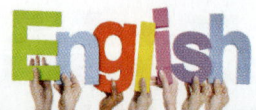

Passage-5

There is an incident which occurred at an examination during Gandhiji's first year at the high school. Mr Giles, the Inspector of schools, had come on a visit of inspection. He gave the students five words to write as a spelling exercise. One of the words was 'Kettle'. Gandhiji had misspelt it. The teacher tried to prompt Gandhiji but he would not be prompted. He would not copy the spelling of his neighbour's slate. The result was that all the boys except Gandhiji were found to have spelt each word correctly. Only he had been stupid. The teacher later tried to bring this stupidity home to him, but without effect. Gandhiji could never learn the art of copying.

Questions

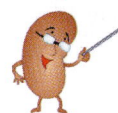

1. Who was Mr Giles?
2. What did he do during his visit to Gandhiji's school?
3. What mistake did Gandhiji make?
4. Was Gandhiji really stupid? What could he not learn?
5. Give a suitable heading to the passage.

Passage-6

Oliver Twist was born in a workhouse and for long time after his birth there was a considerable doubt whether the child would live. He lay breathless for some time, rather unequally balanced between the world and the next. After a few struggles, however, he breathed, sneezed and uttered a loud cry. The pale face of a young woman lying on the bed was raised weakly from the pillow and in a faint voice she said, 'Let me see the child and die.' 'Oh, you must not talk about dying yet,' said the doctor, as he rose from where he was sitting near the fire and advanced towards the bed. 'God bless her,' added the poor old pauper who was acting as the nurse. The doctor placed the child in her mother's arms. She pressed her cold white lips on its forehead, passed her hands over its face, gazed wildly around, fell back and died.

Questions

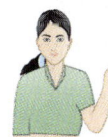

1. Where was Oliver Twist born, and what was the doubt at the time of his birth?
2. What was the mother's conditions at that time?
3. What did she say to the doctor?
4. What did the mother do when the doctor placed the child in her arms?
5. Give a suitable heading to the passage.

Passage-7

Too much importance must not be attached to the wrong acts done by children, particularly if they happen to be of a minor nature. Many boys and girls at a young age are likely to be in the habit of stealing, neglecting their studies, slipping out of their classes, or using bad language. In nearly every case, the root cause of the trouble is the fear that proper care of the child is not taken in the house, or sufficient interest is not shown in him. But if the parents were wise, they would correct the faults of their children by paying more attention to them. Whatever the case, one thing should never be done. The bad thing in the children should never be repressed, that is, they should not be compelled to change for the better under fear of the rod. Physical punishment does not improve them. It only makes worse than before.

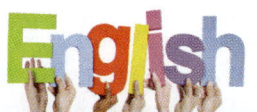

Questions

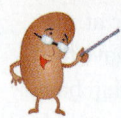

1. What do boys and girls at a young age do?
2. What is the root cause of their misbehavior?
3. What is the duty of a wise parent?
4. Why should not a rod be used to make children better?
5. What is the one thing that should never be done?

Passage-8

Science and technology have relieved mankind of degrading drudgery. They have added to man's comfort, health and enjoyment of existence. The average life span of man on earth has been greatly increased. Science has added to the dignity and stature of the individual. When man is relieved from the battle for physical safety, he becomes a little creator. Every challenge of science has added to man's moral stature. As we find the world is much more wonderful than we ever dream it to be. We are led into new fields of awareness, new ranges of attainment, new realization of destiny. New knowledge is both a challenge and an opportunity. Further, it is not yet known what man may be. He must, without haste and without rest, strive to the quality of human greatness, that is, greatness in humanity.

Questions

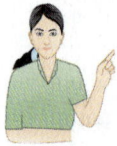

1. What service has science and technology rendered to the modern man?
2. When does man become a little creator?
3. How has science opened up new horizons for man's realization and attainment?
4. What does new knowledge offer to man?
5. Give the meaning of:
    a. Enjoyment
    b. Destiny

Passage-9

In America, which is the most advanced country industrially, and to a lesser in other countries which are approximating to the America condition, it is necessary for the average citizen, if he wishes to make a living, to avoid incurring the hostility of certain big men and these big men have an outlook 'religious, moral and political' with which they expect their employees to agree, at least outwardly. A man who openly dissents from Christianity, or believes in a relaxation of the marriage laws, or objects to the power of the great corporations, finds America a very uncomfortable country, unless he happens to be an eminent writer. Therefore, the safeguarding of liberty in the present world is far more difficult where economic organisation has been carried to the point of monopoly.

Questions

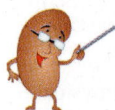

1. What is necessary for the average citizen in America?
2. What do the big men expect of their employees?
3. Who finds America a very uncomfortable country?

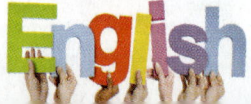

4. Why is it difficult to safeguard liberty in the present world?
5. Give the meaning of:
    a. Liberty
    b. Agree

Passage-10

People travelling long distances frequently have to decide whether they would prefer to go by land, sea or air. Hardly anyone can positively enjoy sitting in a train for more than a few hours. Train compartments soon get cramped and stuffy. It is almost impossible to take your mind off the journey. Reading is only a partial solution, for the monotonous rhythm of the wheels clicking on the rails soon lulls you to sleep. During the day, sleep comes in snatches. At night when you really wish to go to sleep, you rarely manage to do so. If you are lucky enough to get a couchette, you spend half the night staring at the small blue light in the ceiling, or fumbling to find your passport when you cross a frontier. Inevitably you arrive at your destination almost exhausted.

Long car journeys are even less pleasant, for it is quite impossible even to read. On motorways you can at least travel fairly and safely at high speeds, but more often than not the greater part of the journey is spent in narrow, bumpy roads which are crowded with traffic. By comparison, trips by sea offer a great variety of civilized comforts. You can stretch your legs on the spacious decks, play games, swim, meet interesting people and enjoy good food—always assuming, of course, that the sea is calm. If it is not, and you are likely to get sea-sick, no form of transport could be worse, even if you travel in ideal weather, sea-journeys take a long time. Relatively few people are prepared to sacrifice up to a third of their holidays for the pleasure of travelling on a ship.

Aeroplanes have the reputation of being dangerous and even hardened travellers are intimidated by them. They also have the grave disadvantage of being the most expensive form of transport. But nothing can match them for speed and comfort. Travelling at a height of 30,000 feet, far above the clouds, and at over 500 miles an hour is an exhilarating experience. You do not have to devise ways of taking your mind off the journey, for an aeroplane gets you to your destination rapidly. For a few hours. you settle back in a deep armchair to enjoy the flight. The real escapist can watch a free film show and sip a hot or cold drink on some services. But even when such refreshments are not available, there is plenty to keep you occupied.

An aeroplane offers you an unusual breathtaking view of the world. You soar effortlessly over high mountains and deep valleys. You really see the shape of the land. If the landscape is hidden from view, you can enjoy the extraordinary sight of unbroken clouds, plains that stretch out for miles before you, while the sun shines brilliantly in a clear sky. The journey is so smooth that there is nothing to prevent you from reading or sleeping. However you decide to spend your time, one thing is certain: You will arrive at your destination fresh and uncrumpled. You will not have to spend the next few days recovering from a long and arduous journey.

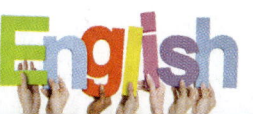

Answer the Following Questions as Briefly as Possible

1. Why is it difficult to read on a train in long distance journeys? Give two reasons.
2. What are the two disadvantages of travelling by sea?
3. What are the two disadvantages of travelling by air?
4. What are the pleasures of air flight, according to the writer?
5. Why does the writer dislike long car journeys?

Find words in the passage which convey a similar meaning as the following:

1. Pieces ....
2. Feel around ....
3. Causing excitement ....

Passage-11

1. Everybody knows that the education given at present in our universities is narrow and strictly intellectual and is confined to giving instruction in the subjects of the set course with an eye only to the students' success in the examination. The physical side of education is neglected, and there are practically no facilities for social life or corporate activities of any kind. Naturally in such narrow grooves, there is little opportunity for training the character of the student and developing his personality. In this connection, it will be wise to look up to America, the most practical country in the world. America possesses democracy in education. Education is not a monopoly of idle rich, or the privilege solely of the bloated and arrogant middle class, but the birth right of every American Child. In Europe primary education is free and compulsory, but higher education is reserved only for a few. No attempt is made by American educationists to dole out education according to social position. It is possible for a student to slit the common school and right up to the University.

2. Education in America is frankly utilitarian as it is not either in England or in India. Metaphysics and Latin and Greek occupy a very subordinate place in the curriculum. The almost miraculous success of American business all over the world is due to the strictly utilitarian ideals of American education. In America businessmen generously give away large sum of money for education. It is not an idealistic generosity which prompts them to do so, but the realization that their education has helped them to make money and so they must give money for giving similar education to others. No American would even dream of encouraging a type of education without direct social utility. A look into an American University Calendar would show that the courses of study offered range from dish-washing to Metaphysics, but dish-washing is given more importance than Aristotle.

3. The difference between American and Indian education is that Indian educationists aim at producing merely glorified clerks while Americans want self-respecting citizens who shall be taught to make an independent living in every walk of life. Our unemployed are consoled by being told that 'man shall not live by bread alone?' This is not true. The truth is that man shall not live by culture alone. He wants bread first. That is recognized by American Universities. So in these two ways we can learn much from America. We must make education cheap, within reach of all who are capable of it and desire it and we must

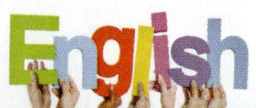

make it utilitarian. A man who can do the job of dish-washing really efficiently is a better citizen than a man who writes Babu Piche Lal's English, and murders Shakespeare. In America, examinations have been completely eliminated. Instead of holding examinations and promoting those who receive a certain percentage of marks, the entire group is promoted. The more slowly developing child is given individual attention, and the brilliant child is not retarded. The gifted child is given more work of a creative nature, and is even encouraged to dream, but is never placed in a class of children older than himself, where he may grow self-conscious and lose confidence.

On the basis of your reading the passage answer the following questions:
1. What is the aim of present system of education in India?
2. What are the two shortcomings of the social life of a student?
3. On what grounds can we say that American education is utilitarian in nature?
4. What is the great distinction between American and Indian education?
5. Americans treat the gifted child on different norms. What are those?

Pick out the words from the passage which mean:
   a.Opportunity ....
   b.Miraculous ....
   c.Eliminated ....

Write three facts from the passage that speak about success of business in America.

Passage-12

Read the following passage and answer the questions which follow:

1. Wolves, jackals and foxes all belong to one family, the family of dogs. They are found on all the continents except Antarctica. They live in the forest and on the steppes, in the mountains and on the plains in the tundra and in the desert.

2. The legs of the animals in this family are long and well-shaped. The paws have strong, blunt claws. All the animals run fast, some at a speed of 65 kilometers an hour!

3. The hair is thick and of various shades of gray or red. Some of the animals are striped. One of the African jackals is called the striped jackal. The African wild dog has black, white and yellow spots. This is the only wild animal that has hair of three colors.

4. The largest and strongest animal in the dog family is the wolf. It can run so fast with a goat or sheep on its shoulder that you can hardly catch up with it even on a good race horse. It is very true to say that the wolf lives by its feet. Sometimes it runs 60 kilometers a day in search of prey. And not always does it find it, even running that distance. It is not easy for an animal in the wild to find food. For this reason, when a wolf makes a good kill, it gorges itself. It can eat 10 kilograms of meat at one time. The wolf has very strong jaws. It can crush large bones easily. The jackal is the most cunning member of the dog family. People don't like it because it is a terrible thief. What cunning it shows! If a jackal wants to catch a crow or a magpie, it lies down by the road and makes it believe it is dead. When the bird sees the jackal, it comes down to peck at the 'dead' flesh. Up jumps the cunning jackal, and that is the end of the bird!

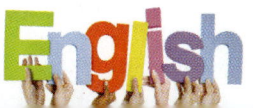

5. There are many tales about the cunning fox, but they are all untrue. The wolf and the jackal are far more cunning than the fox. It is certainly not a greedy animal. It never hunts just to kill. It feeds mainly on barn and field mice. It is a master at catching these rodents that do so much damage to farms.

6. The fennec is the smallest relative of the dog but has the biggest ears. It is as small as a kitten, but its ears would be suitable for a big sheep dog. These charming animals live in the hottest place on earth, the Sahara. All day the fennecs have to hide from the blistering sun in deep and cool burrows. Only towards evening do they all crawl out at once and sit quietly near their burrows waiting for the day to cool off. If the sun still burns, they lie down and cover their heads with their bushy tails, as though the tails were umbrellas. At long last it is pleasantly cool. The fennec suddenly stiffens its big ears. It has heard something! It creeps to where a lizard may have jumped. A desert lark may have stirred in its sleep. Imagine how little noise that would make! But the fennec hears everything. It knows exactly where the bird is hiding. It creeps forward again like a shadow, stops and leaps. There! It has the victim in its teeth.

On the basis of your reading the passage answer the questions given below:

1. When a wolf finds a good kill it gorges itself. Why?
2. What is often wrongly said of the fox?
3. How does the fox help us?
4. How does the fennec use its tail when the sun is hot and burning?
5. Americans treat the gifted child on different norms. What are those?

Find the antonyms of following words from the passage:

 (i) Same (para 5) ....
 (ii) Starves (para 4) ....
(iii) Slightly (para 5).......................

Pick out synonyms from the passage which are similar in meaning to the following:

 (i) Grassland (para 1) ....
 (ii) Harm (para 5) ....
(iii) Moved (para 6) ....

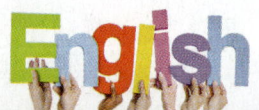

Various Forms of Composition

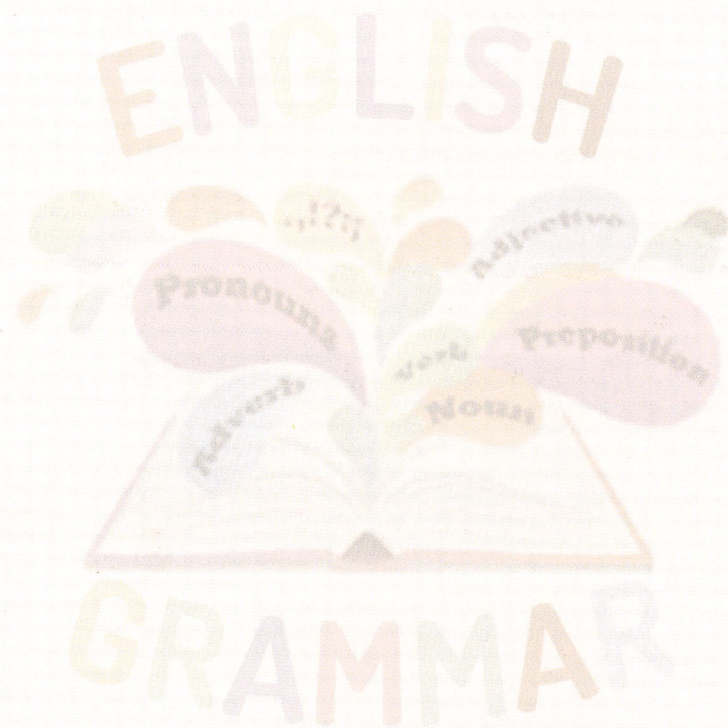

Chapter 22

Letter

INTRODUCTION

Letter writing in an art. In letter one should be respectful to superiors, courteous to inferiors, familiar to friends, affectionate to relatives, simple to children, tender and sympathetic in condolence, lively and joyous in congratulations, forceful and impressive in weighty matter, easy and sprightly on lighter topics.

ART OF LETTER WRITING

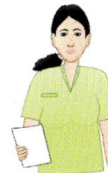 Of all the forms of communication with people at a distance, letters are less commonly used these days than in the days when there were neither mobiles nor any telephones or e-mails. Communication by telephone may be faster and easier but it does not have the advantages of a letter. Letter is a record; one can refer to it as and when one wants. Letter has a personal touch, it has the imprint of the personality of the writer. It strengthens good relations and establishes personal and emotional bonds. It may be used for a variety of purposes making enquiries, replying to enquiries, keeping in touch with people, applying for jobs, asking for things or services, making business deals, complaining news, sharing experiences, enacting transactions, consoling, congratulating, greeting, etc.

There are many kinds of letters—as many as different kinds of people to write, different persons to whom to write, different situations that make people write and different purposes for which letters are written. For practical purposes, which may reduce this great variety into two—informal and formal letters.

I. **Informal letters** are friendly in tone and written generally to persons you know well. They have a specific layout. Under this heading would come (a) letters to close relatives (father, mother, brothers, sisters, uncles, aunts, cousins, etc. and friends) (b) letter to friends of your parents, acquaintances, former headmaster, Principal, teachers, persons who are not known personally but known to you by repute whom you invite to become your chief guest, etc.

Sometimes the letters under (b) group as listed above are classed differently. They are put under the category of semiformal letters. They are less friendly as well as less formal but their layout is that of the informal letters.

II. **Formal letters** are business-like in tone, matter of fact in content and written generally to persons not personally known. They have specific layout. These are letters to persons not personally known, government departments, business firms, public organisations, municipal authorities, local authorities or officials, etc.

Letter can also be classified into the following four kinds:

1. Personal Letters
2. Social Letters
3. Official Letters
4. Business Letters

LETTER WRITING

Introduction to Letter Writing

Letter writing is a great riddle for the people from the time immemorial. There are different types of letters, but it can be classified in two major categories, i.e., formal and informal. The opening paragraph of a letter should state the purpose of the letter. The middle paragraph(s) should explain the details, beginning a new paragraph for each main point. The closing paragraph should state the course of action needed or repeat the purpose of the letter. Always use the appropriate phraseology for opening and closing.

Be clear about the point being made in each paragraph: topic sentences are very important. Also, plan your letter well and in advance. It is very important to use the correct forms of salutation and signature endings should always be appropriate. Note that in the letter writing section of the exam you are not required to write any addresses. The exact number and division of paragraphs may also depend on the specific instructions for each letter writing task.

Register is another important thing in letter writing: always bear in mind whom you are talking to and how this should affect the 'tone' of your letter. Remember to use the appropriate vocabulary for both formal and informal letters.

Make sure that when writing a letter it is well structured and organized. Even if you make mistakes, both the reader and the writer will be more tolerant of these in a letter which is attractively set-out and neatly-written. Another very important point is the use of linking words and phrases.

Formal and Informal Letter

Style

The style of the letter varies depending on who it is addressed to. For instance, a letter to someone you do not know requires a formal style, a letter to someone you know but are not intimate with requires a semiformal style, whereas a letter to a friend requires an informal style.

The characteristics of formal style are:
- The greeting (Dear Sir/Madam, Dear Mr/Mrs/Miss/Ms Lee)
- Frequent use of passive

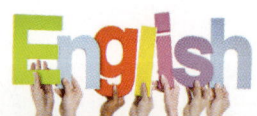

❏ Formal language (complex sentences, noncolloquial english)
❏ No abbreviated forms
❏ The ending (Yours sincerely, Yours faithfully)

Note: Use yours sincerely when you have used Dear Mr Lee and Yours faithfully when you have used Dear Sir/Madam. Use Ms when you do not know whether the woman is married or not.

The characteristic of informal style are:

❏ The greeting (Dear Alex Dear dad)
❏ Informal language and style (idioms, colloquial english)
❏ Abbreviated forms, pronouns omitted
❏ The ending (Yours/Love/Best Wishes/Regards/Anthony)

The characteristics of semiformal style are:

❏ Formal greetings (Dear Mr/Mrs + surname)
❏ Informal endings (Best wishes/Yours + first name/full name)
❏ A respectful tone, depending on the relationship you have with the recipient of the letter. Also, pronouns should not be omitted and idioms should be carefully used.

Transactional Letters

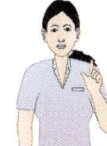

❏ Transactional letters are the letters which respond to writing input (advertisements, other letters, notes, invitations, etc.) and/or visual prompts (maps, drawings, etc).
❏ They can either be formal or informal depending on who you are writing to.
❏ Transactional letters can be of any type (complaint, application, invitation, asking for giving information, etc.)
❏ When you write a transactional letter you should include all the relevant factual information given, using your own words.
❏ You should also make sure that each paragraph deals with only one topic.

LETTERS OF COMPLAINT

Complaint Latters

❏ Complaint letters are normally written in a formal style.
❏ Mild or strong language can be used depending on the feelings of the writer or the seriousness of the complaint, but abusive language must never be used.

Introduction

Paragraph 1: Appropriate opening remarks. State the purpose of the letter and give enough detail for the reader to understand the correct nature of the complaint.

Main Body

Paragraph 2: Give all the detail(s) of the complaint, Make sure you include all necessary dates, times, people involved, the inconvenience you faced, etc.

Paragraph 3: State what you would like to be done about the matter. Suggested action is to be taken.

Conclusion

Appropriate closing remarks.

Useful Language for Letters of Complaint

Opening remarks: (Mild) I am writing to complain about/regarding/on as account of/on the subject of/I am writing to draw your attention to/I am writing in connection with, etc.

(Strong) I was appalled as/I want to express my strong dissatisfaction with/I feel I must protest/complain about, etc.

Closing remarks: Mild/I hope/assume you will replace/I trust the situation will improve/I hope the matter will be resolved/I hope the matter can be sorted out, etc.

(Strong) I insist you replace the item at once/I demand a full refund. I hope that I will not be forced to take further action, etc.

Letter Asking for/Giving Information

Their style can be either formal or informal.

Introduction

Paragraph 1: Appropriate opening remarks. State the purpose of the letter. If you are responding to an advertisement, say where you saw it.

Main Body

Paragraph 2: Make a specific request for information or give the appropriate information.

Paragraph 3: Finish the letter politely (offering or send any more information required if it is a letter *giving* information).

Conclusion

Appropriate closing remarks.

Useful Language for Letters Asking for Information

Opening remarks: (Formal) I am writing to inquire about/in connection with, etc. (Informal) can you let me know/I want you to tell me, etc.

Introducing first request: (Formal) Could you possibly send/I would be grateful if you could/I would appreciate some information about, etc. (Informal) can you send/tell me, etc.

Introducing further requests: (Formal) Could you also please send me/Another matter I also need information is (informal) can you also find out, etc.

Closing remarks: (Formal) I look forward to receiving/I would appreciate it if you could inform me as soon as possible, etc. (Informal) Please, let me know/Send me the details, etc.

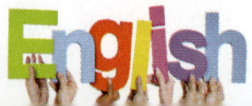

Useful Language for Letters Giving Information

Opening remarks: (Formal) I am writing in reply to your letter asking for information about/I am writing to inform you about/In reply to your query, etc. (Informal) You wanted me to tell you a few things about/This is what I found out, etc.

Closing remarks: (Formal) I hope that I have been of some assistance to you/Please inform me if I could be of any further assistance/Please do not hesitate to contact me if you need any further information, etc. (Informal) I hope this will help you/Please, let me know if you need any more help, etc.

LETTERS OF OPINION

- ❑ They regard a person's concern about and views on a certain matter and usually contain suggestions on how to tackle a problem. You need to state the nature of the problem and its causes and effects. Letters of opinion are usually letters to the authorities/editors of newspapers and are formal pieces of writing.
- ❑ They are written when we wish to express our approval or disapproval of something which is of interest to the general public or when we wish to reply to letters or articles previously published and on which we have strong views.
- ❑ Letters of this type tend to contain a combination of formal and informal languages such as idioms, phrasal verbs and rhetorical questions. This is done in order to have a more persuasive effect on the readers.
- ❑ When writing a letter to the editor it is necessary to refer to what other people may think of the subject we are expressing our views on. Each point should be presented in a separate paragraph containing a clear topic sentence supported by examples and/or justification.

Introduction

Paragraph 1: Appropriate opening remarks. State what subject you are going to give your opinion on and reason(s) for writing.

Main Body

Paragraph 2: Describe the problems(s) and consequences giving arguments to support your opinion.

Paragraph 3: Present opposing viewpoint and contradict it.

Paragraph 4: Suggest solutions/measures to be taken.

Conclusion

Sum up stating final conclusion and closing remarks.

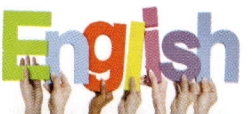

Useful Language for Letter of Opinion

Opening remarks: I am writing to draw your attention to/I am writing to you in my capacity as/I am writing to express my approval/disapproval of, etc.

To state your opinion: In my opinion/view, I feel/believe, I am totally opposed to/in favor of, It is my firm belief/conviction that/I am convinced that.... etc.

To express cause: Owing to the fact that/On the grounds that/In view of/For this reason, etc.

To express effect: Therefore/consequently/As a result

Closing remarks: I hope you will give this matter your urgent consideration/attention looking forward to hear from you.

LETTERS OF APPLICATION

- A formal letter of application is written when applying for a job or a place on an educational course.
- A letter of application should be similar in style to the advertisement; that is, if the job advertisement is written in a less formal style, the letter could also be written in a less formal style. On the other hand, if the job advertisement is written in a formal style, the letter must be formal, too.
- Advertisements for temporary jobs (holiday or summer jobs) may be written in a less formal style. A letter of application for such a job may not include extensive reference to experience, qualifications or skills.

Letters Applying for a Job

Introduction

Paragraph 1: Appropriate opening remarks, state reason for writing mentioning the position you would like to apply for and where and when you were informed about the vacancy.

Main Body

Paragraph 2: Give details of age, qualifications, present/past employment, qualities and skills and any other details you consider relevant.

Paragraph 3: Express your interest and suitability for the job and give your present/past employers' opinions of you. Appropriate closing remarks.

Conclusion

State that you are willing to attend an interview and look forward to a favorable reply.

Useful Language for Letters of Application (for a Job)

Opening remarks: I am writing with regard to your advertisement/I am writing to apply for the post/job/position of/which I saw advertised in, etc.

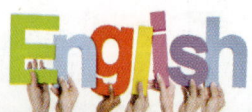

Reference to experience: ... for the past/last year/I have been working as/Two years ago I was employed as/I worked as/I have had experience of ... etc.

Closing remarks: I would appreciate a reply at your earliest convenience/Please contact me regarding any queries you might have/I enclose my curriculum vitae and I would be glad to attend an interview at any time convenient to you/I look forward to hearing from you in due course, etc.

Useful Language for Letters of Applications (for a Course)

Opening remarks: I would like to apply for admission to the beginning/I would like to be considered for, etc.

Reference to experience: I hold a certificate/degree in/I am due to take examinations in/I have completed the following courses/My degree is in English, etc.

Closing remarks: I would appreciate a prompt reply at your earliest convenience/I look forward to meeting you/I enclose, further details regarding my education and qualifications to date/I hope that you will consider me for entry/I look forward to receiving your response in the near future, etc.

LETTERS OF RECOMMENDATION

- ❑ In this type of letters you are usually requested to express your opinion on a certain matter and also to provide suggestions supported by expected results/consequences.
- ❑ In this type you might either be asked to recommend someone for a job or what might be done to further improve existing standards.

Introduction

Paragraph 1: Appropriate opening phrases. State reasons for writing.

Main Body

Paragraph 2: State who the person that you would like to recommend is and what you are recommending him/her for/give an overall opinion of the subject.

Paragraph 3: Give details of the person and the reason for recommending him/her/further actions to be taken making suggestions and commenting on the expected results.

Conclusion

Express your hope that he/she will be a suitable applicant offering to give further details upon request/final suggestion/recommendations on the subject.

Useful Languages for Letters of Recommendation

Introducing suggestions: To begin/start with, firstly, secondly, additionally, finally, etc.

Introducing the expected results: Thus, as a result, consequently, therefore, hence, etc.

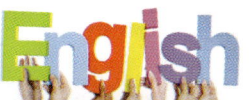

LETTERS OF ADVICE

- ❏ Letters asking for or giving advice can be formal, semiformal or informal depending on the situation. A letter asking for advice can be sent to a friend, a consultant or an advice column in a magazine.

Details of the problem should be mentioned.

- ❏ A letter giving advice should contain suggestions introduced with appropriate language.
- ❏ Letters of advice are usually written in response to a request or an enquiry.

Asking for Advice

Introduction

Paragraph 1: Appropriate opening remarks. State reasons for writing establishing friendly contact.

Main Body

Paragraph 2: Describe the circumstances.

Paragraph 3: Ask for a prompt reply making a final request for advice.

Conclusion

Appropriate closing remarks.

Useful Language for Letters for Advice

Opening remarks: (Formal) I would appreciate it if you could give me some advice about/I would be grateful if you could offer some advice/I wonder if you could help me with a problem, etc. (Informal) I am writing to ask for your advice/I have got a problem and I need your advice about … etc.

Closing remarks: (Formal) I would appreciate it if you could give me your advice as soon as possible/It would be of great help if you could advise me … etc. (Informal) Please let me know what you think I should do.

IMPORTANCE AND FUNCTION OF LETTER WRITING

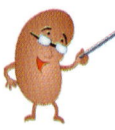

In both academic writing and professional writing, your goal is to convey information clearly and concisely, if not to convert the reader to your way of thinking. Transitions help you to achieve these goals by establishing logical connections between sentences, paragraphs and sections of your papers. In other words, transitions tell readers what to do with the information you present them. Whether single words, quick phrases or full sentences, they function as signs for readers that tell them how to think about, organize and react to old and new ideas as they read through what you have written.

Transitions signal relationships between ideas such as: Another example coming up-stay alert! or "Here's an exception to my previous statement" or "Although this idea appears to

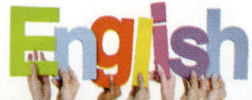

be true. Here's the real story." Basically transitions provide the reader with directions for how to piece together your ideas into a logically coherent argument. Transitions are not just "window dressing" that embellish your paper by making it sound or read better. There are words with particular meanings that tell the reader to think and react in a particular way to your ideas. In providing the reader with these important cues, transitions help readers understand the logic of how your ideas fit together.

Since the clarity and effectiveness of your transitions will depend greatly on how well you have organized your paper, you may want to evaluate your papers organization before you work on transitions. In the margins of your draft, summarize in a word or short phrase what each paragraph is about or how it fits into your analysis as a whole. This exercise should help you to see the order of and connection between your ideas more clearly.

If after doing this exercise you find that you still have difficulty linking your ideas together in a coherent fashion, your problem may not be with transitions but with organization.

BUSINESS LETTERS/ELEMENTS OF STRUCTURE

A **business letter** is more formal than a personal letter. It should have a margin of at least one inch on all four edges. It is always written on 8 (or metric equivalent) unlined stationery. There are six parts to a business letter.

1. *The heading:* This contains the return address (usually two or three lines) with the date on the last line.

    Sometimes it may be necessary to include a line alter the address and before the date for a phone number, fax number, Email address, or something similar.

    Often a line is skipped between the address and date. That should always be done if the heading is next to the left margin. It is not necessary to type the return address if you are using stationery with the return address already imprinted. Always include the date.

2. *The inside address:* This is the address you are sending your letter to make it as complete as possible. Include titles and names if you know them.

    This is always on the left margin. If an 0″ papcr is folded in thirds to fit in a standard 9″ business envelope, the inside address can appear through the window in the envelope.

    An inside address also helps the recipient route the letter properly and can help the envelope be damaged and the address become unreadable. Skip a line after the heading before the inside address. Skip another line after the inside address before the greeting.

3. *The greeting:* Also called the salutation. The greeting in a business letter is always formal. It normally begins with the word "Dear" and always includes the person's last name.

    It normally has a title. Use a first name only if the title is unclear. For example, you are writing to someone turned "Leslie" but do not know whether the person is male or female. For more on the form of titles, see the greeting in a business letter always ends in a colon. (You know you are in trouble if you get a letter from a boyfriend or girlfriend and the greeting ends in a colon—it is not going to be friendly.)

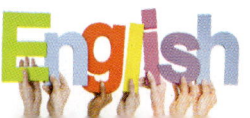

4. *The body:* The body is written as text. A business letter is never hand written. Depending on the letter style you choose, paragraphs may be indented. Regardless of format, skip a line between paragraphs. Skip a line between the greeting and the body. Skip a line between the body and the close.

5. *The complimentary close:* This short, polite closing ends with a comma. It is either at the left margin or its left edge is in the centre depending on the business letter style that you use. It begins at the same column the heading does.

   The block style is becoming more widely used because there is no indenting to bother with in the whole letter.

6. *The signature line:* Skip two lines (unless you have unusually wide or narrow lines) and type out the name to be signed. This customarily includes a middle initial, but does not have to. Women may indicate how they wish to be addressed by planning **Miss, Mrs, Ms** or similar title in parentheses before their name. The signature line may include a second line for a title if appropriate. The term "By direction" in the second line means that a superior is authorizing the signer.

   The signature should start directly above the first letter of the signature line in the space between the close and the signature line. Use blue or black ink.

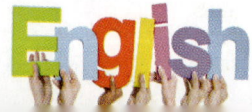

OFFICIAL LETTERS AND APPLICATIONS

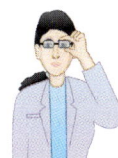

1. Write an application to your principal for remission of fine.

The Principal

Nursing College

Chandigarh

Sub: Remission of fine.

Sir/Madam

As I could not sit for the monthly test in English held yesterday, my English Teacher Mr AK Sharma, has fined me ₹200/- for that absence. I am extremely sorry for not taking the test, madam. But it happened because of circumstances over which I had no control.

I was just getting ready for school when my mother got a heart attack. As my father was not at home, I had to attend her. I had to arrange her medical aid on the spur of the moment, as all the members of the family were upset to see dear mother under the attack. In confusion, I could not send my application even for leave to my worthy teacher. Thank God that timely medical assistance saved life of my dear mother.

Thus my absence was not at all a studied happening but an unavoidable incident. I request your honor to remit the fine imposed on me by my worthy teacher. I assure you madam, that I will be extremely careful in future.

Thanking you

Yours obediently

Reena BSc 1st year   12/08/2021

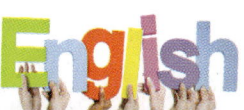

2. Write a letter to the Postmaster of your town complaining against the wrong delivery of your mail.

C-105, Vikaspuri
New Delhi
July 20, 2021
The Postmaster
Hira Nagar Post Office
New Delhi-110 018

Sub: Complaint against the wrong delivery of mail.

Sir

Please refer to my letter No. S.B./121/K.S.S./13, dated 29th June, 2021 in which I requested you to arrange the delivery of my mail at C-105, Vikaspuri, New Delhi-18. It is a new built two-storey house and I occupied its first floor in February 2021.

1 am sorry to bring to your kind notice that my mail is still delivered at my old residence A-250, Vikaspuri, New Delhi-18 where I used to reside before shifting to my present residence. To my good luck my previous landlord takes the trouble of sending my letters to me through his children.

Sir, you can well imagine the inconvenience and the unnecessary delay caused to me because of the misdelivery of my mail by your postoffice.

May I request you to consider my complaint sympathetically at your earliest and arrange for the correct delivery of my post at my present address?

Yours sincerely
IS Johar

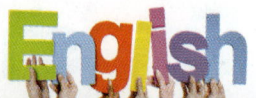

3. Write a letter to the Health Officer of the municipality of your town complaining against the poor sanitary conditions of your locality.

528, Green Avenue
Rajpura
July 18, 2021
The Health Officer
Municipal Committee
Rajpura

Sub: Complaining against the poor sanitary conditions.

Sir

May I draw your kind attention toward the poor sanitary condition of our area "Green Avenue" with the hope that necessary action will be taken to improve it as early as possible. I venture to say that you have never paid a visit to this area for the last one year at least otherwise the necessity of this complaint would not have been there.

Through this letter, I am going to voice the grievances of the residents of the above-named area. Several oral complaints to the sanitary inspector of this area have failed to bring about the desired result.

There are some old buildings on either side of the narrow lane No. 50. They are almost in ruins and lying uninhabited for years. Whenever there are rains, one part or the other of any of these buildings collapses. The debris blocks the way as well as all the drains. As a result, the dirty water overflows to push the area in an insanitary condition. Not only this, the falling buildings are danger to life also.

In short, the sanitary condition of our area is awfully bad. People use these old buildings as public latrines. The pigs make the matters still worse. The rains cause a foul smell to arise from those buildings and it spreads over the entire area. It is very much feared that some dangerous diseases may break out shortly.

I earnestly pray to you to take immediate steps to demolish these old buildings and improve the sanitary conditions through necessary instructions to your sanitary staff.

Thanking you
Yours sincerely
Garish Sharma

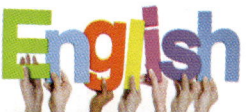

4. About increase in Thefts

You are Tarun Jain of 28, Sector 20A, Chandigarh. Write a letter to the Police Commissioner complaining about the number of thefts in your area.

28, Sector 20A
Chandigarh
June 2, 2021
The Police Commissioner
Chandigarh

Sub: Complaint against number of thefts.

Sir

Recently there has been an alarming increase in the number of thefts in the crowded area of this city. Hardly a day passes when there is no theft or burglary. Cases are regularly reported to the nearest Police Divisions but no headway has so far been made in apprehending the culprits. To be quite frank, people have started doubting that the policemen are mixed up with these thefts and burglaries. Though it is a wild charge, the fact remains that the culprits always go scot free. There is a danger to the life of the residents also since the burglars come armed with knives and pistols.

It is requested that night patrolling in this area should be intensified and all-out efforts should be made to nab the culprits.

Yours sincerely
Tarun Jain

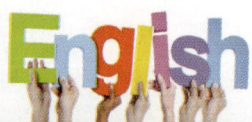

5. About law and order situation

You are Deepika of MS Nagar, Khanna. Write a letter to the SHO Mandi Road, Khanna, complaining about bad law and order situation in your area.

16, MS Nagar
Khanna
July 16, 2021
The SHO
Mandi Road
Khanna

Sub: Complaint against bad law and order situation.

Sir

The law and order situation in our area has gravely deteriorated during the past few months. Hardly a day passes when there is no incident of rowdyism. Some antisocial elements have sprung up in the absence of an effective check on them. They also extort money from petty shopkeepers in the area. Nobody dares to stand against them because of some musclemen at their back. They feel free to do any damn thing they like. They tease young girls going to or coming back from their school or college. People have started suspecting that some policemen are patronising them. It may not be true but the fact remains that these people have become a big trouble and nuisance for the residents. It is requested that some hard steps should be taken to curb the activities of these antisocial elements.

Yours sincerely

Deepika

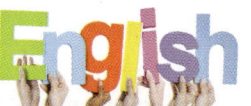

6. **Write a letter to the President of the Municipal Committee of your town requesting him to provide a park for children.**

17, Phase-7
Mohali
June 20, 2021
The President
Municipal Committee
Chandigarh

Sub: Provision of park for children.

Sir

It is a matter of regret that there is no park for children in our area. Children have no proper place to play in. They play either in the streets or on the road-sides. There always remains a danger of their being run over by some speeding vehicle. It is the duty of the civic authorities to look to this need of their tiny citizens.

Children have an inborn love of beauty and nature. They love flowers, trees, parks and gardens. This love of beautiful objects changes into a love of beautiful thoughts when they grow up. So we must provide children with beautiful surroundings if we want them to grow into men and women of refined tastes.

Parks are necessary from another point of view also. They add to the beauty of a town. Children can play there while the elders can refresh their weary minds. So, it is requested that at least one big park should be provided for children.

Yours sincerely
Hari Sharma
President
Mohali
Welfare Society

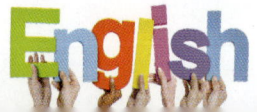

7. Write a letter of complaint to a firm that the goods sent by it are defective and asking for a free replacement.

\# 7, Sector 71
Mohali
June 14, 2021

M/s Ram Nath & Sons
Daryaganj
New Delhi

Sub: Regarding order No. R-620.

Dear Sir

The forty Computer keyboards that we ordered on 5th March were delivered yesterday. I regret that eight of them are defective and damaged.

The packet containing the keyboards appeared to be in perfect condition. Therefore, I accepted the delivery and signed for it. I unpacked the keyboards myself with great care. I can only say that the defect or damage must have been caused due to careless handling by your men. I have sent back the defective keyboards through the local Akal Transport Company.

It is requested that all these keyboards should be replaced free of keyboards cost.

Yours sincerely
Ram Nath

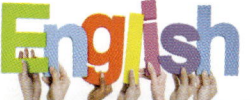

8. **Write a letter to your bankers requesting for a short-term loan explaining the circumstances why you require it, and assuring them of an early repayment.**

Evershine Garments
Industrial Area, Patiala
January 3, 2021
The Manager
State Bank of Patiala
The Mall Patiala

Sub: Request for short-term loan.

Dear Sir

As you know, our firm has been keeping a current account with your branch for the past several years. Our past record is absolutely clean. We have never over-drafted nor has any of our cheques ever bounced.

Now we are in need of short-term loan for the purpose of expanding our factory. We want to buy some new machinery which is estimated at about rupees two lakh. It will increase our production manifold and we hope to make good its cost in less than a year's time.

We request you to grant us a loan of rupees two lakh for a period of one year and we promise to repay it with interest. Possibly even before the due date.

Yours sincerely

SP Sharma

MD

Evershine Garments

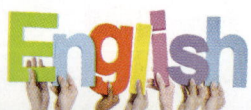

9. Write a letter to the Deputy Commissioner requesting for a government hospital in your area.

5, Model Town
Ramesh Nagar
Patiala
March 20, 2021
The Deputy Commissioner
ABC City

Sub: Request for a Government Hospital.

Sir

It is strange but true that our town, with a population of fifty thousand is without a Government hospital. This causes great hardship to the residents.

There are some private physicians and surgeons in the town, but their charges are very high. Consequently, a large number of patients have to go to a hospital which is at a distance of 5 kilometers. Only the other day a patient died on the way.

The town has the distinction of supplying to the Indian Army quite a large number of jawans and officers. So it has a greater claim on the civil authorities. The residents of our town have already contacted the local MLA in this connection. He has kindly assured us to consider our request sympathetically.

1 would request you to take up the matter with the higher authorities for favorable consideration of our genuine demand.

I am enclosing the signatures of 500 residents of the town in support of my request.

Yours sincerely
Rakesh Chander

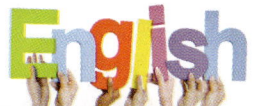

10. **Write to the Editor of a daily newspaper about improvement in the bus service in your town.**

117, Model Town
Amritsar
January 12, 2021
The Editor
The Tribune
Amritsar

Sub: Regarding improvement in the bus service.

Sir

Please permit me to bring to the notice of the transport authorities of the State, the deplorable condition of the local bus service in our town. The bus service in this town has been going from bad to worse from the last six months or so. Previously it was satisfactory but recently it has crossed all the limits of tolerance. It has touched the rock bottom of the efficiency. First of all the number of buses is very few. The population of our town has been increasing rapidly. But the number of buses has remained unchanged for the last so many years. While the fares have been going up, the difficulties of the people have been increasing.

I would request the General Manager to travel in a bus for some time and see for himself how the passengers have to suffer. The overcrowding has reached a point of suffocation. People at the bus stops have to wait because the buses come overloaded from the previous stops. The conductors have also become rude because of such crowds. There is much pushing and jostling by the people trying to come in or go out of the buses at various stops. The students and the office goers are particularly in trouble. They cannot reach their destinations on time. Many of them can often be seen running after the buses hanging on the foot boards. I hope that the authorities would look into the matter before there is some violent agitation. The people are really sick of the local bus service.

Yours truly
Raj Kumar

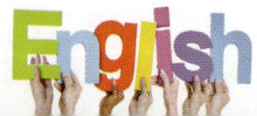

11. Write a letter to the Editor of a newspaper commenting on the increasing display of violence and sex in Indian films.

119, Street No 1
Sirhindi Gate
Patiala
July 23, 2021
The Editor
The Indian Express
Chandigarh

Sub: Increasing display of violence and sex in Indian films.

Sir

I shall be thankful if you allow me to air my views about the increasing display of violence and sex in Indian films.

The increasing display of violence and sex in Indian films is highly disturbing and objectionable. The producers feel that the success of their film can be ensured only with liberal inclusion of semi-naked beauties swaying their hips in all kinds of vulgar ways. Bed-room scenes, bathing scenes, rape scenes, whether or not the story demands them, are inserted at every odd place. As a result, most of the Indian films now are full of scenes which are disgustingly lewd and utterly unsuitable for mass viewing.

Another menace on the increase is the use of violence. The fight composer has acquired a far greater importance than the director himself. He is constantly trying to discover clever ways of perpetrating cruelty. Torture and persecution are being raised to the level of art. The ill effect of this indulgence in violence on the minds of young boys and girls who feel exalted in intimating their heroes cannot be underestimated. Their entire sensibility is being gradually contaminated. They now think that violence not only enjoys social sanction but is something to gloat over and they claim license to indulge in it. The situation has become too grave to be neglected any longer.

But the solution does not lie in a kind of blanket directive that all scenes depicting violence should be strictly excluded from films. Sex, the physical manifestation of love, if treated artistically, becomes a source of pleasure. Violence is one way in which evil is objected to and any medium that aims at a faithful representation of life cannot exclude evil altogether. All that is needed is just this, the depiction of sex be freed from vulgarity and lust and violence depicted in such a manner that it appears hateful rather than glorious.

Yours truly
Sunil Kapoor

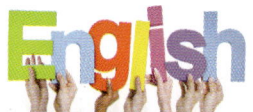

12. Write a letter to the Editor of a daily newspaper expressing your views about the evil of eve-teasing at all the public places. Suggest some remedies and measures to curb the evil.

1197, Sector 18-C
Chandigarh
July 16, 2021
The Editor
The Hindustan Times
Chandigarh

Sub: Regarding evil of eve-teasing at public places.

Sir

I shall be thankful if you allow me to express my views through the columns of your newspaper regarding the increasing incidents of eve-teasing in our town. Eve-teasing has become very common in buses on the road-side in front of cinema and other public places. Road-side romeos are always on the prowl to pass indecent remarks at girls and young women who happen to pass by them. Bottom pitching is common in overcrowded buses in big cities. Loafers are always ready to say something vulgar and obscene if an unescorted girl happens to travel in a bus or goes along a road. The increasing incidents of eve-teasing is a telling commentary on the hopeless law and order situation. Even when a girl makes a report to a policeman standing by, he simply shuts his eyes. Incidents of eve-teasing can also be seen in front of girl's colleges. Recently a cricketer turned politician's wife was subjected to eve-teasing by the men in a Maruti car when she was taking a walk on a city road. Sexy scenes in films and obscene posters also encourage the boys to resort to eve-teasing. Moreover, some girls are also to blame. They wear provocative dresses and thus invite comments from the rowdies.

Remedial measures should be taken by posting policemen in plain clothes in front of girl's institutions. Surprise checks must be carried out in public places. Young men found guilty of eve-teasing must be booked and punished immediately. In buses, seats for women should be reserved. No male should be allowed to sit there. Such steps would curb the evil of eve-teasing to a considerable extent.

Yours truly
Shiva

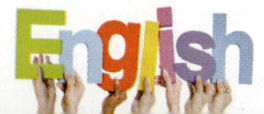

13. Write a letter to the Editor of a newspaper appealing for the help of the victims of flood.

12, Model Town
Jalandhar City
July 21, 2021
The Editor
The Tribune
Chandigarh

Sub: Appeal for help for the victims of flood.

Sir

I shall feel obliged if you kindly publish my following appeal to help the victims of recent floods that have destroyed the best area in the Jalandhar district.

No doubt the people are already familiar with the terrible tragedy that has overtaken the poor inhabitants of this part. But I have visited the scenes of recent victims and I must appeal to the people of the State to contribute liberally for the help of sufferers. The sad plight of the victims is hard to describe. Hundreds of villages have been completely destroyed, a large number of cattle have been swept away, the crops over large areas have been destroyed and thousands of people have been rendered homeless. Some are living in temporary shelters, exposed to the harsh weather many of them are suffering from lack of food and clothing. Moreover, the swampy area is an unhealthy breeding ground for mosquitoes and other disease germs resulting in the breaking out of diseases, like malaria, typhoid and cholera. The Government is doing all it can, to relieve the suffering of the victims but much larger funds are needed for their rehabilitation. Without the cooperation of the public tremendous task of relieving the distress of the people cannot be coped with by the Government alone.

I, therefore, strongly appeal to the public to rise to the occasion and help the Government in this humanitarian task of relief of flood victims. By their liberal contribution to Prime Minister's Flood Relief Fund, the people will earn the gratitude of the poor suffering fellow men.

Yours truly
Ramesh Kumar

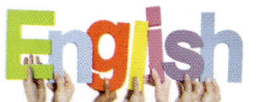

14. Write a letter to the Editor of a newspaper complaining against reckless driving.

15, Sector 15-A
Chandigarh
July 12, 2021
The Editor
The Tribune
Chandigarh

Sub: Complaint against reckless driving.

Sir

I shall feel grateful if you allow me some space, in your esteemed paper. I want to draw the attention of the authorities concerned toward the reckless driving in Jalandhar.

Jalandhar has wide roads and chances of accidents are very less here. But, probably a terrific speed, trucks carrying sand, stones or bricks are seen moving at a very fast speed. Carts pass by you whizzing even at turnings. Young college boys drive motorcycles and scooters without caring for their own or anybody else's life. It poses a danger to school-going children, to old men and women who cannot cross the road quickly.

The rash driving is a regular nuisance and is responsible for fatal accidents which take place daily. Not a single day passes when we do not hear of some accidents. Yesterday a young man, who was on the left side, was run over by a motor cycle. The motor-cyclist sped away at a great speed and nobody could even take down number of his motorcycle. Speed limits are not strictly enforced. Many a time defaulters bribe the policeman on duty and get away unbooked.

The need of the hour is that a speed limit should be fixed and the offenders be severely dealt with.

Yours truly
Rajesh

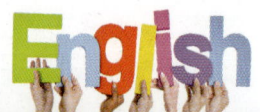

15. Write a letter to the Editor of a newspaper expressing your views regarding the nuisance of stray cattle in Punjab cities.

125, Ranjit Avenue
Batala
July 12, 2021
The Editor
The Indian Express
Chandigarh

Sub: Regarding nuisance of stray cattle.

Sir

I shall be thankful if you allow me to express my views about the nuisance of stray cattle on the roads of Punjab towns through the columns of your newspaper.

Cows, bulls, buffaloes and stray dogs have become a terrific hazard on our state city roads. Cattle squat on the roads and throw traffic out of gear. The presence of stray cattle often leads to accidents.

Some crossings are always crowded with cattle, when the lights turn red, the pedestrians cannot cross. When the lights turn green, vehicles cannot pass because of the stubborn presence of the cattle.

Cattle and dogs often excrete on the roads. This causes filth and stench all around. Such excreta is a breeding ground for bacteria which can spread various diseases.

Some remedial steps are urgently needed to check the nuisance.

Yours truly
Ravi Malhotra

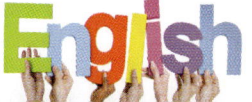

16. Write a letter to the Editor of a newspaper appealing to the public in general and students in particular not to burst crackers on Diwali.

145, Urban Estate
Patiala
May 16, 2021
The Editor
The Tribune
Chandigarh

Sub: Regarding not to burst crackers on Diwali.

Sir

Kindly allow me to express my views about the bursting crackers on Diwali through the columns of your newspaper.

Bursting of crackers has become a regular feature of celebration of Diwali in our state and country. Diwali is actually a festival of lights. It should be celebrated by the lightning of lamps or 'diyas'. Unfortunately, the young and the old join one another in celebrating Diwali with the bursting of dangerous and very noisy crackers. Such a practice adds to the air pollution in our already congested and overcrowded towns and cities. Incidents of acute asthma, bronchitis and heart attack are often reported. In certain cases, deafness is caused by crackers. Mischievous boys take delight in bursting crackers when passers-by happen to pass by them. Thus these crackers become hazards for life. Sometimes shops dealing in crackers catch fire by care-less bursting of crackers near these very shops.

I appeal to the public and youth not to burst crackers on Diwali. They should celebrate it as a festival of lights.

Yours truly
Kapil

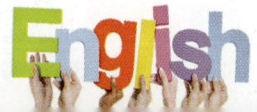

17. Write a letter to the Editor of a newspaper against the municipal council of your town who is not performing duties properly.

104, Nehru Street
Subhash Nagar
Barnala
April 6, 2021
The Editor
The Times of India
Chandigarh

Sub: Complaint against municipal council.

Sir

The municipal council of our town seems to be very indifferent to the hopeless condition of our street. Otherwise it must have attended to our genuine grievances brought to its notice from time to time.

We are fed up with the attitude of the council particularly for three things. First, the roads of our street are in poor shape. They are full of dangerous pits, which cause accidents and breed mosquitoes during the rainy season. Moreover, the street presents the very picture of ugliness with the heaps of refuse lying here and there. This is due to the careless attitude of the sweeper, who rarely visits the street. And whenever he comes he behaves like a bully. As if this were not bad enough, the street is poorly lit. The electric bulbs or tubes, once damaged, are replaced after months. This results in accidents and thefts on dark nights.

So I would like to request the authorities concerned to wake up to their obligations to the residents of our street and set things right.

Yours truly
Kamala

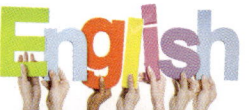

18. Write a letter to the Editor of a newspaper expressing your concern at the cruelty against animals, people's attitude to it and how this menace can be checked.

7, Model Enclave
Janipur Road
Rohtak
May 10, 2021
The Editor
The Times of India
Delhi

Sub: Cruelty against animals.

Dear Sir

The Prevention of Cruelty to Animals Act exists only on paper. The Times of India on Tuesday carried a photograph of a horse dangling precariously in the air, simply because the cart it was pulling was so overloaded that it had tipped over. The agony of the animal haunts the mind for long and the dramatic photograph highlights how cruel and callous society is toward animals. It is obvious that the cart had been carrying more weight than the 750 kg limit fixed by law.

Animal rights activists say that even this limit is too high, and that in any case, most owners overload the carts, especially those carrying goods like steel bars and spiked objects. Any policeman above the rank of a constable is empowered to take action against such violations, but often, they take a lenient view since owners are often poor. In general, society's attitude toward animals, with the specific exception of pets, has been indifferent or negative. Circuses continued to use animals in their acts, till they were forced to desist. Now without the animals also, the circuses run well. There are regular reports of stray animals, especially cows and bulls, facing hardship.

Most of the time, the concern merely amounts to lip service. As a society, we need to be more aware of the conditions around us and be more responsive toward these hapless creatures who cannot articulate their pain. After all, a society is judged by how it treats animals.

Yours truly
Brijesh Khattar

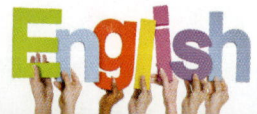

INFORMAL LETTERS

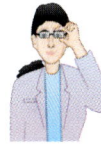

1. **Write a letter to your younger brother advising him to pay proper attention to his health.**

#1220, Sector 18-C
II Chandigarh
July 23, 2021

Dear Avish

I received your progress report only yesterday and was very glad to go through it. You have secured 82% marks in aggregate and distinction in almost all subjects. This is very heartening and I am sure that a little more effort on your part is sure to win you a very high position in the Board Examination. We all are very happy here to know of your brilliant progress in studies.

But one thing is very sad and alarming. You have lost weight during the last two months. How is it? It shows you have not been paying any attention to your health. Certainly you stay away from games and sports. At the same time you do not seem to be taking regular exercise and healthy food. This is not proper at all. Achievement in studies at the cost of health is of no use. So, I would advise you to pay proper attention to your health through exercise, wholesome food and proper rest and sleep.

With love and best wishes.

Yours affectionately
Parth

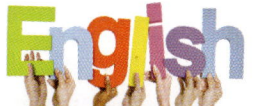

2. Write a letter to your friend on his recovery from serious illness.

#589, Sector 20-A

Chandigarh

March 16, 2021

Dear Mohit

It is indeed heartening to note that you have survived the worst ordeal of attack of influenza and are now on a fair way to recovery.

Your father must have told you of my visit to your house about a fortnight back. You were then suffering from high fever and could not recognize me at all. It was certainly a period of very great anxiety for your family and friends. We prayed to the Almighty to spare your promising life.

Please accept my heartiest congratulations on your recovery. Please be careful not to overwork.

With love and best wishes:

Yours sincerely

Manish

3. Write a letter to your father asking him for money and explaining why you need it.

R.No. 15

GSCON Hostel

Ram Nagar

March 23, 2021

Dear Dad

I have received your affectionate letter in which you have advised me to pay attention to my studies. I venture to confess that I have not been working according to any time table so far. I always studied by fits and starts with the result that my progress has always been discouraging.

Dad, I have now resolved to observe regularity at my studies devoting my full attention to them according to a time table. You will appreciate to learn that I need an alarm clock for this purpose. It will help me to rise early and also to study regularly.

I have enquired from the market that a good alarm clock costs ₹300/-. Moreover, I need some good books also to prepare myself for the annual examination. I think ₹1500/- will do for the books. So, be kind enough to send me ₹1800/- at the earliest. I assure you that the next report from my college will please you.

With deepest regards

Your loving daughter

Sheena

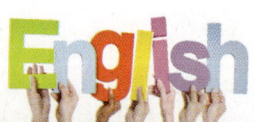

4. Write a letter to your friend describing him a horrible dream.

100 Lower Bazaar
Shimla
July 12, 2021

Dear Sheeba

Last night, 1 saw a horror film on the TV. It was about ghosts and witches. After the film, I took my meal and lay on the bed. I do not know when sleep overpowered me. In my sleep, I passed through strange regions. I met an old man who was a magician, he said that he could command airy spirits to do anything he liked. I laughed at him saying that he was an imposter. The old man grew angry with me. He lifted both his hands up in the air and muttered some strange words.

Immediately, two big cobras appeared in his hands. He let loose these cobras toward me. I lifted my feet off the ground. I gave a loud cry of fear. My father, who was sleeping by my side got up. He shook me and asked what the matter was. I told him about my horrible dream.

Yours sincerely

Parth

5. Write a letter to your neighbor about the nuisance caused by his dog.

#1187, Sector 18-C
Chandigarh
April 12, 2021

Dear Mr Suresh

It sounds very strange that I should approach my neighbor a letter instead of talking to him personally. But sir, you are hardly ever seen at your house. Moreover, your dog restrains me from calling at your house. It was on this score that I wanted to talk to you.

Dear Mr Suresh I know that you are a very gentle and soft spoken person. But perhaps you do not know the mischief your dog is doing to your good name. All the people in the street are scared of your dog. Your servant keeps him unchained. He keeps roaming about in the street and barks at little children. Poor children cannot play in the street. No sooner do they step into the street then your dog chases them back into their houses.

None can deny your right to keeping a dog. But at the same time you must consider that others too have the right to live in peace. Please ask your servant to keep the dog chained so that the residents may be able to move about freely.

Yours sincerely

Manish

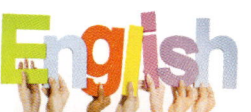

6. Write a letter to a friend whom you have offended by saying unkind words in a fit of anger.

#126, Street No-I

Banur

April 12, 2021

Dear Varinder

I am extremely sorry for what happened yesterday in the recess period. I thought that you intentionally pushed me against the wall. I got some bruises on my arm. So I lost my temper.

I spoke many harsh and insulting words to you. In that fit of anger, I thought you deserved all that and even much more.

But now I have realized my mistake. Anil came to my house this morning. He was present at the time of the incident. He told me that a naughty boy had pushed you. You lost your balance and fell on me. So, you were not at all to blame.

Varinder dear, I am ashamed of my rude behavior. I am really sorry for it. I hope you will forgive me. Please do not let this incident affect our friendship.

Yours sincerely

Mohan

7. Write a letter to your father informing him about a prize which you have won by standing first in the house examination.

Nehru Street

Manali

May 14, 2021

My dear father

The prize-distribution function of our college was held on the seventh of this month. The Chief Minister presided over the function.

Dear father, you will be glad to know that I have won a prize by standing first in the house examination. There were many prize winners, but I was the first to be called for getting the prize. I went to the dais and shook hands with the Chief Minister. The students and the teachers gave loud cheers. The Chief Minister gave me the prize and took me in his embrace. After this I came back to my seat. 1 wish, papa, you had been there on that day.

After giving away the prizes, the President made a speech. He advised the students to work hard and to remain away from politics. After this our Principal thanked the President and the function came to a close. All my friends gathered round me and asked for a party. I entertained them with sweets and cold drinks.

With regards

Your loving son

Jagan Nath

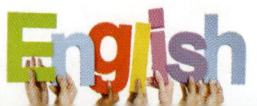

8. Write a letter to your friend describing some interesting details of your sister's marriage.

1098, Seem 22-A

Chandigarh

June 18, 2021

My dear Avish

I missed you badly at the time of my elder sister's marriage. It was an occasion of fun and joy. We ate, drank and made merry. I want to tell you some interesting details of this marriage.

The marriage party came from Panchkula. There were men, women and children in the marriage party. They came dancing to the beat of drums. We gave them a warm reception. Dinner was served to them.

After dinner, the bridegroom was taken inside the house. He was teased much by my sister's friends. They asked him many odd questions. The poor fellow only smiled them off. When the wedding rites were being performed, some girls gave him hard pinches. The elders blessed the new couple after the marriage ceremony was over.

The scene of partying was very touching. Nothing could console my parents. There were tears in every eye. The bride and the bridegroom sat in a decorated car. They went away leaving us all in tears.

With love

Your friend

Vishal

9. Write a letter to your friend, telling him some details of a marriage party that you attended.

18, Kidwai Street

Ludhiana

May 18, 2021

My dear Mohan

Last Sunday, I joined the marriage party of my friend's elder brother. The marriage party consisted of ten members only. We reached the bride's house at 10 am. We were given a warm reception. However, no formalities were observed. It was all a very simple but impressive affair.

The bride and the bridegroom garlanded each other. A priest solemnised the marriage ceremony. He recited 'mantras'. The bride and the bridegroom made seven rounds of the holy fire. The two were now husband and wife. The elders blessed the new couple.

After this we were served with lunch. There were no costly dishes. The meals were simple but tasty. We prepared to leave at 4 pm. No dowry was taken. Everybody praised the boy and his father who had set an example for others. It was really an ideal marriage. If only all young men could follow this example.

Your friend

Mahesh

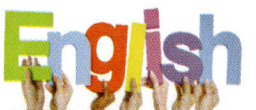

10. **Write a letter to your father asking him for permitting you to join an educational tour of your college.**

GSCON Hostel

Banur

June 20, 2021

My dear father

Our college is breaking up for Christmas holidays on the 24th of this month. Some students of our college are going on an educational tour. The tour has been organised by our Principal. It will be a seven-day tour, from December 25 to December 31. The students shall be taken to some places of historical interest. They shall visit Jaipur, Agra and Delhi. Dear father, I have a great desire to join this tour. It is only rarely that such tours are organised. It will give me a chance to learn about India's glorious past.

I request you to allow me to go on this tour. I shall not spend much. Each student has to deposit ₹2,500 for this tour. I shall do with only ₹500 for my pocket expenses. Kindly send me ₹3,000 as soon as possible. I hope you will not disappoint me. You are my sweet dear father, aren't you?

With regards

Your loving daughter

Manisha

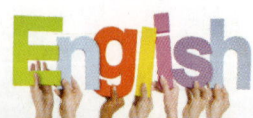

Practice Exercises

I. Write a letter to your pen friend who is coming to meet you for the first time. How he/she should recognise you. You will be waiting to receive him/her at the railway station.

II. Your younger brother, Suresh, needs your advice for the preparation of his secondary school exams. Write a letter to him giving some tips in brief. You are Ramesh/Reena staying in Kotagiri Public School hostel, Kotagiri.

III. You could not visit your sister at Nepal due to certain unavoidable circumstances. Write a letter to your sister explaining and regretting your inability. You are Madhu/Madhvan of Kerala.

IV. Your sister has not been able to qualify her entrance test for PhD. Write a letter to console her as she is very upset.

V. Write a letter to the Editor of the Indian Express drawing the attention of the concerned authorities toward indiscipline in the universities. Also give suggestions.

VI. You are upset to find the only public garden of your locality has been grabbed by the local self- styled 'Netas'. Write a letter to the Editor of 'The Hindu' drawing the attention of the government to this unauthorized occupation.

VII. Write a letter to the Editor of "The Times of India" about the poor attention and the negligence on the part of the medical staff in some of the government hospitals of Chennai.

VIII. You are Supriya of Indira Nagar Ludhiana. Write a letter to the Editor of "The Tribune" Chandigarh about the misuse and poor maintenance of public parks in your city.

IX. Write a letter to the Editor of the "The Indian Express" about the impact of watching too much television on the health and studies of the school going children.

X. You are worried that in spite of a legal ban on child marriages in the state Bhopal. Thousands of child marriages are performed. Write a letter to the Editor, "The Bhopal Times" expressing strong views against child marriages and advocating some immediate steps to get rid of this social evil.

XI. Write a letter to the Editor of a national daily expressing your views on our present system of examinations.

XII. Write a letter to your father telling him what you plan to do after completing your studies.

XIII. Write an encouraging letter to a friend who has suffered a loss in business.

XIV. Write an application to the Principal of a school for the post of a teacher.

XV. Write a letter to your mother about restrictions in the college hostel.

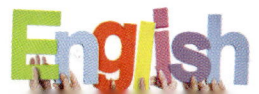

NOTES

Chapter 23

Note Taking and Note Making

NOTE TAKING

Note-taking is an important skill for students, especially at the college level. In some contexts, such as college lectures, the main purpose of taking notes may be to implant the material in the mind, the written notes themselves being of secondary importance.

Note-taking is a central aspect of a complex human behavior related to information management involving a range of underlying mental processes and their interactions with other cognitive functions. The person taking notes must acquire and filter the incoming sources, organize and restructure existing knowledge structures, comprehend and write down their explanation of the information, and ultimately store and integrate the freshly processed material. The result is a knowledge representation, and a memory storage. Studies comparing the performance of students who took handwritten notes to students who typed their notes found that students who took handwritten notes performed better on examinations, hypothetically due to the deeper processing of learned material through selective rephrasing instead of word-for-word transcription which is common when typing notes.

Note making is useful. It involves a useful exercise and practice for the reader, it enables a person to summarize relevant information from a given text. The condensed form can be there whenever needed. Thus note–making will prove handy not only for examination but help in life as well.

Importance of Notes

- ❏ Notes help in remembering the information collected.
- ❏ Notes come in handy for a quick revision before the examination.
- ❏ Notes help in understanding the texts better.
- ❏ Lengthy lessons can be condensed into short relevant pieces by making notes.
- ❏ Notes help in storing supplementary material taken from reference books or journals.
- ❏ Notes help in making a speech or writing an article.

How to Make Notes?

In order to make clear and concise notes quickly you must be methodical, follow these steps:

- ❏ Read the passage from beginning to end. Try to grasp the gist of the passage, ask your-self: What is it about?' This will provide you the theme and subject of the passage.
- ❏ Read the passage again very carefully, underline (Or mentally make a note of) the main idea.
- ❏ Make a note of the main ideas.
- ❏ Try to find out allied ideas to the main ideas, these will form the sub points as they supplement the main points.
- ❏ The sub-heading or allied ideas may have one or more ideas, find these. These will form sub-sub headings.

What do you Notice?

- ❏ The points are numbered in different ways, but the numbering is uniform.
- ❏ The sub points as well as the sub-sub points are also numbered, they also indent.
- ❏ **Title:** Underline with double lines, it should be a phrase. Avoid verbs and use a short title.

Form of Sentences

Use brief, clear phrases or words, complete sentences are not needed. Use symbols and abbreviations

Universal Symbols

for and	% for per cent
sub for subject sub	100 for hundred
acc for according.	e.g., for example

Important Note

1. Write notes in phrases/words.
2. Eliminate all examples and figurative speeches.

NOTE MAKING

However note-taking is an art and one needs to be very critical while taking notes. Different techniques such as SQ3R approach or a more visual approach, i.e., a spray diagram can be made use of while taking notes. As far as note making is concerned, the knowledge of organizational skills is very important. The lecturer or the author organizes his/her material in a logical way, so the students should try to utilize their organizational skills while taking the notes. This helps one in giving the final shape to one's notes when one is in the process of giving final touch by making the notes. Effective note taking along with its final make-up reduces one's study time, increases one's retention of knowledge and provides one with a summarized list of resources for one's future projects.

Now before we proceed further, it is worthwhile to make a distinction between the two concepts, i.e., Note-taking and note-making can be done from lectures and reading.

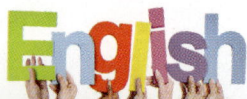

Note-taking is a preliminary process where the person tries to pen down the overall impression of a lecture or a preliminary reading. Though various methods are available for taking notes, involving various strategies, yet more or less, this is a primary exercise to have a track of the material listened to or read.

Note-making, however, is an advanced exercise as it comes after has taken notes. It is the process of consciously organizing the haphazard information in order to give it a final shape. Thus it involves an analysis, synthesis and proper outlining of the gathered material so that it may be consulted for future reference or grasp.

The Purpose of Notes Making

One should focus on note making because:
- ❏ Notes trigger memories of lecture/reading.
- ❏ Notes are often a source of valuable clues for what information the instructor thinks is the most important.
- ❏ Notes inscribe information kinesthetically.
- ❏ Taking notes help one to concentrate in class.
- ❏ Notes create a resource for test preparation.
- ❏ Notes often contain information that cannot be found elsewhere.
- ❏ Notes build up an understanding of the topic. Taking notes forces one to make sense of the text so that one can paraphrase in one's own notes.
- ❏ Notes prompt questions and debate.
- ❏ Notes act as a Symbol of Progress. They are a testimony to the fact that one has worked so much to aid one's understanding and thus it greatly boosts one's morale.

Phases of Note Taking

- ❏ Before the class
  - Read assigned material and highlight important information.
  - Review notes from previous session.
  - Begin notes for each lecture on a new page.
  - Date each page of your notebook as well as date and number each handout.
  - Identify the chapter being covered at the top of the page.
- ❏ During the class
  - Don't let your mind wander and stay focused.
  - Participate in the class.
  - Watch for clues to identify the important information.
  - Highlight the information that the instructor states as it is important.
  - Use symbols or abbreviations for commonly used words by writing the first few letters.
- ❏ After the class
  - Review, revise, or edit your notes as soon as possible after the lecture by filling in the gaps, clarifying words or ideas, adding any missing information, or adding any details to clarify a point.
  - Use your textbook or a friend's notes to clarify points
  - Rewrite notes if necessary.

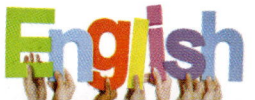

NOTES

Chapter 24

Précis Writing

INTRODUCTION

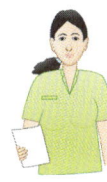

Précis-writing is an exercise in comprehension. A précis is a summary and précis writing means summarizing. A précis is the gist or substance or main theme of a given passage in as few words as possible. Thus précis-writing is an exercise in expression and includes all the essential facts of the passage to be summarized. All unnecessary details are to be left out. Although no strict rules can be laid down for the length of précis, but usually it should not contain more than one-third of the number of the words in the original. Précis-writing is a very fine exercise in reading. Most of the people read carelessly, and retain only a vague idea of what they have read. It is a very useful exercise in comprehension (understanding), in order to get the real idea of the passage. This is very important otherwise the summary will not present the salient features of the passage given. The following procedure may be followed while attempting a précis:

- Read the passage carefully, several times, if necessary, to get the real idea of the passage. The more you go through it, the clearer will be its subject and what is said about the subject.
- Go through the passage again and underline all that seems relevant to the passage and number them at the margin.
- Arrange the marked lines in the best possible manner to make an outline summary.
- Go through the summary again and strike out those points or portions, which have no bearing on the topic.
- Avoid repetition and illustrations.
- Write summary in your own words. Never try to copy out words or phrases from the original otherwise your summary will present a look of disjoined piece. You may, of course, retain the most important words of the original.
- Write your summary in the indirect form of speech and in third person.
- Use the same tense throughout.
- If the summary is too long, you should try to remove some words which do not seem to be very important or which can be expressed in fewer words. Write it out again.
- Supply a short title which might express the subject of the passage.

A GOOD PRÉCIS

A good précis comprises the following essentials:

- ❑ Accuracy
- ❑ Clearness
- ❑ Completeness
- ❑ Coherence
- ❑ Conciseness

In compressing three hundred words into hundred words, it is obvious that much must be deleted. Hence, the art of précis-writing lies in making the right omissions and in combining skillfully what is left.

ART OF COMPRESSION

Generally, you are supposed to follow the order of original but you are not bound to follow the same, if you can express its meaning more clearly and concisely by transporting any of its parts. The art of compression aims rather at remodeling than mere omissions. The following are a few examples:

- ❑ The rain continued unabated and did not cease until it was day dawn. The rain continued till dawn.
- ❑ George was hard up for money and was being pressed by his creditors. George was in financial difficulties.
- ❑ Sham fell into the river and before help could reach him, he sank. Sham drowned in the river.
- ❑ Mahatma Gandhi lived the life of an ascetic, abstaining from all luxuries and comforts, drinking the goat's milk and never caring for fashionable dresses. Mahatma Gandhi lived like an ascetic, shunning all luxuries of the world.
- ❑ Science has been having a harmful effect upon religion. Science is the negation of religion.
- ❑ The courage of Arjuna in battle might, without exaggeration be called lion like. Arjuna fought like a lion.
- ❑ Those days when most of the people used to keep cows and buffaloes for milk are now dead and gone.
  In olden days, people used to keep buffaloes and cows.
- ❑ Zoo is a place where all kinds of fish, flesh and fowl, harmless birds, animals and those that are dangerous, tame and wild are kept. Zoo is a place for beasts and fowls.
- ❑ When sorrows come, they do not come alone but in battalions. Calamities do not come alone.

SOME PRACTICAL SUGGESTIONS FOR WRITING PRÉCIS

The student should go through the following suggestions carefully. These are no magic formulas or short-cuts, but a careful study of these suggestions will prepare the student better to attempt the question on précis-writing.

- ❑ **Try to use one word for a group of words as:**
  - • 'That which cannot be seen' can be replaced by 'invisible'.

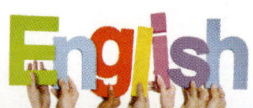

- 'Something that cannot be heard' can be replaced by 'inaudible'.

Example:

This is a state of affairs that cannot be tolerated by a man who has the capacity to see beyond the immediate present.

This can be summarized as:

This state of affairs is intolerable for a far-sighted man.

□ **Replace clauses by phrases and phrases by words:**

- *In a suitable manner* can be replaced by *suitably.*
- Sardar Patel, who was known as the iron man of India and who was a man of a very well-known strong will, set all the princes right by just one stroke of the pen in no time.

This can be summarized as:

Sardar Patel, a strong-willed man, set the princes right in no time.

Example:

The coming of machines has enabled people to produce a far greater quantity of goods than they had done in the past. Because of machines there are many more things of all kinds that people have in the world today than ever had before.

This above passage can be summarized as:

Machines have increased production considerably and the modern man has a greater variety of things available to him.

□ **Similarly passages can be condensed into a single sentence or shorter passages.**

Example:

The world has received its leaders and philosophers from the cottages of the poor only. Poverty has always been the breeding ground for greatness in life. Lal Bahadur Shastri was born in a poor home; he became the Prime Minister of India. Same was the case with Abraham Lincoln. Thomas Alva Edison was not born with a silver spoon in his mouth but he became one of the greatest inventors of his time.

This can be summarized as:

It is from the homes of the poor only that the world has received her great leaders. Lal Bahadur Shastri, Abraham Lincoln and Thomas Alva Edison are glaring examples of men who rose in life from a state of extreme poverty.

□ **Avoid irrelevant matter and unnecessary repetition.**

Example:

- I kept waiting for him all through the day and could not go anywhere.

  In this sentence *and could not go anywhere* is unnecessary repetition.

- India is a country of many communities. People of various religions live here. We have Muslims, Hindus, Parsis, Sikhs, Christians and the like.

Unless we learn to live in harmony with each other, respecting each other's beliefs and habits, allowing everybody freedom in his mode of worship, we cannot build up a strong nation.

This can be summarized as follows:

India is a land of several communities. The nation cannot prosper unless people learn to respect each other's ways and beliefs.

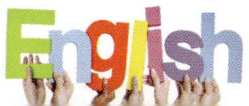

❏ **Wherever possible, form one sentence out of two or three.**

Example:

It was a dark night. It was pitch dark in the jungle. A tiger suddenly appeared on the scene. We were terribly afraid.

This can be written as:

We were terribly afraid to see a tiger coming suddenly out of the jungle in that dark night.

❏ **Avoid examples, stories, illustrations and details.**

For example, here, refers to the solved exercises that follows:

Original Passage/Sentence	Précis
• He is the manager of a place of shelter and support for such children who have lost their parents.	• He is the manager of an orphanage.
• It was a conclusion that anybody could foresee and that appeared to have been arrived at beforehand.	• It was a foregone conclusion.
• I have received a complaint which does not carry the name or address of the complainant.	• I have received an anonymous complaint.
• Many people consider poverty to be a great curse. They believe that unlucky is the man who is born in a poor family.	• Many people feel that poverty is a curse.
• It is natural that prosperity should attract friends. The friends of a prosperous man come to him as bees come to rose to suck honey from its petals.	• Prosperity attracts selfish friends.
• Like any other instrument that man has invented, sports can be used either for good or for evil purposes. Like a surgeon's knife, they can be used for healing a wound as well as for causing an injury.	• Sports can be used for good as well as for bad ends.
• Really good talk is a source of great pleasure. It gives joy whenever one finds one-self lucky enough to hear one. But it is only rarely that one comes across a good talk.	• Really good talk, even though it is rare, is always very pleasing.
• There is a difference of earth and sky between conquering by power and conquering by kindness; the two are, as it were, diametrically opposed to each other and more so, when we consider their final effect.	• There is a big difference between conquering by power and conquering by kindness.
• The unpunctual man is a general disturber of other's peace and serenity. Everybody with whom he has to do is thrown from time to time into a state of fever and impatience.	• An unpunctual man generally disturbs others.
• Many people foolishly look upon manual labour as something humiliating and insulting. They do not consider the wielding of a spade, or the driving of plough or the drawing of water from a well, as honorable.	• There are people who look down upon manual labour.

USES OF PRÉCIS WRITING

Précis-writing is a very fine exercise in *reading*. Most people read carelessly, and retain only a vague idea of what they have read. You can easily test the value of your reading. Read in your usual way a chapter, or even a page, of a book; and then, having closed the book try to put down briefly the substance of what you have just read. You will probably find your memory is weak. No; it is because your attention was not centered on the passage while you were reading it. The memory cannot retain what was never given it to hold; you did not remember the passage

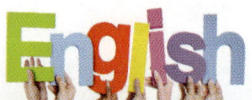

properly because you did not properly grasp it as you read it. Now précis-writing forces you to pay attention to what you read; for no one can write a summary of any passage unless he has clearly grasped its meaning. So, summarising is an excellent training in concentration of attention. It teaches one to read with the mind, as well as with the eye, on the page.

Précis-writing is also a very good exercise in *writing* a composition. It teaches one how to express one's thoughts clearly, concisely and effectively. It is a splendid corrective of the common tendency to vague and disorderly thinking and loose and diffuse writing. Have you noticed how an uneducated person tells a story? He repeats himself, brings in a lot of irrelevant matter, omits from its proper place what is essential and drags it in a latter matter as an afterthought, and takes twenty minutes to say what a trained thinker would express in five. The whole effect is muddled and tedious. In a précis you have to work within strict limits.

You must express a certain meaning in a fixed number of words. So you learn to choose your words carefully, to construct your sentences with an eye to fullness combined with brevity, and to put your matter in a strictly logical order.

So practice in précis-writing is of great value for practical life. In any position of life the ability to grasp quickly and accurately what is read or heard and to reproduce it clearly and concisely, is of the utmost value. For lawyers, businessmen and government officials it is essential.

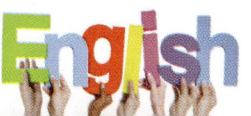

Solved Examples

Passage-1

To be a good teacher, you need some of the gifts of the good actor; you must be able to hold the attention and interest of your audience; you must be clear speaker; with a good, strong, pleasing voice which is fully under your control and you must be able to act what you are teaching in order to make its meaning clear. Watch a good teacher and you will see that he does not sit motionless, he stands the whole time he is teaching, he walks about using his arms, hands, fingers to help in his explanation and face to express his feelings. The fact, a good teacher has some of the gifts of a good actor does not mean that he will indeed be able to act well on the stage, for there are very important differences between the teacher's work and the actor's. The actor has to speak the sentences which he has learnt by heart. A good teacher works in quite a different way. His audience takes an active part in his play. They ask and answer questions. The teacher has, therefore to suit his acts to all needs of his audience, i.e., his class. He cannot learn his part by heart; he must invent it as he goes along.

Good Teacher

A good teacher has the talent of an actor. He expresses through the movements of his organs and gestures. A good teacher has well-modulated yet powerful and pleasant voice. This holds the attention and interest of his pupils. He moves about in the class although he is different from an actor as his success depends on adaptability of methods to the need of his pupils. On the other hand, an actor has to stick to the role assigned to him.

Passage-2

It is physically impossible for a well-educated intellectual or brave man to make chief object of his thoughts; just as it is for him to make his dinner the principal object of them. All healthy people like their dinner, but dinner is not the main object of their lives. So all healthy-minded people like making money, ought to like it, and enjoy the sensation of winning it, but the main object of their life is not money, it is something better than money. A soldier, for instance, mainly wishes to do his fighting well. He is glad of his pay - very properly so, and justly grumbles when you keep him ten years without it - still, his main notion of life is to win battles not to be paid for winning them. So of the doctors. They like fees no doubt, ought to like them; yet if they are brave and well-educated, the entire object of their lives is not fee. They on the whole desire to cure the sick, and if they are good doctors, and the choice were fairly put to them they would rather cure their patient, and lose the fee than kill him and get it. And so with all other brave and rightly trained men; their work is first priority and their fee second, very important no doubt but still second. But in every nation, as I said, there are vast numbers of people who are ill-educated, cowardly and more or less stupid. And with these people just as certainly the fee comes first and the work second.

Money Making

Money making can never be the object of a cultured or brave person. For all healthy-minded people work comes first, their fee second. The fee is important, no doubt, yet it is second. For a soldier, a clergyman and a doctor the sensation of doing their duty is always more satisfying than the earning of money. A doctor would lose rather his fee than the life of his patient. But sadly every nation has some ill-educated, cowardly and stupid people with whom the fee comes first and the work second.

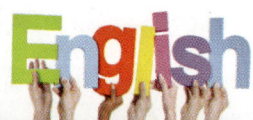

Practice Exercises

I. Information technology and library services are two faces of the same coin. In village set-up, mostly the young and the old use libraries and the middle-aged make little use of these libraries. They need job-related information to update their skills and knowledge. The library and information services play a dominant role in catering to education, information and recreational requirements of the society. Library is an instrument of social change. All along, the concept library has been associated with literacy and books, and the librarian was considered the keeper of the books. Concurrent with the changes in society, the concept of library has changed. It is a multimedia centre and a place for learning resources for the literates as well as the illiterates. Education is the key to individual achievement and national strength.

II. In recent decades there have been many advances, one of the most important of these advances has been the mobile telephone. The mobile telephone is a particularly important invention because it enables people to contact other people by means of a device that they can carry around. Before invention people who wanted to be in telephone contact with someone had to make a call either from a telephone in a private house or from a public telephone box. Being able to make a call from a telephone that you can carry about has revolutionized communication by telephone. If you need to contact someone on a business matter, you can use your mobile. There is no danger of your missing out on an important business opportunity because of communication difficulties.

III. Environmental pollution is an outcome of modernisation. It is much prevalent in metropolitan cities. There are millions of vehicles plying on the roads in them. They consume petrol and diesel which produce toxic smoke on burning. Besides this, factories belch out smoke. This poisons the air. Carbon dioxide, carbon monoxide and other particles are plenty in the air. When the people breathe in such air, these poisonous substances are inhaled. Thus, people contract many diseases like bronchitis, asthma, sore throat and irritation in eyes. Not only this, some chemical factories discharge effluents in the rivers. These effluents contain many poisonous substances and other dangerous chemicals. The soil gets contaminated. Nothing grows on it. The marine life is also harmed to a greater extent. The Chernobyl disaster is an example in this direction.

IV. If we look back at India's long history we find that our forefathers made wonderful progress whenever they looked out on the world with clear and fearless eyes and kept the windows of their minds open to give and receive. And, in later periods, when they grew narrowly in outlook and shrank from outside influences, India suffered a setback, politically and culturally. What a magnificent inheritance we have, though we have abused it often enough. India has been and is a vital nation, in spite of all the misery and sufferings that she has experienced. That vitality in the realms of constructive and creative effort spread to many parts of the Asian world and elsewhere and brought splendid conquests in its train. Those conquests were not so much of the sword, but of the mind and heart which bring healing and which endure when the men of the sword and their work are forgotten. But that very vitality if not rightly and creatively directed, may turn inward and destroy and degrade.

V. Newspapers keep us in constant touch with the whole of mankind. They, in fact, make us a citizen of the whole world. In olden days, a man's world consisted of his own village and one or two neighbouring villages. It was difficult for him to know what was going in other parts of the country. But the press, assisted with rapid means of communication brings us news from the farthest corner of the globe. The press is also responsible for educating public opinion. It is true to say that newspapers

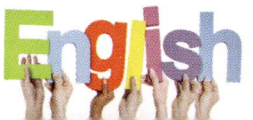

rule the world. Once a wise man said, "Let me control the press and I do not care who governs the country." The laws of the nation are really shaped by its press. The press leads and the people follow.

VI. There are more literate people in India today than ever before. But there are also more illiterates than ever before. More children go to school than any time in the past. But more children today are out of school than any time in the past. But it is not enough to blame the high birth rate for the state of affairs. Indeed, it can be reasonably argued that continued mass literacy is not the result but the cause of the high birth rate. Consequently, spread of literacy can be a potent weapon of socio-economic development. Unfortunately, official thought and planning on this regard has betrayed a failure of perception. The problem of illiteracy is related to but not the same as that of education. And while it is colossal task to provide proper and full academic education to all children and youth in the country, the problem of eradicating illiteracy calls for a different and less leisurely blue print. The following measures will be in the right direction: more primary schools, new part-time educational centres for those who cannot attend regular schools and functional literacy centres for adult, especially in semi-urban and rural areas.

VII. We can neither take rational decisions nor can we reach definite conclusions unless we give a serious consideration to various aspects of the problems and issues before us. So it is imperative that we develop thinking efficiency to make clear our decisions about the dilemmas of life. We should also keep in mind that much depends upon our viewpoint about something when we pass our judgments upon it. It is rightly said that nothing is good or bad. It is only our thinking which makes it so. We should, therefore, try to make our thinking positive, constructive and optimistic. In this way, we will be confident enough to resolve our problems in a better manner.

VIII. Lack of moral values, character-building incentives and good cultural values accounts for the present crisis prevalent in Indian scenario. Today, we find that even the persons in the most powerful positions have become an accomplice corrupt culture even though they are well-educated and well-reputed for scholarship. The tragedy is that even after independence, Indian society could not lay down the foundations strong enough to evolve an effective leadership which could give a new direction to the people. The perennial fact still remains that no system of the government can be successful until strong emphasis is placed on moral values in the society. It can be done through creating a proper climate—an environment where these values can grow fully and are not in the cruel grasp of corruption.

IX. The children of today are the future of tomorrow. The responsibilities of nation will lie on their shoulders in future. We should help our children in developing happy, healthy and wholesome personalities. We should give a patient hearing to their small queries and respond calmly and in the best possible way we can think of to whatever they ask. We should not suppress their curiosity rather we should encourage them to express themselves so that when they grow up, they will become self- confident and self-reliant. If as parents, teachers, guardians and their well-wishers, we channelize their unbridled energies in the right direction and if we can give them right perspective, only then can we be optimistic about their constructive role in national life.

X. Growing up is not a simple process. Generally people take it as growing in age. It in fact, means psychological maturity. Growing up actually gets reflected in our behavior, our attitude to life and our reactions to different odd situations. We are really grown up when we become mentally and emotionally mature enough to encounter the hardships and challenges of life smilingly. If we are mature, we do not break under the pressure of defeat but we face it with fortitude. Growing up, indeed, is a continuous process which gets strength from our experience, our self-confidence and strong will and thus we learn to face our life boldly and confidently.

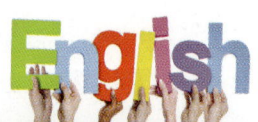

XI. If there is one custom that might be assumed to be beyond criticism, it is the custom of shaking hands; but it seems that even this innocent and amiable practice is upon its trial. A heavy indictment has been directed against it in the Press on hygienic grounds, and we are urged to adopt some more healthy mode of expressing our mutual emotion when we meet or part. I think it would need a pretty stiff Act of Parliament and a heavy code of penalties to break us of so ingrained a habit. Of course, there are many people in the world who go through life without ever shaking hands. Probably most people in the world manage to do. The Japanese bows, and the Indian says 'Namaste', and the Chinese makes a grave motion of the hand, and the Arab touches the breast of his friend at parting with the tips of his fingers. By comparison with these modes of salutation, it may be that our Western custom of shaking each other by the hand seems coarse and rustic, but I cannot conceive that Englishmen will ever be argued out of shaking hands with each other. A greeting which we really feel without the grip of the hand to accompany it would seem like a repulse, or a sacrilege. It would be a bond without the seal—as cold as a step-mother's breath as official as a type-written signature. It would be like denying our hands their natural office.

XII. There is perhaps a certain conflict always between the idea of progress and that of stability. The two do not fit in; the .former wants change, the latter a safe unchanging and continuation of things as they are. The idea of progress is modern and relatively even in the West; the ancient and mediaeval civilization thought far more in terms of a golden past and of subsequent decay. In India also the past has always been glorified. The civilisation that was built up here was essentially based on stability and security and from this point of view it was far more successful than any that arose in the West. The social structure based on the caste system and joint families, served this purpose and was successful in providing social security for the group and a kind of insurance for the individual who by reason of age, infirmity, or any other incapacity, was unable to provide for himself. Such an arrangement, while favoring the weak, hinders, to some extent, the strong. It encourages the average type at the cost of the abnormal, the bad or the gifted. It levels up or down and individualism has less play in it. It is interesting to note that while Indian philosophy is highly individualistic and deals almost entirely with the individual's growth to some kind of inner perfection, the Indian structure was communal and paid attention to groups only. The individual was allowed freedom to think and believe what he liked, but he had to conform strictly to social and communal usage.

XIII. The vision of a world in which all people will live together in peace and brotherhood may be far from realization, but it remains the noblest ideal of human existence. It is the ideal of all the great religions. It is the ideal which the United Nations embraces. Today it assumes a significance more imperative than ever known. For the instruments of destruction now available to war make of mankind's ability to approach this ideal in his day-to-day relationships the decisive challenge. It is a blunt challenge—learn to live together or perish together. Let me repeat—in meeting this challenge, and it can be met, the individual bears a crucial responsibility. It is, after all, in understanding the attitudes, the enlightened self-interest of the people of the world, that the riddle of the future is locked. As we maintain faith and confidence, in ourselves and in our fellow-men, as we heed reason and live by the good in our hearts, we contribute mightily to that security of the future, that peaceful and better world towards which all mankind aspires.

XIV. One of the most frightened and destructive phenomena of nature is a severe earthquake and its terrible after effects. An earthquake is a sudden movement of the earth, caused by the abrupt release of strain that has accumulated over a long time. For hundreds of millions of years, the forces of plate tectonics have shaped the earth as the huge plates that form the earth's surface slowly move

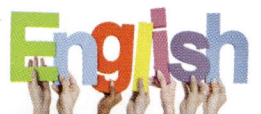

over, under and past each other. Sometimes the movement is gradual. At other times the plates are locked together and are unable to release the accumulating energy. When the accumulated energy grows strong enough, the plates break free. If the earthquake occurs in a populated area, it may cause many deaths and injuries and extensive damage to property.

XV. Valentine's Day is celebrated on February 14 every year to honour St. Valentine. The association of St. Valentine's Day with love and courtship rose from coincidence of the date with the Roman festival of Lupercalia. The festival is believed to have been in honour of Faunus, the Roman God of flocks and fertility. Also known as Lupercus, he was worshipped in a temple on Palatine Hill, and the festival was celebrated on February 14. The festival survived until the 5th Century AD. The Christian Church ended the feast of Lupercalia, transforming it into the feast of St. Valentine. The name St. Valentine is given to two legendary Christian martyrs whose feasts were formerly observed on February 14. One was a Roman priest martyred in 269 AD. The second was a Bishop of Terni martyred in Rome. In 1969, the feast day was dropped from the Vatican calendar.

XVI. It took just seventy years till 1914 for all the passenger pigeons in the World to disappear. The last moa was one of the hundreds eaten year by year, by the first settlers in New Zealand. The last elephant bird probably lived over three hundred years ago. And the hunters of South Africa shot the very last Quagga in 1883. All these animals, and countless others are as dead as the dodo that waddled its last on the island of Mauritius in 1681. When we see pictures of these fabulous creatures in books it sends a shiver down the spine to know that it was man who plundered their habitats or hunted them all to extinction, only to satisfy his selfish and insatiable greed. Could this happen to all that remains of our planet? Could there ever be a last tiger or elephant, rhinoceros or any

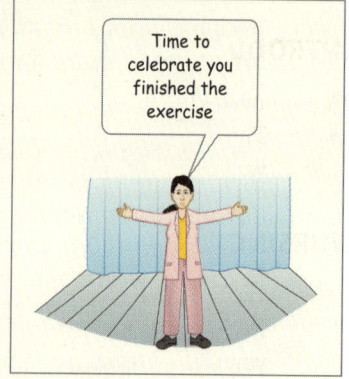

Time to celebrate you finished the exercise

other animal or even a last tree? Yes, there could. Today, thousands of species are endangered. And because man not only hunts them for their meat and skin but also destroys their habitat, one of the species that is doomed to face extinction is man himself. In a World where other animals can't live, man can't live.

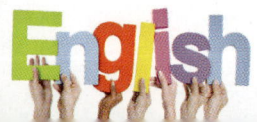

Chapter 25

Nurses Notes

INTRODUCTION

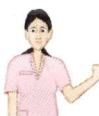

Accurate record keeping and careful documentation is an essential part of nursing practice. The Nursing and Midwifery Council (NMC) state that good record keeping helps to protect the welfare of patients and clients—which of course is a fundamental aim for nurses everywhere.

NURSING DOCUMENTATION AND RECORD KEEPING

High quality record keeping will help you give skilled and safe care wherever you are working. Registered nurses have a legal and professional duty of care. According to the NMC guidelines your record keeping and documentation should demonstrate:

- ❐ A full description of your assessment and the care planned and given relevant information about your patient or client at any given time and what you did in response to their needs.
- ❐ That you have understood and fulfilled your duty of care, that you have taken all reasonable steps to care for the patient or client and that any of your actions or things you failed to do have not compromised their safety in any way.
- ❐ A record of any arrangement you have made for the continuing care of a patient or client. Investigations into complaints about care will look at and use the patient/client documents and records as evidence, so high quality record keeping is essential. The hospital or care home, the NMC, a court of law or the Health Service Commissioner may investigate the complaint, so it makes sense to get the records right. A court of law will tend to assume that if care has not been recorded then it has not been given.
- ❐ **Documentation:** You will see lots of different charts, forms and documentation. Every hospital, care home and community nursing service will have the same basic ones, but with small variations that work best locally. The common documents that you will use include some of the following:
  - • **Nursing assessment sheet (NAS):** The nursing assessment sheet contains the patient's biographical details (e.g., name and age), the reason for admission, the nursing needs and problems identified for the care plan, medication, allergies and medical history.

NURSING CARE PLAN

The documents of the care plan will have space for:

- Patient/client needs and problems.
- Sometimes, nursing diagnoses will be documented but these are not used as frequently as in North America.
- Planning to set care priorities and goals. Goal-setting should follow the SMART system, i.e., the goal will be specific, measurable, achievable and realistic, and time-oriented. For example, a SMART goal would be that 'Mr John will be able to drink 1.5 L of fluid by 22.00 hours'. Some goals, such as reducing anxiety, are not easily measured and it is usual to ask patients to describe how they feel about a problem that was causing anxiety.
- The care/nursing interventions needed to achieve the goals.
- An evaluation of progress and the review date. This might include evaluation notes, continuation sheets and discharge plans. In some care areas you might record progress using a Kardex system along with the care plan.
- Reassessing patient/client needs and changing the care plan as needed.

VITAL SIGNS

The basic chart is used to record temperature, pulse, respiration and possibly blood pressure. Sometimes the patient's blood pressure is recorded on a separate chart. Basic charts may also have space to record urinalysis, weight, bowel action and the 24-hour totals for fluid intake and output. More complex charts, such as neurological observation charts, are used for recording vital signs plus other specific observations.

FLUID BALANCE CHART

This is often called a 'fluid intake and output chart' or sometimes just 'fluid chart'. It is used to record all fluid intake and fluid output over a 24-hour period. The amounts may be totaled and the balance calculated at 24:00 hours (midnight), or at 6:00 or 8:00 hours. Sometimes the amounts are totaled twice in every 24 hours (i.e., every 12 hours). Fluid intake includes oral, nasogastric, via a gastrostomy feeding tube, and infusions given intravenously, subcutaneously and rectally. Fluid output from urine, vomit, aspirate from a nasogastric tube, diarrhea and fluid from a stoma or wound drain are all recorded.

MEDICINE/DRUG CHART

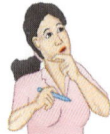

It is important for you to become familiar with the medicine/drug-related documents used in your area of practice. A basic medication record will contain the patient's biographical information, weight, history of allergies and previous adverse drug reactions. There will be separate areas on the chart for different types of drug orders. These include:

- Drugs to be given once only at a specified time, such as a sedative before an invasive procedure.
- Drugs to be given immediately as a single dose and only once, such as adrenalin (epinephrine) in an emergency.

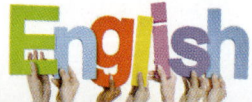

- Drugs to be given when required, such as laxatives or analgesics (pain killers).
- Drugs given regularly, such as a 7-day course of an antibiotic or a drug taken for longer periods (e.g., a diuretic or a drug to prevent seizures).

All drugs, except a very few, are ordered using the British Approved Name, and the order (or prescription) will include the dose, route, frequency (with times), start date and sometimes a finish date. There is space for the signature of the nurse giving the drug and in some cases, the witness. It is vital to record when you give a drug. This is done at the time so that all staff knows that it has been given, and do not repeat the dose. Likewise, if you cannot give the drug for some reason (e.g., patient is in another department or their physical condition contraindicates giving the drug), make sure that this fact is recorded on the medicine/drug chart and the doctor is informed if necessary.

Remember that in some situations you will need to record in the nursing notes when you give patients a drug, (e.g., if you give analgesic drugs (pain killers).

INFORMED CONSENT

Responsibility for making sure that the person or the parents of a child have all the information needed for them to give informed written consent rests with the health practitioner (usually a doctor or nurse) who is undertaking the procedure or operation. This information will include:

- Information about the procedure/operation
- The benefits and likely results
- The risks of the procedure/operation
- The other treatments that could be used instead
- That the patient/parent can consult another health practitioner
- That the patient/parent can change their mind

INCIDENT/ACCIDENT FORM

Any non-routine incident or accident involving a patient/client, relative, visitor or member of staff must be recorded by the nurse who witnesses (sees) the incident or finds the patient/client after the incident happened. Incidents include falls, drug errors, a visitor fainting or a patient attacking a member of staff in any way.

An incident/accident form should be completed as soon as possible after the event. Careful documentation of incidents is important for clinical governance (continuous quality improvement, learning from mistakes and managing risk, etc.) and in case of a complaint or legal action (see above).

The following points provide you with some guidance:

- Be concise, accurate and objective.
- Record what you saw and describe the care you gave, who else was involved and the person's condition.
- Do not try to guess or explain what happened (e.g., you should record that side rails were not in place, but you should not write that this was the reason the patient fell out of bed).
- Record the actions taken by other nurses and doctors at the time.

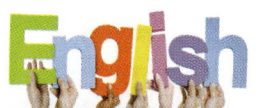

❑ Do not blame individuals in the report.

❑ Always record the full facts.

GUIDELINES FOR DOCUMENTATION AND RECORD KEEPING

The basic guidelines for good practice in documentation and record keeping apply equally to written records and to computer held records.

    The Nursing and Midwifery Council has said that patient and client records should:

❑ Be based on fact, correct and consistent.

❑ Be written as soon as possible after an event has happened to provide current (up-to-date) information about the care and condition of the patient or client.

❑ Be written clearly and in such a way that the text cannot be erased (rubbed out or obliterated).

❑ Be written in such a way that any alterations or additions are dated, timed and signed, so that the original entry is still clear.

❑ Be accurately dated, timed and signed, with the signature printed alongside the first entry.

❑ Not include abbreviations, jargon, meaningless phrases, irrelevant speculation and offensive subjective objective statements.

❑ Be readable on any photocopies.

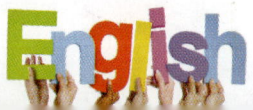

Chapter 26

Anecdotal Behavior Records

RECORD

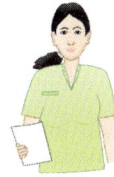

One of the best aids which a head nurse can use in evaluating the work of the nurse and describing her personality traits is the anecdotal Behavior record. An anecdote is a brief account of some incident. An anecdotal Behavior record is a compilation of anecdotes which describe Behavior. If anecdotes are accurate, well selected, and well written, the anecdotal record gives a clear picture of typical Behavior which serves as an aid in understanding the individual. When the number of anecdotes is large, they may be used in evaluating the work of nurse and gaining a concept of her attitudes.

ANECDOTAL RECORD

'An anecdotal record is a running description of actual examples of behavior of a student as observed by teachers and the counsel or it is followed by his comments. These are descriptive accounts of episodes or occurrences in the daily life of the student.'   **—Brown and Martin**
Thus an anecdotal record is a report of a significant episode in the life of a student.
'Anecdotal record is a record of some significant items of conduct, a record of an episode in the life of student, a word picture of the student in action ... a word snapshot at the moment of the incident, any narration of events which may be significant about her/his personality.'

—Randell

'Anecdotal record, as the name implies, involves setting down an anecdote concerning some aspects of student behavior which seems significant to the observer.'   **—Tandler**

It is a simple statement of an incident deemed by the observer to be significant with respect to a given student.

CHOICE OF ANECDOTES

The keeping of anecdotal records can become exceedingly cumbersome and time consuming both in their writing and summarizing the material for use. Of the many incidents which are constantly occurring, the head nurse must learn to choose those which have meaning and value. Some incidents are trivial and some are significant. In general those which portray the personality of the nurse should be selected.

CHARACTERISTICS OF ANECDOTAL RECORDS

These are records of specific incidents, factual description of important and meaningful event or behavior of students on informal occasions. Each event or behavior is described shortly after it occurs.

Anecdotal records must possess the following characteristics:

- They should contain a factual descriptions of what happened, when it happened, and under what circumstances the behavior occurred.
- The interpretations and recommended action should be noted separately from the description
- Each anecdotal record should contain a record of a single incident.
- The incident recorded should be that which is considered to be significant to the student's growth and development.

MERITS OF ANECDOTAL RECORDS

- These records help in clinical service practices.
- If properly used, they provide a factual record of our observation of a simple, significant incident in the student behavior.
- They stimulate teacher to use the records and contribute to them.
- They record critical incidents of spontaneous behavior in natural setting.
- They provide the teacher with objective description.
- They are very good for young children, who are unable to use paper-pencil test.
- They direct the teachers' attention to a single student.
- They provide cumulative record of growth and developments.
- They can be used by the counselor as a source of information for giving evidence.
- They provide specific and exact description of personality and minimize generalizations.
- They provide more complete descriptions of behavior better suited to understanding and guiding students than the other observational tools available.
- They can be used as a supplement to quantitative data.
- The new members may use these records and acquaint themselves with the students.

DEMERITS OF ANECDOTAL RECORDS

- They tend to be less reliable than other observational tools as they tend to be less formal and systematic.
- They are time-consuming to write.
- It is difficult for the observer to maintain objectivity when he/she records the incidence observed.
- When incidents are noted and read out of context, they may lose their meaning.

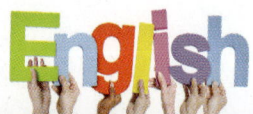

◻ The observer tends to record only undesirable incidents and neglect the positive incidents.

◻ They present only a verbal description of the incident. They do not reveal causes.

ANECDOTAL NOTES

Anecdotal notes are frequently used in nursing education for recording data about the student's practice and reliability. The concerns expressed here relate to the format of the note, the system of collecting the notes and the use made of the information collected. Perhaps some teachers expect too much from anecdotal notes simply because they do not understand their function fully. An anecdotal note is a recorded description of the behaviors and activities of the learner during a particular performance of short duration. It is a vignette of the learner's practice experience. The note itself is usually written informally without modifying expressions and contains only data that clarify the image of the event.

Opportunities for Observation and Behavior

The head nurse has many opportunities to observe the nurse. Her best field of observation is at bedside of the patient. She also sees the nurse and observes her behavior in the workrooms and kitchen as she prepares for treatments, cares for equipment, serves diets or nourishments. The head nurse includes in her anecdotal records evidence of interest, judgment and other important characteristics which she observes in the nurse outside her regular duty time. Significant Behavior may be observed in the dining room, the corridors of the hospital, the library or nurses' residence. Perhaps the nurse may be overheard talking about patients in the elevator or in the bus.

CONTENT OF ANECDOTAL RECORDS

There is some disagreement as to whether the report of an incident should be wholly objective or whether it should include some interpretation. It is fairly well agreed that any interpretation which accompanies an anecdote should be separate from the facts and that the observer should be well aware that she is using interpretation. Records are more valid if it is necessary to interpret only a few of the incidents. Nursing activities which are not performed well, if important in the nurse's development, are recorded. For example, the unwise handling of a patient's worries or complaints, the failure to record important information or to take needed precautions are significant. Following a poor performance, the head nurse makes a point of observing the nurse in similar situations to determine whether improvement has been made.

METHOD OF RECORDING ANECDOTES

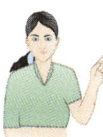

The anecdotal record for each individual is kept in chronological order on cards or in a notebook. Needless to say, anecdotal records are highly confidential and must be kept in safe place, preferably under lock and key, where they will not be a temptation to inquisitive individuals. The clinical instructor, ward supervisor, assistant head nurse, team leader, the evening and night supervisors as well as the head nurse should write anecdotal records. It is important that

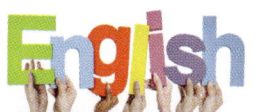

the head nurse keeps records regardless of how much direct teaching responsibility she has or how many other people are also keeping them.

Anecdotes must be written promptly if they are to be accurate. The head nurse in all probability will not have time or opportunity to write up an incident the moment it occurs. Anecdotes will not be written on every nurse, each day. It is advisable in the beginning of her experience in writing anecdotal records for the head nurse and to plan to write two or three anecdotes on each nurse every week.

Value of Anecdotal Records

Anecdotal records take time and they take thought. It is often very difficult for the head nurse to find time to write them. However they are invaluable aids in understanding and helping the nurses and the head nurse cannot afford to omit them. Practice makes it easier to simplify them and to include only the essentials. The more skill the head nurse develops in observing behavior and recognising its importance, the easier the task becomes.

USES OF ANECDOTAL RECORDS

Three groups of individuals will find rich use for anecdotal records: written by the head nurse, the school of nursing (for students) or nursing service (for staff nurses), and the nurse herself.

1. *Use by the head nurse:* Primarily, records are kept for the use of the head nurse in evaluating the work and characteristics of individual nurses and in turn for evaluating her teaching and quality of nursing care. To help the individual nurse recognize her strengths and needs, the head nurse studies her anecdotal record prior to every planned individual conference.

2. *Use by the student or staff nurse:* Nurses, especially students, should be encouraged to write anecdotal records on themselves and to evaluate them in terms of good performance and satisfactory Behavior.

3. *Use by the school of nursing:* Well-written anecdotal records provide source material for evaluation of the entire educational program of the school. Even though the time may not have arrived when wide use can be made of anecdotal records; the head nurse, the staff nurse, and the student nurse will still find them invaluable aids in achieving their goals.

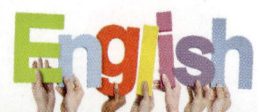

Chapter 27

Diary Writing

INTRODUCTION

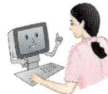 Unlike other types of writing, a diary is generally not meant to be read by anyone else. So if nobody else is going to read it, why to write it? There are many reasons why people keep a diary. For some people, it's a way to nurture their creativity. Writing in a diary can help spark new ideas or develop thoughts. For other people, keeping a diary is a way to stay emotionally healthy. Writing in a safe space can help you to process past experiences. A diary is also a way of keeping a record of what happened and when. Others keep a diary of things that they're thankful for, as a way to be more grateful for the good things in their life. Also, some people keep a diary as a way to improve themselves or the follow through the changes they're trying to make. You can keep a diary for any reason that interests you in any manner.

A diary can take many different forms—one can use it as a regular notebook. One can also buy a specially designed diary, some of them even come with small ped locks. But how do you keep a diary? If there are no rules, how do you know what to do? First of all, there are no hard and fast rules to keeping a diary; there are conventions that many diary keepers follow. A convention is a way or a style in which something is usually done or accomplished. Following conventions can make things easier, because you don't need to reinvent the wheel rather you can benefit from the experiences of other people.

FORMAT

One common convention which need to be followed when keeping a diary is to write the date at the top of each entry. Some people are very specific when writing the date, including the exact time of day that it is. Other people might simply write the month or year. The main idea here is that diaries are often organized chronologically by date. After date, time and day is mentioned. The time should be noted. Usually dairy should be written at the night time, before going to sleep.

Diaries are great ways to keep on track of your past and think about your future. You can make predictions about what will happen and can see if they come true and you can see how you have changed over the time of period and can read over memories, having a laugh.

Understand that eventually the diary will become your best friend, silent confessor or witness. You will eventually trust your diary for anything, even for your biggest secrets. Try to write your diary at night because in that way, you can describe the entire day schedule. There is no point of writing a diary when you wake up in the morning because the only thing you can write about is your dreams. You can write about any celebration or disaster that happened that day and you can write freely too. Put your pen to the page and write whatever is in your mind. Write cool facts, important information, advice, tips, ideas, recipes anything you want to keep as your secret. The list goes on and on.

Describe how your day went and do not leave out any detail. If you want your day to go better write how and why. If you have a special grudge against somebody, have no fear in expressing it. Move on to the afternoon, then the evening and finally the night. It should always be written truthfully. Your diary will always listen, never forget, never judge and nor it will ever reveal your secrets. So do not worry about writing the truth in it no matter how horrible it is.

Diaries in intensive care unit (ICU) support patients and relatives during and after a stay in the ICU. Writing a diary for patients and relatives means an additional amount of time and workload, but according to the enhanced of nursing the time favors to be feasible for implementation of this idea of diary writing. Diary helps student nurses in learning and is also useful for developing a habit of writing. Diary is an effective tool to assess the clinical activities of students enrolled nursing education. Personal diaries record the experiences of the writers and the student nurses diaries have useful information regarding services provided to patients. They have important date which is gathered during their community visits outside the hospital. In a diary, all the events are recorded in a chronological order and thus provides a daily record of activities.

The instructors get the information that has not been given to them at times from the diaries of the student nurses. With diary entry the student nurses are forced to jog their memory as they have to recall the events of the day at the end of the day. Writing a diary encourages students to be truthful always as people usually do not lie to their diary. Nurses become disciplined by themselves as they sit down every day and write a page or two in their diary. They come to know how much time they are utilizing in clinical area. It could be important for student nurses to write in their diary about emotionally challenging situations faced by them.

As a nurse who has recently joined her duty, write a diary entry.

Wednesday   10 pm
November 4, 2015

After 4 years of training I am now qualified to be a nurse. I love being a nurse. I am keen to take care of people when they are sick and admitted in hospital. When I reported for duty in the morning the first thing I did was listening to the night nurse who told me all that happened during the night. I looked at the charts and carefully noted everything she said. Then I went on a quick round to greet every patient I was assigned to. After that, I made their beds. This was one of the first thing I learnt as a student—how to make a hospital bed, to tuck the sheets in firmly. Then I took patient's temperature, blood pressure and samples at specific time. I also provided information about patients to the doctors when they came on rounds.

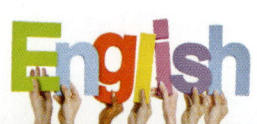

Practice Exercises

I. Suppose you are working as a Nurse in Rajindra Hospital, Patiala. You had a very bitter experience with one of the patients so felt disturbed. Write a diary expressing yourself.

II. You are a Nursing student of Gian Sagar College of Nursing. You have recently joined BSc. Write a Diary entry at the end of the week.

III. You are a Nursing Tutor in Swift College of Nursing. Write a Diary entry expressing your feelings.

IV. Imagine you stood First in the examination and prize distribution was done today in the evening. Write a diary entry of how you spent the day today with excitement.

V. You had a Fresher's Party today. Write a diary entry describing your enjoyment whole day.

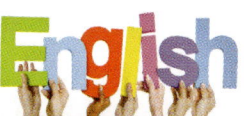

NOTES

Chapter 28

Report on Client's Health Status

WHAT IS REPORT?

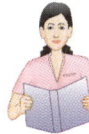

According to J Staney Jones *a report is a special form of narrative which aims chiefly at conveying information based upon facts.* If we analyze the above-quoted definition we come to the following aspects:

- ❑ Report is a form of narrative.
- ❑ But it is not an ordinary type of narrative.
- ❑ Its chief aim is to convey information that should be based upon facts.

The aim of a report is to convey information. This implies that no fact should be left out. Sometimes the speaker gives irrelevant material, we should trim it in accordance with the main topic.

TYPES OF REPORTS

- ❑ Oral
- ❑ Written

Oral report: Oral report is made by the nurse who is assigned to the patient care to another nurse who is planning to relieve her.

Written reports: Written reports are written when information is to be used by several people or is more or less of permanent value. Included in this are day and night reports and incident reports and assessment/evaluation reports.

Advantages of maintenance of records and reports:

- ❑ Helps is sound decision making, acts as effective channel of communication.
- ❑ Serves as tools for performance evaluation.
- ❑ Promotes accountability and efficiency.
- ❑ Serves as legal documents, provides data or research and vital statistics.

Oral Reports

Reports between the Head Nurse and her Assistant

The assistant head nurse should know everything pertinent to the management to the ward even though she may never be concerned with parts of the information. She is expected to take over the management of the ward in the event of the enforced absence of the head nurse. There can be a great deal of confusion if the head nurse possesses important information which she has failed to tell to her assistant because she is expected to handle the situation herself. The assistant needs to be informed also when the head nurse is away from the ward for her daily hours or weekly day of rest.

The well-informed assistant head nurse knows the condition of all patients, the treatment they are receiving, observations which are to be made, problems of staffing the plans for meeting them, questions relating to equipment and supplies, expected admissions, discharges and treatments, plans for student experience, changes in hospital or ward routine. In other words she has all the information she needs to keep the ward running smoothly without interruption or waste of time.

When the head nurse returns to the ward after hours or days of absence the assistant head nurse reports to her all changes in the situation including the condition of patients and the happenings during her absence.

Reports between Nurses Who are Assigned to Bedside Care

Content

Reports of students and staff nurses to those who are to relieve them include the condition of all patients assigned to their care; treatments and medications which have been given and those which are due; adaptations in method required by each patient, information about the patient as a person and his diagnosis if these are not already known to the relieving nurse. Sometimes this information is put in writing.

Methods

These reports are probably best given if the two nurses together go through the plan for each patient's care. If there is no plan, the doctor's orders, treatment and medicine cards or lists may be substituted. When nurses read the orders together, no doubt is left about their meaning or whether they have been carried out to date. Questions are asked and answered immediately. Effective reports are organized, given promptly in a place free from interruption and out of the hearing of patients and visitors. When possible it is advisable for the two nurses to go together to see the patients, to check on their condition and the status of their care. This also gives an opportunity to let patients know to whom they may look for care while their regular nurse is away.

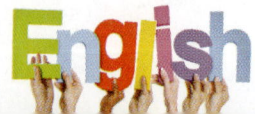

Reports of Staff Members to the Charge Nurse

During the Day

The head nurse or the nurse in charge looks to the bedside nurse to keep her informed throughout the day of changes in patients' condition and results of treatments if they are unusual or significant. She expects from the bed side nurse to let her know whether she has insufficient or too much time to carry out the assignments. She also expects to be told of problems relating to supplies and equipment and those in relation to patients, such as the nurse's inability to give the care ordered, patients complaints or their difficulties in adjustment.

When Reporting off Duty

When the nurse is ready to go off duty the head nurse receives a brief concise report on each patient and unfulfilled assignments. At this time the head nurse has an opportunity to help the nurse learn what is important to report and how to do it in a way to avoid unnecessary expenditure of time. It is an excellent practice to have nurses, particularly students, bring to the head nurse for her review the nurse's notes for the day and the records of treatments and medications which have been given and of fluid intake and elimination. In this way questions are raised in the mind of the head nurse which she clears before the nurse leaves the floor.

Charge Nurse's Report to Bedside Nurses

The information which the charge nurse needs, especially to report to the nurses who are caring for patients relates to changes in orders. In the patient and team methods of assignment the nurse carries the responsibility for the total care of a group of patients. It is impossible for her to learn of changes in orders without frequent reading of the doctors' order book unless the charge nurse assumes the responsibility for informing her of new or discontinued orders.

Report of the Head Nurse to Administrative Supervisor

The administrative supervisor needs to receive from the head nurse an overview of the ward in sufficient detail to understand its problems and needs. This includes the name, diagnosis, condition and treatment of each patient, plans for their nursing care, difficulties in providing the care which is needed including those relating to staffing and equipment problems in securing privacy or arranging congenial company for patients. She is told about complaints of patients, visitors, doctors and members of the nursing staff as well as accidents and mistakes. The latter are reported immediately by telephone if serious. She is told of the head nurse's plans for changes in ward practice end for building a constructive program to improve nursing care.

Reports to the Clinical Instructor

Reports to the clinical instructor include everything in the ward situation which affects the educational process. Hence she receives the same report relating to patients as that given to the administrative supervisor.

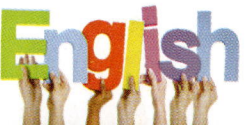

Report of the Head Nurse to the Director of Nursing or her Assistant

In small hospitals one of these individuals may assume direct responsibility for the supervision of the wards in which case she will need the full report which has been described. In large institutions it is impossible for the director or even for her assistant to be in such close contact with the details of ward administration and teaching. It is very stimulating to the head nurse when the director of the nursing service makes rounds. When she does so she receives a direct report. At other times the ward report is transmitted through the supervisor to the nursing office. The director of nursing usually wishes to receive a general picture of the ward, to learn the condition of the sickest patients, to be told of new treatments and the difficulties in giving nursing care including problems of staffing. She is also told of accidents, mistakes or complaints and any other problems of an administrative nature which involve patients, visitors or personnel. She should know the individuals to whom such reports have already been given and how the situation has been handled.

Report of the Charge Nurse to the Physician

Reports Related to his Patients

The specific information which every doctor expects to receive from the nurse in charge of the ward relates to his patients under her care. He wishes to be told of the symptoms which they show, the results of treatment, inability to carry out his orders and difficulties or mistakes in doing so. He is also interested in complaints of patients or their families about their care, attending patients, and their personal problems which may require the assistance of a medical social worker.

Reports on Policy Changes

The doctor is also informed of changes in administrative routine which affect the care of the patient or the functioning of the doctor in the ward. Preferably this information reaches him through other channels such as the chief of the medical staff, the medical board, or the director of the hospital. Unfortunately it often does not. The head nurse may acquire information related to policy change which the doctor has not received. Therefore she is wise to assure herself that he is informed before making any changes. For example, the hospital may institute a new form for recording temperature, pulse, respiration in place of the book formerly used. The physician who is accustomed to finding the temperatures of his patients recorded in a particular place should be informed by the head nurse of the change in system before it is instituted.

Change-of-Shift Report

The change-of-shift report occurs at least twice a day in all types of nursing units. At the end of each shift, information about your assigned clients is given to nurses working on the next shift. The purpose of the report is to provide better continuity and individualized care for clients. For example, if you find that a certain position increases a client's breathing, you relay that information to the next nurse caring for the client.

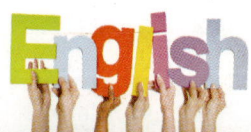

Change-of-shift reports are given orally in person, by audiotape recordings, or during rounds at the client's bedside. Oral reports are given in person, with staff members from both shifts participating. Audiotape reports may be done before the end of the shift which can increase efficiency and minimize social interactions. An opportunity for a last minute update on events that occur after taping and for classification when there are questions essential. Reports given in person or during rounds allow you to obtain immediate feedback when questions are raised about a client's case. When you make rounds, the client and family members also have the opportunity to participate in any decision.

The change-of-shift report should be given quickly and efficiently. A good report provides a baseline for comparison and indicates the kind of care to be anticipated for the next shift. An organized and concise approach helps you set ground and anticipate client needs and lessens the chance of important information being overlooked. A sample format is as follows: background information (name, age and medical dialysis), primary health problem, nursing diagnoses, observation of the client's condition and response to therapies, pro with teaching, interventions, and family involvement. It is especially important to report any recent changes or priorities in situations concerning the client's condition.

When giving a report, you must maintain a professional manner. Describe interactions in objective terms, avoid such judgmental labels as "uncooperative," "difficult", "bad" when describing client behaviors. This kind of language can contribute to prejudicial opinions about the judgmental statements overheard by the client or could also lead to legal charge.

Telephone Reports and Orders

Telephone Orders

When significant events or incidents in a client's condition have occurred, a telephone report is made to include clear, accurate and concise information. When the phone call includes when the call was made, who made it (if you did not make the call), who was called, to whom the information was given, what information was given, and what information was received?

Transfer Reports

Client may be transferred from one unit to another or to another facility to receive different levels of care. For example, the transfer of patient from intensive care unit to general nursing unit when the level of care no longer requires intense monitoring. A transfer report involves communication of information about clients from the nurse on the sending unit to the nurse on the receiving unit. Transfer reports may be given by phone or in person. When giving a transfer report, the following informations are included:

- Client's name, age, primary physician and medical diagnosis.
- Summary of medical progress up to the time of transfer.
- Current health status (physical and psychosocial).
- Allergies.
- Emergency code status.
- Family support.
- Current nursing diagnoses or problems and care plan.

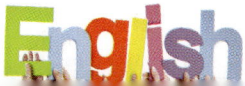

❑ Any critical assessments or interventions to be completed shortly after transfer (helps receiving nurse to establish priorities of care).

❑ Need for any special equipment.

At the completion of the transfer report, the receiving nurse may clarify information by asking questions about the client's status.

Written Reports

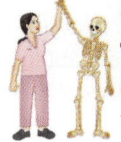

Day, Evening, and Night Reports

The purpose of interval reports is to provide a means of transferring pertinent information about patients to the head nurse, the ward evening and night nurses, to the nursing office and to the evening and night supervisors. Only that information which is necessary to give a general picture of the ward needs to be included, such as the census, the names, diagnoses and general condition of patients, the patients, admitted and discharged. Detailed information is available on charts and order sheets. Some institutions include only the sickest patients in the written report, others include them all. It may help the day nurses to start the day more easily if the night nurse includes in her report a list of the patients on whom new orders have been written.

Incident Reports

An incident is any event not consistent with the routine operation of a health care unit or routine care of a client. Examples include client falls, needle-stick injuries, a visitor becoming ill and medication errors. An **incident report** is filed when there is an actual or potential injury and is not a part of the patient record. Therefore an objective description of what was observed and follow-up actions taken are documented in the client's medical record without reference to the existence of the incident report. It becomes necessary to complete an **incident report** when anything unusual happens that could potentially cause harm to the client, visitor or employee or when you make an error. For example, if you administer an incorrect medication to a client and a client suffers a fall in the hospital, an incident report should be prepared. Most institutions provide specific forms for this purpose. You should objectively record the details of the incident and any statements made by the client. An example follows: "Mrs Jones found lying on floor on right side. Abrasion on right forehead. Client stated, "I fell and hit my head". At the time of an incident, always contact the physician to examine the client. After examining the client, the physician should document assessment findings and treatment plans in the progress notes. Any untoward effects caused by the incident must also be documented. Subjective assumptions and statements assigning blame or fault should not be included in the chart or the incident report.

Incident reports are not a part of the client's medical record. The reports are generally not admissible in court and in some jurisdictions are considered privileged documents. Know your employing institution's policies and procedures on incident reports. Incident reports are also used by employing institutions for quality improvement and risk management. By reviewing incident reports, administrators can determine areas of client risk. For example, if a certain kind of problem has occurred repeatedly, such as client falls when being transferred to X-ray carts, educational methods can be used to help, prevent the problem in the future.

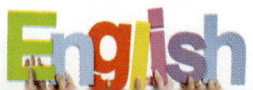

GENERAL FORMAT OF REPORT

Name:
Father's Name:
Sex:
Age:
Diagnosis:
Operation done:
Date of Operation:
Unit Head/Consultant in charge:

Assessment: General condition, cleanliness, level of consciousness, vital signs, emotional and psychological status, pain/any discomfort, diet, eliminations bowel and bladder, any specific exercises.

Investigation Done

Treatment: IV fluids, transfusion, feeding, medication, any other.

Accurate Report: A report should be precise and short but easy to read:
- ❏ It should be objective.
- ❏ Nothing should be left to guessing.
- ❏ There should be no personal opinion.
- ❏ There should be no bias.
- ❏ State the time, date and place.
- ❏ Do not include each and every detail to avoid lengthy report.

Nursing measures carried out with their outcomes—Hygiene measures, comfort measures, feeding, exercise and recreation, etc. specific observations, specific reports maintained.

REPORT OF A PATIENT SUFFERING FROM JAUNDICE

Name:
Father's Name:
Sex:
Age:
Ward No.:
Bed No.:

Signs and symptoms: The patients came to the hospital with fever, yellow eyes, complained of loss in appetite, nausea, lethargy.

Diagnosis: The patient was advised blood tests, liver function tests, abdominal X-rays, urine test, ultrasound. Tests confirmed the patient was suffering from jaundice.

Treatment: The consumption of fats and oils, chilies, sour foods, meat, fish are restricted, rich carbohydrate diet advised. Medicine given in the afternoon and is now to be given before sleeping.

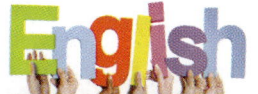

Transfer Reports

Transfer reports involve communication of information about clients from the nurse on sending units to the nurse on the receiving unit. Nurse should include the following information.

- ❑ Client's name, age, primary doctor, and medical diagnosis.
- ❑ Summary of medical progress up to the time of transfer.
- ❑ Current health status-physical and psychosocial.
- ❑ Current nursing diagnosis or problems and care plan.
- ❑ Any critical assessment or interventions to be completed shortly.
- ❑ Needs for any special equipment, etc.

Incident Reports

- ❑ The nurse who witnessed the incident or who found the client at the time of incident should file the report.
- ❑ The nurse describes in concise what happened specifically objective terms, etc.
- ❑ The nurse does not interpret or attempt to explain the cause of the incident.
- ❑ The nurse describes objectively the client's, conditions when the incident was discovered.
- ❑ Any measures taken by the nurse, other nurses, or doctors at the time of the incident are reported.
- ❑ No nurse is blamed in an incident report.
- ❑ The report is submitted as soon as possible.
- ❑ The nurse should never make photocopy of the incident report.

Census Reports

It is a report compiled daily for the number of patients. Very often it is done at midnight and the norms are collected by the night supervisor. The report will show the total number of patients the number of admissions, discharges, transfers, births and deaths. The nurses should remember that a single mistake in the census figures made buy one of the nurses make the census report of the entire institution incorrect.

Birth and Death Reports

The nurses are responsible for sending the birth and death reports to government authorities within the specified time.

Anecdotal Reports

An anecdotal is brief account of some incident. Incident reports and reports on accidents, mistakes and complaints are legal in nature. A written record concerning some observation about a person or about her work is called an anecdotal note.

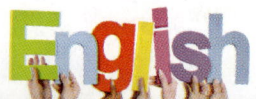

SAMPLE OF AN ACCIDENT REPORT

Name: Age: Address:

Bed no.   Ward no.:   C.R. No.:

Date & time of accident:

Description of how the accident occurred:

Safety precautions:

Condition of the patient before and after the accident:

Doctor's examination finding:

Treatment ordered: witness to accident:

Signature of the doctor:

Signature of the nurse:

Unit:

Date of report:

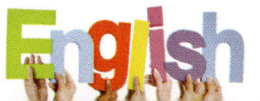

NOTES

Chapter 29

Story Writing

WRITING STORIES

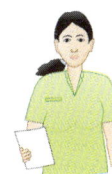

❑ You already know how to write stories based on outlines. In the present chapter you learn:
  • Retelling in detail a brief story
  • Developing stories from incomplete outlines
  • Completing incomplete stories

❑ All the three types of exercises require:
  • Use of imagination in tune with the material provided
  • Observance of rules of grammar
  • Logical development of thought or ideas
  • Judicious use of direct and indirect narration
  • Liveliness
  • The art of giving flesh and blood to a skeleton

Here are the details of stories:

RETELLING A STORY

Read the following story which is briefly told:

STORY IN BRIEF

A poor young girl was passing through a street. She wanted to sell her clothes. She was forced to take this step because she was very poor. Her mother was sick and aged. Her father had died poor as a loyal officer in the service of the king. She was disappointed when she found that nobody came forward to buy her clothes. At last she came across a gentleman whom she told the whole story. He was, in fact, the king. He felt sorry and realized his fault in neglecting the girl's father. He did what was right for the family.

Now read the same story in detail.

STORY IN DETAIL

There was a young girl passing through the streets of a city. She was empty-handed. But what on earth made her take this extreme step? She was the only child of her widowed mother, who was aged and sick. The girl did not mind her own hunger. She was too brave to shed a tear on this account. But what made her heart ache was the miserable condition of her mother. The mother and the daughter had inherited only poverty from the head of the family. He had died poor as a loyal officer in the service of the king of the country.

The people whom she met were stunned when they learnt that the young girl wanted to sell her clothes. They sympathised with her, but nobody came forward to accept her offer. She was disappointed.

But as she turned her steps homeward, she came across a gentleman. She requested him to buy her clothes.

With tears in her eyes, the girl related to him the circumstances which had driven her to extreme poverty. At the end, she said, "If my father had served God with the zeal with which he served the king, he would not have neglected him."

On hearing these words, the gentleman's eyes became moist. In fact, he was no other than the king himself. He was in disguise going about to acquaint himself with the real condition of his subjects.

With folded hands, he said, "Pardon me, I am the thankless king who ignored your father."

The young girl could not believe her ears. But the king went on: "Please offer my sincerest apologies to your unhappy mother. I hereby grant her a pension of ₹500 per month. I shall arrange a suitable match for you, self-sacrificing girl, and bear all the expenses on your marriage."

What more could the poor girl have wished for? She thanked God for this sudden good luck. She thanked the king too.

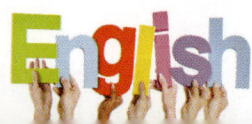

Practice Exercises

I. **Develop stories from incomplete outlines:**

1. A snake frozen in cold _____ found by a farmer _____ takes pity _____ snake taken home _____ warmed near the fire _____ snake gets life _____ rushes towards the children _____ gets killed. (*The Snake and the Farmer*)

2. Two beggars _____ one blind, one lame _____ both helpless_____ cripple's proposal _____ the blind man to carry him and he to lead _____ agreed _____ result and moral. (*Two Beggarts*)

3. A wolf at a stream_____ a little down stream a lamb drinking _____ his mouth waters _____ wants to find an excuse _____ Says, "Why do you make the water muddy _____ the lamb surprised _____ the water runs from the wolf to the lamb _____ the wolf finds an other excuse _____ devours it.
(*A wicked man find an excuse to do mischief*)

4. A clear pool _____ stag drinking _____ admires his horns _____ despises his thin legs _____ hunter and hounds _____ stag flees _____ horns caught in a bush _____ stag pulled down _____ dying thoughts. (*The Foolish Stag*)

5. An old man and his son _____ taking a donkey to the fair _____ none riding _____ are laughed at _____ son asked to ride _____ is rebuked by the people _____ father rides _____ he is rebuked also _____ both ride _____ are laughed at _____ decide to carry the donkey _____ the donkey is frightened on a bridge _____ jumps into the river _____ drowned.
Moral. (*Try to please everyone and you please no one*)

6. Wolf hungry _____ sheep too well guarded _____ wolfs plan _____ put on sheep's skin _____ mingles with the flock _____ sheep bleating _____ wolf tries to bleat _____ only howls _____ detected _____ killed by shepherd. (*A Wolf in Sheep's Clothing*)

7. A country mouse invites a town mouse and serves a simple food which the town mouse does not like; after some days the town mouse invites the country mouse and sets rich food before it; but a cat comes up and the two run for their lives. _____

8. A child returns home from school, bubbling over with Arithmetic learnt during the day _____ family at dinner _____ two fowls served _____ the child declares they are three fowls, 'This is two; and two and one make three'_____ father says, 'Your mother will have the first, I shall have the second, and you will have the third.

9. Hare mocks tortoise for slowness _____ tortoise challenges for a race _____ one mile fixed _____ start made _____ hare far ahead _____ takes a nap _____ sleeps too long _____ awakes_ looks round for tortoise _____ tortoise at the winning post. (*Hare and the Tortoise*)

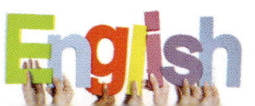

10. A boy falls into bad company _____ father gives him a few good apples _____ places a rotten apple among them _____ a few days later _____ the rotten apple spoils the good ones _____ lessons learnt.

11. A lion asleep in a forest _____ a mouse jumps over his body _____ caught by the lion _____ begs for mercy _____ the lion spares its life _____ the lion caught in a net _____ roars _____ the mouse helps _____ nibbles the net _____ lion set free _____ moral. *(The Lion and the Mouse)*

12. An old man _____ dyes his beard _____ hair of the head white _____ once questioned _____ says the hair of his head was twenty years older than his beard explanation. *(The Dyed Beard)*

13. A bee _____ falls into a tank _____ a dove flies past drops a large leaf into the water _____ the bee climbs on to the leaf` flies away _____ a hunter takes aim at the dove _____ the bee stings him _____ the dove saved. *(One Good Tarn Deserves Another)*

14. Two friends travelling in a forest _____ a bear appears _____ one hastily climbs up a tree _____ the other lies down, motionless_ the bear sniffs _____ prowls off _____ the friend on the tree climbs down _____ enquires from the other _____ Don't trust a false friend was the reply _____ Moral.

15. A fat merchant _____ wishes to see the cinema_ sends a servant to arrange for a seat _____ gets two seats booked _____ one seat too small _____ one in the front row and the other in the back row_____ merchant angry _____ servant dismissed. *(The Fat Merchant)*

16. A fox, a wolf and a lion _____ chase a prey _____ begin to share _____ wolfs suggestion _____ makes the lion angry _____ wolf killed _____ fox makes a good suggestion _____ the lion very pleased _____ the fox questioned _____ reply. *(Division of Share)*

17. A traveller reaches an inn _____ knocks at the door_ the innkeeper says he has lost the key _____ the traveller pushes in a rupee _____ the inn-keeper asked to bring a bag from outside _____ shuts the door_ gets back the same rupee _____ moral. *(The Silver Key)*

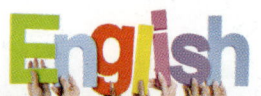

Chapter 30

Essay Writing

WHAT IS AN ESSAY?

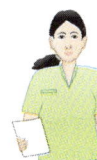

The word essay means 'an attempt'. But in grammar it means a composition made up of paragraphs to deal with a topic. These paragraphs make a connected logical reading.

An essay is a literary composition in prose, written in correct beautiful English to discuss a given topic in detail.

The word 'Essay' is defined in 'The Concise Oxford Dictionary' as a literary composition (usually prose and short) on any subject. Properly speaking, it is a written composition giving expression to one's own personal ideas or opinions on some topic; but the term usually covers any written composition also, whether it expresses personal opinions, gives information on any given subject, or details of a narrative or description.

Essay-writing is an art that requires careful planning on the part of the writer. Firstly, the subject or topic for the essay should be selected very wisely so that the writer may be able to collect a good number of ideas about it and he is in a position to discuss them in a suitable way. Secondly, he must be able to express himself or herself through suitable words and well constructed sentences. In other words, he must have a good command of the language. Here are adduced some hints for writing:

- Try to understand the topic clearly from all angles.
- Concentrate coolly and carefully and jot down all the ideas related to the topic of the essay.
- These ideas must be discussed logically and supplemented by the original ideas of the writer.
- Chalk out a plan, i.e., outline of the essay giving the chief points to be discussed.
- Arrange these points in a logical order.
- Discuss each point in a separate paragraph which should be complete by itself.
- The language should be simple, clear, direct and idiomatic.
- After writing the essay it is necessary to go through it carefully and correct all the errors of spelling or structure, etc.

There are three other points that need attention while writing an essay. First, you should understand the scope of the topic. Second, you should observe proportion dealing with the different aspects of the topic. Third, you should divide the essay in different paragraphs. This is called paragraphing. Now we will disease these one by one.

THE SCOPE OF THE TOPIC

Study the following topics, which concern an examination hall:
- The scene at an examination hall
- The scene outside an examination hall before the examination
- The scene inside an examination hall
- The scene outside an examination hall after the examination
- Suppose you found a question paper very tough. State how you felt in the examination hall. How did you face the situation?
- Suppose a candidate was caught red-handed while copying from a few torn pages of a book. Describe how he behaved, disturbing everybody in the examination hall.

You will notice that each topic is to be handled differently according to its scope.

PROPORTION

Suppose you are asked to write an essay entitled, "My Father". Suppose further that your father is a doctor. It will be perfectly right if you make a reference to your father as doctor and deal with other sides of his personality in proportion to their importance. Your essay will be disproportionate if you describe your father as a doctor in detail. Putting it differently you know salt is a very essential part of certain dishes, without which they are tasteless. But if you add too much salt, these dishes would taste bitter. Would you like them in that case?

So give proportionate importance to the different aspects of a topic.

PARAGRAPHING

Paragraphing means dividing a piece of writing into groups of several sentences, each group dealing with one main idea. Paragraphing in fact indicates the different stages in the development of any piece of writing.

The different paragraphs must be united in the matter of ideas. One idea must naturally refer to what has gone before or is going to follow. This unity may be achieved by using relevant linking devices.

TYPES OF ESSAYS

Essays are of four main types:
1. **Descriptive essays** describe persons, things, places, animals, plants, minerals or machines, buildings, etc.
2. **Narrative essays** narrate some event or events as visits, matches, journeys, fights, robberies, or some accidents, etc. They also narrate stories or legends and biographies.

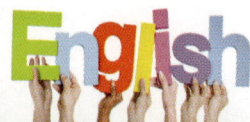

3. **Reflexive essays** deal with abstract topics such as habits, feelings, qualities and social topics, etc.
4. **Imaginative essays** attempt topics about which the writer has little experience. Only imagination can help him to write down such an essay. For example:

    'If I were a principal', 'The Story of a dog' and 'The Adventures of Bunny, these are all imaginative essays.

STRUCTURE OF AN ESSAY

An essay can be divided into three chief parts:

1. Beginning or Introduction
2. Body
3. End or Conclusion

The beginning of an essay should be very brief but catchy and interesting. It may form a short paragraph. It must state the main topic in a befitting way. The topic must be defined and introduced, if possible, through a pithy saying or quotation. The beginning must not be lengthy at all.

The body of the essay forms the essay proper. It should have two or three good paragraphs discussing the different aspects of the topic. The length of each paragraph should be according to the idea discussed in it. The language should be idiomatic and fluent. Do not use unnecessary words and irrelevant points.

The conclusion of the essay should be again very striking. It should sum up the subject in a natural and effective manner. The end should not be abrupt but quite natural.

EXAMPLES OF PARAGRAPHS AND ESSAYS

A Morning Walk

Morning walk is the best form of exercise. It costs nothing. It is very useful for health. It refreshes our mind. It strengthens our body. It prolongs our life. It saves from many diseases. It is equally good for the young and the old. Morning walk makes us fresh for the whole day. It develops in us the habit of rising early. It awakens in love for nature. The dew drops, the fresh flowers, the chirping birds and the leaves charm our mind. We start loving these objects of natural beauty. Thus morning walk is useful not only for our body but for our mind also.

A Picnic

There is a beautiful canal outside our town. Last Sunday, my friends and I decided to go for a picnic. We bought some fruits and sweets. We reached the canal and sat under a tree on its bank. There was a small tea-shed nearby. One of us went there and brought tea. We took tea with fruits and sweets. After this we played a game of cards. Mohan entertained us by singing songs. Many groups of men, women and children had come to the canal. The children played hide and seek. The parents found it hard to keep the children away from water. Everydody was in a holiday mood. We took way back home in the evening. It was a lovely picnic.

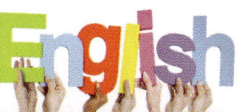

Advantages of Hostel Life

Hostel life has many advantages. It gives one a chance to develop some good habits. Hostellers live like the members of one family. They learn lessons of love, sympathy and tolerance. A hosteller has to help himself in many ways. He has to make his bed. He has to polish his own shoes. Sometimes he has to wash his clothes also. He himself has to look after his things. In this way he learns to self-dependent. Life in a hostel is very calm and quiet. A student can study as much as he likes. These are some of the advantages of hostel life.

Exploitation of Women

This world has always been a man-dominated world. A man never treated woman as an equal partner in his life rather he treated her as a mere slave. Woman is for him the weaker vessel. He has given her many beautiful names. A man calls his wife as better-half. Women are known as the fair sex. We call them devils. But all these are mere sugar-coated words. Man uses such words as a bait to beguile this beautiful creation of God. He abuses her physically, sexually, morally, economically and also politically. But times are beginning to change now. Women are becoming alive to their rights. Education has gone a long way to improve their lot. But still much remains to be done.

The Dowry System

The dowry system is a stigma on our society. It is an insult to women. It is a matter of shame for humans. The greed of dowry has taken the lives of many innocent girls. They are tortured physically as well as mentally. Many a time they are even burnt alive. Though we have a law which disallows the giving and taking of dowry, yet this evil is spreading day by day. We cannot end it merely by shouting slogans and holding demonstrations. Women will have to become bold. They should have education and become economically self-dependent. They should refuse to marry dowry-seekers. Men should also try to wash off this dirty stigma. They should take a vow not to demand or accept any dowry at the time of their marriage. It is only by exercising a strong will power that this evil can end.

Horrors of War

War brings only death and destruction. Science has placed deadly weapons of attack in the hands of man. Modern wars are a danger to civilization. They bring untold misery to humanity. They are indeed very horrible. Two world wars have been fought in the history. They tell us how destructive modern wars can be. The use of bombs, tanks, guns and shells is a common thing in modern wars. They leave behind desolated fields, factories and towns. If there is a Third World War, only God knows what will be left of the world after it.

Fashions

Most of the time of our young boys and girls is spent in front of the mirror. They want to embellish themselves in such a way as to attract every eye. In their desire to look modern and attractive they go crazy for new fashions. They dress themselves in the latest styles. With every change in fashions, their hair-styles also change. To be in the latest fashion seems to be the

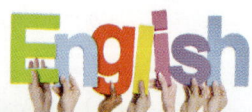

only care of our young boys and girls. They care so much for their exteriors that they have no time to attend to their interiors. They frequently visit the beautician for facials but never visit the library for books, jobs or periodicals. If ever they carry some book or journals in their hand that too is never meant for reading. It is merely for the sake of fashion. I hate these modern clowns.

Need for Fighting Against Corruption

Corruption means dishonesty or immorality in any form. But generally it means the accepting of bribes. This evil has become so common in our society that we feel bad about it. In all walks of life now, it is only money that can make the mare go. There is no section of society that has remained untouched by trade, commerce, industry, education, administration, police, judiciary you name any department the one common thing that will certainly be found in each one of them is CORRUPTION. This evil has made us dead to all sense of shame. We have bankrupted morally and spiritually. All of us have become mammon-worshippers. Only God knows where we are heading. The situation has become so alarming that the structure of our society seems to be shaking. Every successive government makes promises to root out this evil, but is ultimately itself devoured by it. Everyone does feel that the evil of corruption should be fought against, but no one can tell how to go about it. A corruption-free society has gone beyond our dreams.

All That Glitters is Not Gold

This proverb means that all things are not what they seem to be. We should not be misled by the outward appearance of things. Appearances are often deceptive. Many things appear to be charming and attractive outwardly, but they are in fact worthless and even harmful. A snake has a glossy body, but it is one of the most dreaded reptiles. Similarly many wicked men pass for noble and virtuous men. They are like a wolf in sheep's clothing. Shakespeare says in 'Hamlet' that one may smile and smile and yet be a villain. So, we should not go after external looks. We should judge things by their inner worth. We should not be led by the outward appearance of things since all that glitters is not gold.

A Thing of Beauty is a Joy for Ever

Beauty in any form is a source of great joy. The appeal of beauty is eternal and universal. Charming looks, noble deeds, sweet songs, great works of art—are all things of beauty. Beauty lies not only in man-made things but also in objects of nature. The moon-lit night, the multi-colored rainbow, the green valleys, the snow-covered mountains, the sweet smelling flowers have all been sources of great joy to man. A thing of beauty gives us joy not only for the present moment but for the future use also. It gives us an endless source of joy from which we can draw whatever we like. A pretty girl with rosy cheeks and red lips arouses desire in the heart of the beholder. But she lives in our imagination even after she has retired from our view. Great works of art and beautiful objects of nature are ever lasting sources of joy. It is only beauty that sustains the world. Without it the world would have been a dull place not worth living in.

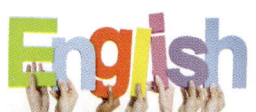

Watching Television

What's that crowd in front of a TV showroom in the market? Oh! They are those who do not have a TV set of their own but still are interested in seeing a live cricket match being telecast. Wait for another day and you will find a similar crowd viewing a popular TV serial. Who can deny the hold of such serials as **Ramayan** or **Mahabharat** on the Indian heart?

Those who think it below their dignity to stand before a TV showroom are always on the look-out for a chance to buy a set of their own. Time was when only the well-to-do had TV sets. Their immediate neighbors or relatives used to visit them to view such programmes as a feature film or **Chitrahaar**. But today, TV has become as common as the radio. Black and White has yielded to color. Even domestic servants, if given a choice, prefer to work with employers who have TV sets of a superior quality.

Today the nation seems to be under the spell of TV. It is watched with equal interest by the grandson and the grandmother, the student and the teacher, the subordinate and the boss, or the villager and the citizen. Some viewers go to the length of adjusting their daily programmes according to what TV has to offer them.

True, TV is a great source of entertainment and education. But is it proper to be watching it all the time? Let us watch TV but not at the cost of our work. Let us not do it even at the cost of play. Games and sports have their own importance.

Newspapers

You wait for your newspaper as you wait for your letters. Both bring you news. Letters bring you news only about your personal or private affairs. But newspapers bring you news about the whole world. When you cannot get your favorite paper, you feel restless.

Newspapers are a source of information about all walks of life. They tell you every morning what has happened in the world even a short time before their publication. The news caters to all interests—political, social, economic, etc.

Newspapers offer you not only news but views also. They contain the views of editors and prominent writers. They also carry letters to the editor on matters of public interest. Again, if you have anything to advertise, newspapers are there to help you.

Almost every newspaper has its magazine section on Sunday, which contains a rich and varied feast of reading material. Sometimes it has special features for women and children.

Newspapers are in your hands, thanks to the inventions of science. The inventions of the printing press and transport facilities have made newspapers popular as an easy and quick means of communication. Thousands of people owe their living to the newspaper industry.

Newspapers can play an important role in a democratic country like India. They can raise their voice against evil in all its shapes. They can guide both the people and their representatives in the law-making bodies.

In short, newspapers have become an indispensable part of modern life. They should remain ever awake to their role in a civilized society.

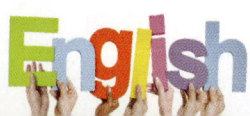

Good Manners

The word 'manners' simply means habits and customs or social behavior. So manners may be either good or bad. But saying that a person has no manners, means that he is very badly behaved.

Whether a person is well~mannered or ill-mannered depends upon his own nature or training. An illiterate person may show good manners while an educated one may show bad ones. But usually a truly educated person is supposed to be pleasant in his behavior towards his fellow human beings.

Good manners are best learnt in childhood. When somebody gives a child something or does something for him, the child is told by his parents to say 'Thank you.' When he asks for something, he is taught to say 'Please.' When he does or says something wrong, he is taught to say 'Sorry.' This is direct teaching. The also child learns good manners from similar situations around him.

These are some of the simple formulas of courtesy. There are many others. But all of them are a mark of good upbringing. Good manners cost nothing. But they win the hearts of those to whom they are shown. The person who shows them too feels pleased. In short, good manners are the basic qualities which make human life pleasant.

Not only that good manners are very paying in our professional life. Once a young man was selected for a job for showing good manners at an interview though he had no recommendation. A shopkeeper who is courteous attracts more customers.

The Place of English in India

English has remained with us so long that now it has become a part and parcel of our daily life. It is such an inexhaustible treasure of knowledge that we will only impoverish ourselves if we decide to go without it. The slogans against English are coined by those who are narrow-minded and pseudo-nationalists. By their diseased thinking they are doing more harm than good to the nation.

It is advocated by the Hindi zealots that the use of English should be banned in India. All education in schools and colleges should be given through the medium of the national language. And if one says that no good books on science and technology are available in Hindi, they say that we should translate the available English books into the national language. They forget that by the time we translate one book into Hindi, ten new will be published and our work shall never be completed. We shall merely turn ourselves into a nation of translators. It would be ridiculous to translate all the scientific and technical terms into the Hindi language.

However, all this is not to suggest that pride of place in India should go to the English language. We must honor our national language and take all steps for its development. All work, as far as possible, should be done in the national and regional languages. But we should have no prejudice against the English language if we are not to deprive ourselves of the latest developments in the field of science and technology.

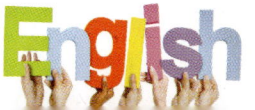

Our System of Education

The greatest defect in our present system of education is that it is too theoretical. An educated man has only bookish knowledge. He knows nothing about practical things.

The present system of education gives too much importance to English. At many places it is the medium of instruction. English may be an international language. It may have rich treasures of science and literature. But it can never be our national language. Education must be in mother tongue. This will save much talent of the country from going waste.

Vocational education is the need of the hour. We need more and more technicians, engineers and doctors. But the number of vocational institutions—Engineering and Medical Colleges, Polytechnics and ITI is limited. A large number of men and women, who cannot do well as technicians are deprived of technical or vocational knowledge. The 10 + 2 + 3 system was designed to vocationalize education and to channelize the talent to different fields. But, different states have taken to it only half-heartedly. As the things stand today, the 10 + 2 + 3 system has become a riddle. No one knows what exactly it is, our system of education really needs to be overhauled and made purposeful.

Population Explosion

The population of India is increasing at a very fast rate. We can call it 'population explosion'. It is very harmful for the country. At present the population of our country is approximately 1.27 billion. Control over disease is one of the causes of this fast increase. Medical science has made a great progress. Powerful drugs have been invented. We have better medical services. There are no epidemics now. The fear of disease has almost ended. So death by disease famine or flood is a thing of the past now. It is good that death rate has decreased. But we should check the birth rate also. We must take steps to control the fast growth of our population. People should be educated about the need of family planning. They should be educated about the advantages of small families. The most important task before the nation is to check the increase of the population.

It is never possible for any father to bring up a large number of children well and properly. He cannot supply all their needs. He cannot give them good education. Thus he spoils not only his own life but also the future of his children. A big family is a curse not only for an individual but also for the nation.

It is not at all difficult to restrict the size of one's family. It merely requires a bit of confidence and will-power. One must come out of the shell of worn-out ideas and customs. Medical science has come to the help of man in planning his family.

The Evil of Drug-Addiction

Drug-addiction is becoming very common among our youth. The evil is more rampant in big cities than in small towns. Perhaps the youth find this life too tiring and burdensome, and as an escape from it they take to drugs. Now, look what happens. Very often, love of fun and new thrills make the beginning. Sometimes parents themselves become the cause of pushing their children into this evil. They are either too strict, or have no time to look after them. The young ones feel neglected. It may be also that they find their education purposeless. In most cases, parents lay high hopes on their sons and daughters. They use bitter words when their wards

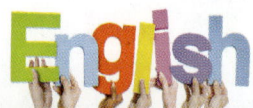

fall short of their expectations. Even those who do well in their studies are not able to get any good jobs. It leads to bitter disappointment.

In utter despair, they take to drugs. Thus they try to forget their problems and miseries. They little realize that by doing so they are inviting their doom. Drug-addiction has become a big social problem. It cannot be checked or prevented by the police alone. Drug-addiction is an illness almost an epidemic. It cannot and should not be treated as a crime. It cannot be ended merely by opening rehabilitation centres. It must be clearly understood that there is no readymade short-cut cure for drug abuse. We often complain that our youth are going wrong. But, hardly do anything to understand their problems. The best way to keep our youth away from drugs is to use their energies in constructive ways.

Florence Nightingale

The pioneer of nursing and reformer of hospital sanitation methods, Florence Nightingale was born in Italy on May 12, 1820 and was named after the city she was born in. So whenever the pious job of a nurse is remembered, only one name clicks in mind and that is 'Florence Nightingale'. She was raised mostly in Derbyshire, England and received a thorough classical education from her father. Her parents William Edward and Frances Nightingale were quite rich. They lived at Lea Hurst in Derbyshire during summer and Embley in Hampshire during winter. Now Lea Hurst has been converted into a retirement home and Embley as a school.

Florence and her elder sister Parthenope were taught at home by their father. Florence was good at studies while her sister was interested in painting and needlework. When Florence grew up she was very beautiful and it was expected that she would make a good marriage, but she had other callings that she heard in 1837 as, the voice of God. Till that time she did not have any ideas what that work would be.

She started, finding answers to the social questions and started visiting the homes of the sick and investigating hospitals and nursing. In those days nursing was not considered a reputed profession for the girls of educated families. While visiting Europe with her two friends, Florence visited Partor Theodor Fliedner's Hospital and School for Deccanesses at Kaiserwerth, near Dusseldorf. The next year she returned to Kaiserwerth, and received three months nursing training which enabled her to take a vacancy as superintendent of the Establishment for. Gentlewomen during illness at No-1 Harley street, London in 1853.

In March 1854, Britain, France and Turkey declared a war on Russia. Russia was defeated but Aeparts in the Times criticized the British medical facilities for the wounded. Nightingale was stirred by the reports of the promotive sanitation methods and grossly inadequate nursing facilities at the large British barracks in hospital at Vskudar in Turkey. Florence Nightingale was appointed to oversee the introduction of female nurses into hospitals in Turkey. On November 4, 1854, she went at the Barrack Hospital in Scutari, with a party of 38 nurses. In the beginning, the doctors did not want the nurses and they did not seek their help but within ten days fresh casualties arrived and the nurses proved to be help.

She was called 'The Lady-in-Chief' by the soldiers. This lady wrote home on behalf of the soldiers. She acted as banker, sending their wages home and introducing reading homes in the hospital. Whatever she did was reciprocated by the soldiers with immense love and regard. The introduction of female nurses to the military hospital was a great success and to show the

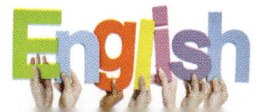

nation's gratitude for Florence Nightingale's hard work, a public subscription was organized in 1855. With the money thus collected, she continued with the reforms in the hospital of Britain.

She was the first woman to be elected as a 'Fellow of the Statistical Society' for her contribution to army statistics in 1860. Her greatest achievement was to raise nursing to the level of a respectable profession for woman. In 1860, she established the Nightingale Training School for nurses at St. Thomas Hospital. The probationer nurses received one year's training under the supervision of the ward sister 'Miss, Nightingale'. In the same year her best known work, 'Notes on Nursing', was published. It laid down the principles of nursing, careful observation and sensitivity to the patient's requirements. These notes later on were translated into eleven foreign languages and are still painted today.

Florence Nightingale's writings on hospital planning and organization had a deep impact on England and across the world. She was the principal advocate of the 'pavilion' plan for hospitals in Britain.

Through her tireless efforts, the mortality rate among the sick and the wounded was, greatly reduced. At the close of the war in 1860, with a fund raised in tribute to her services, Nightingale opened a school and home for nurses at St. Thomas's Hospital in London. The opening of this school marked the beginning of professional education in nursing. Though bedridden for many years 'The lady with the lamp' as she was called by the wounded soldiers, of Crimean War, campaigned without tiring to improve health standards, publishing 200 books, reports and pamphlets. For her extraordinary contribution she was awarded Royal Red Cross, in 1853 by Queen Victoria. She was honoured with the order of merit in 1903 and she was the first woman to receive it. She breathed her last on August 18, 1910 and was buried at St. Margaret's East Wellow, near her parent's home Embley Park in Hampshire.

Ragging

Ragging has not always been the nightmare it has now become. Ragging originated in the west as a sort of initiation rites. The fresh entrants to colleges/hostels were initiated into the manner and way of life of the hostel by their seniors. The latter had also gone through their share of ragging at the time of entry. It was now their turn to have some amusement at the cost of the freshers. They would tease the freshers about their looks or about their manners. Abnormally tall or short students would be easy targets as also the fat and the lean. Students wearing glasses would have their glasses snatched away and made to read without them. Some freshers would be asked to run errands for the seniors. Sometimes the seniors would insist that the freshers bow before them and greet them with folded hands. The freshers would face a major calamity when eatables brought by them from home would be consumed by a group of senior students within a few minutes in their presence. Their protests would invite teasing, ridicule and charge of selfishness.

Ragging frequently consists of mock-interview and mock-trials of the freshers. The seniors would constitute themselves into an interview board and would interview the freshers one by one. The latter would be asked detailed questions. There would be probing questions about the sexual experience or exploits of the freshers. Any attempt to evade the question will invite snubs and ridicule. A fresher who resists the attempts of his senior to ridicule him would become a target for special harassment. He might be charged of stealing an article of a senior and would be put

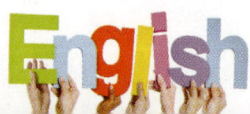

on a mock-trial. The jury constituted by the seniors would act as the accuser, the judge and the punishing authority. The accused may be pressurised by verbal instructions or physical threats into admitting his guilt. The convict would be asked to polish the shoes of his senior for a week or clean their clothes. A boarder who dares complain to the warden would become a target of guerrilla warfare. He could be constantly harassed by some gang of the seniors.

Ragging is indeed a nightmare for the subjects as they go through the ordeal. But it does have some positive effects on the freshers. Those who endure it with courage get emboldened. They get used to facing hardships and unpleasant situations. Many activities, which go under the guise of ragging are extremely questionable practices. It is hard to defend them or to say that they would smoothen the angularities of behavior of the persons and socialise them into the behavior patterns of the majority of the boarders. Such might have the case when higher education was the exclusive preserve of some privileged classes and ragging was limited to a certain extent.

Of late ragging has degenerated into simple torture of the innocent at the hands of Dadas who run the show in the hostels and nobody—neither the principal nor the warden, dares to interfere with the ways of the "Dadas". Such sadists have sometimes locked up the freshers in bathrooms for over 24 hours or have physically beaten them. Cases have been reported in the press of ragging leading to death. Some authorities have reached strongly to tackle the menace of unstrained ragging. Ragging an amusing practice in the olden days, has degenerated into torture and an unmitigated evil. It can no longer be put back on rails. Trails of many educationists try to temper ragging but of no avail. Ragging should be banned in campuses.

Terrorism

A terrorist is a person who creates fear and panic among the people to gain his own ends of the organisation to which he belongs. Terrorism refers to extortion, kidnapping and killing to attract wider attention, to a particular cause by creating fear on a large scale. Thus, terrorism as the Chamber's Twentieth Century Dictionary explains it as means, of an organised system of intimidation especially for political ends. Political terrorism is much more dangerous, and its consequences can be disastrous. Political terrorists are well organised and well trained and it often becomes difficult for the law-enforcing agencies to arrest them in time. They indulge in senseless violence on a large scale in order to intimidate the people and the government. Hijacking of aeroplanes, arsons, robberies, murder of eminent personality, shooting down of innocent people indiscriminately, use of transistor bombs and other explosives, spreading of rumours etc., are the various devices used by terrorist organisations in order to achieve their political ends. Terrorists constantly change their hide-outs, as their tactics in order to escape arrest and punishment. When arrested, they try to commit suicide or are killed by their own close associates. They may think that they are patriots, but in reality they are antisocial or criminal elements, who are exploited by clever politicians to achieve their own ends.

Terrorism is a world-wide problem. It is there in the Middle East and in most countries of Europe. When a group or community feels that the preservation of its identity or way of life is threatened by a stronger group, community or state and no normal or usual method of redressing its grievance will be effective, it takes resort to violence or terrorism to achieve its cherished objectives. Irish Catholics resorted to terror against Protestant England when they

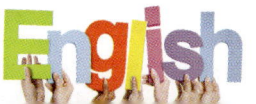

failed to have their way in Northern Ireland. Palestinians took to terrorism when the state of Israel wars established on their land by displacing them.

Terrorists are usually young while the brains behind them are old, seasoned politicians who coordinate and guide their activities. They are fanatics and extremists who act with great fervour and zeal, but studies reveal that if apprehended alive, a terrorist loses his fervour as quickly as he had acquired it. When he has time to think, he feels he has been stupid or that he was misled. We have to disabuse our minds that terrorists who belong to the political class are patriots.

Worsening economic conditions and growing unemployment in Border States enable the terrorists to get a ready crop of fresh recruits. Educated and unemployed youth often swell the ranks of the terrorists. They join them not always out of conviction. Very often they are fed up with their unproductive, unemployed status and join the militants for money and adventure. Bureaucracy is neither sensitive to people's problems, nor responsive to their needs and demands. People, therefore hardly identify with the state. They either remain indifferent when some section of restive population takes up arms against the repressive authorities or provide them with moral or financial support.

There are no short-cuts in the difficult task of combining terrorism. The authorities should analyse the cause of growing disaffection against the establishment with an open mind. The genuine problem should be taken up immediately and earnestly for finding their short term and long term solution. Such a sincere response will bring the people sitting on the fence to the side of establishment thus eroding the support for the terrorists substantially. When the right thinking and patriotic citizens are enlisted on the side of the government, the obstinate, antinational terrorists can be defeated in their designs.

Cheating in Examinations

Cheating in examinations has become very common. Those who indulge in it, feel no shame. Rather they proudly declare how well they could cheat in the examination.

Students start arming themselves for this purpose long before the examination. They prepare chits for all the expected questions and even arrange them serially with an index written on a rate chit. They preserve these chits carefully till the day of examination. Some students don't even take the trouble of writing these chits. They tear out whole pages from help-books to use in the examination-hall. But why spoil a costly book! So the wiser ones carry the entire book to the hall.

The scene in front of an examination hall can leave one in no doubt about the activities of students during the examination. They can be seen tucking up pages of books in their sleeves, socks; shoes or in any other crevices in their dress or body. They try to grease the palm of some peon or water-man working in the hall so that he might help them to smuggle in answers during the examination. The cleverer ones work out contacts with the members of the supervisory staff.

Thus there can be no denying about the curse of copying in examinations. A student who is able to copy out some answers in the examination hall, gets only superficial joy and satisfaction. Even if he scores good marks by virtue of this cheating methods, he does know in his heart of hearts the truth behind this inflated index of his ability and can have no real sense of achievement. In actual life, only real knowledge pays and not the knowledge-tags.

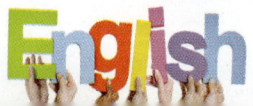

The curse of cheating in examinations has brought a very bad name to our temples of learning. It is a curse that has debased us morally, intellectually and spiritually. But to be frank about it, there seems no way to eliminate it in the near future. Thanks to the defective and purposeless policy of education designed by our nation's architects. Since independence, our system of education has been in an experimental stage. Every year we hear of new schemes being implemented but each of them fails miserably because the architects of these schemes and policies are unimaginative and know nothing about the hard ground realities.

Superstitions

One universal element in human nature observed by me is the belief in superstitions. A superstition is an irrational belief. Every religious system has a web of superstitions woven round it. A Christian, for example, may believe that in time of trouble he will be guided by the Bible if he opens it at random and reads the text that first strikes his eye. Often one man's religion is another man's superstition. All religious beliefs and practices may seem superstitious to a person without religion.

Nearly all persons, in nearly all times have held seriously or half-seriously irrational beliefs concerning methods of warding off evil or bringing good. A few specific beliefs, such as that in the efficacy of amulets, have been found in most periods of history and in most parts of the world. Others may be limited to one country, region or village, to one family or to one social or vocational group.

I have observed some very interesting superstitious beliefs among the people in my neighbourhood. My landlady dreads the sight of a black dog. She says that it always brings her bad luck. Her son, Mohan, has a pen. He calls it a lucky pen. He always writes his examination papers with that very pen. One Mr Malhotra lives next door to me. He always takes curd before leaving his house for some business. He says that the curd protects a man from evil spirits. He has instructed all the members of his family not to call at his back while he is leaving the house. He comes back if some cat happens to cross the path by which he is going. He considers it a bad omen. His wife is also very superstitious. She has a little son. She always puts a black mark on the child's forehead as a safeguard against the evil eye.

I have seen that even highly educated persons are superstitious. Being irrational, superstition should recede before education and especially science. Nevertheless, even in these days of science, there are few people who would, if pressed, admit to cherishing at least one or two superstitions. There is one Prof. Bhalla in our street. He teaches Physics in our college. He says that one should be beware of men with brown eyes and women with moustaches. I don't mind people having superstitions as long as they don't harm others.

Students and Politics

Student life is the best pan of one's life. It is the most enjoyable period in one's life. It is tune to study and play. The physical mental and moral development of a man takes shape in this period. A student should not be a mere bookworm. He should be well informed. He should keep himself in touch with what is happening around him. He should know about the political and economic problems the country is facing.

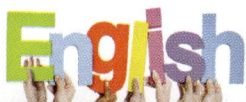

It is advocated by some that a student should take an active part in politics. They think that the education of a man is incomplete if he is not trained in facing the current national problems. In India's struggle for freedom the students played a very important role. Students can prove a very potent force against the wrong policies of the government. Students cannot remain silent when the country is facing serious problems.

But there is an opposite view also. According to this view, students should remain above politics. The primary business of a student is to study. If he takes part in politics his studies will suffer. He will waste the hard earned money of his parents. A student should devote self to his studies with heart and soul. He should learn so that he is able to earn in future. He should acquire all the qualities that go to make a good citizen.

Moreover the mind of a student is immature. Corrupt politicians can mislead him to gain their own selfish ends. Schools and colleges are the temples of learning. Politics is a dirty game. It brings with it strikes, demonstrations and indiscipline in all its ugly forms. It pollutes atmosphere of our schools and colleges. It makes the students rude and irresponsible. They no longer remain obedient and gentle. They become a problem for their teachers and parents. They spoil their future. But the truth dawns on them only when it is too late. It is, therefore in the interest of students to remain away from politics. They should follow Gandhiji's advice in this respect:

'A student cannot be an active politician and pursue his studies at the same time. But at the time of national upheaval he must suspend his studies'.

Generation Gap

The gap between old people and young boys and girls is called the generation gap. The young people are inexperienced, rash and impatient. While the elders are endowed with wisdom prudence and caution. This gap between the two generations is not a new question. It has existed since time immemorial.

The people belonging to the older generation always wonder as to what has gone wrong with the new generation. They feel that during their time young boys and girls used to be much better in their behavior. They had greater respect for their elders. They feel that the young lack respect for their elders. They feel that this lack of respect will bring ruin for the young. Young people, on the other hand feel that they are capable enough to take their own decisions. They donot like to be spoon-fed by their elders. This gap is widening day by day due to various reasons. First of all, the present system of education is little relevant to the realities of life. It is not job-oriented. The result is that after completing their education young people are not able to find any employment. They feel highly disillusioned.

Secondly, life has become very busy and fast. Parents find little time to devote to the children.

Thirdly, tradition is still dominant in India. It kills the initiative of the younger generation. In order to express their resentment, young people behave in a very unconventional manner. They have no respect for traditions, customs, manners, etc.

The generation gap has widened to a great extent. The old and the young people appear to be living in two separate worlds without any interaction. In order to bridge this generation gap, elders should adopt a more sympathetic approach towards the young. They should try to

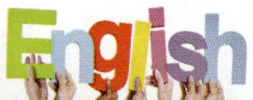

understand the emotions, the aspirations and the problems of the young. The youth should realize that they have no experience of life. They should, therefore, value the advice and counsel of the elders. If the youth have any difference of opinion, they should put across their viewpoint before the elders in a very polite and respectful manner.

In the western countries of Europe and America the generation gap is so wide that the young and the old do not like to live together. They have started living separately. Thus this generation gap results in the break up of homes and joint families.

In India the problem is not so serious. It is due to the influence of the joint family system prevailing in India. There are definitely a lot of advantages in the joint family system. Therefore we should not follow the western system blindly at the cost of the well-tried Indian 'social and family tradition'. It is the duty of both generations to try to understand and respect one another's views. Only then this problem can be solved.

Increasing Indiscipline Among Students

Schools and colleges were once thought to be temples of learning. Students went there to get knowledge. They pursued their studies seriously and wholeheartedly. But modern students have profaned the sanctity of these temples. They have defiled their atmosphere. Schools and colleges have now become hot-beds of indiscipline.

Student life is the most formative period in a man's life. A student can make or mar himself in this period. But the modern student does not recognise this fact. He does not care a fig about his studies. He behaves most irresponsibly. He is not serious in the class-room. He has no respect for his teachers. He has no love for knowledge. He simply wants to pass examinations by fair or foul means. Mass-scale copying during examinations has become very common. Modern students are strike-mongers. They indulge in acts of indiscipline and violence. They look for excuses to create violence. They take part in politics and neglect their studies. The corrupt politicians make them scapegoats to gain their own ends.

The modern student has no aim in life. He is like a rudderless boat. He keeps drifting here and there. But the student alone is not to blame for this ugly state of affairs. The student learns from the example of his teachers. The modern teachers are not dedicated to their job. They run after money. They too, go on strikes quite often. Therefore, it is nothing strange if the students imitate their teachers. We can't expect any discipline from our students if there is corruption, lawlessness and disorder all around.

In order to bring discipline among the students, the teachers must realise their responsibility. They should display high standards of discipline in their own life. Only then their teaching can have any effect on the students. Only good and devoted persons should be allowed to continue in this profession. Schools and colleges should be made real temples of learning. The authorities should try to save them from politicians and hired political workers.

Wonders of Science
or
Science in the Service of Mankind

Science has made man the master of this world. It has brought marvellous changes in man's life. It has made our life-easy and comfortable. It has, in fact, proved a blessing for man.

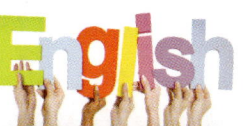

It has translated our dreams into realities. It has brought a revolution in the fields of agriculture, industry, communication and transportation.

Science has helped to bring this world closer. The present-day world is almost a single unit. Space and time have lost their previous limitations. Science has placed at man's disposal quick and safe means of transportation. The days of bullock-carts and horse-driven carriages are over now. Cars, buses, trains and aeroplanes have made journeys faster, easier and more comfortable.

Science has greatly reduced human suffering. Great progress has been made in the fields of medicine and surgery. Diseases, once thought fatal, can now be cured very easily. Small pox, cholera, plague and malaria do not threaten us now. Medicines and injections that can work wonders have been discovered. Operations can be performed without giving any pain to the patient. X-rays can detect ailments inside human body. It has become possible to give eyes to the blind and legs to the lame.

Science has given us many articles of daily use. These articles have made our life easy and comfortable. Gas-stoves, cookers, heaters, washing-machines, etc. have made the job of a housewife much easier.

Science has added to man's knowledge by inventing the printing press. We can now get reading material at very cheap rates. Newspapers and periodicals bring us news from all parts of the world. Radio, television and telephone have made communication quite fast and easy. Science has literally landed man on the moon.

Science has also helped to multiply our agricultural and industrial production. We can now produce in our fields and factories as much as we like. In fact, science has made it possible to meet all the demands of humanity.

But science has its darker side also. It has given man the power fit for gods, but man does not know its proper use. He has invented dangerous weapons like the atom bomb. Science is a good servant but a bad master. Man should, therefore, not let it go off his hands. He should not use science for the destruction of humanity. He should use it to make this world a better place to live in.

Role of Computers in Modern Life

A computer is a machine with a brain. We can call it a thinking machine. It works under instruction or data (or information) that has been fed into it. For example, it can do calculations with numbers. It can point out the mistakes in your spellings. It can mark your answer books.

It can play a game of chess with you, guide a spacecraft, check fingerprints and draw a map of your country. It can do all these things and many more. It can do millions of calculations in a second and normally the results are always exactly correct.

Because computers are electronic machines, they don't have moving parts (for example, a car engine). Therefore, computers do not wear out and hardly ever go wrong: Most computers can carry out a very wide range of tasks, and they can easily switch from one job to another. Because of all these abilities, computers are playing a bigger and bigger part in the modern world. They can perform amazing feats of calculation that are far beyond 'man's mental ability'. They can also do a task over and over again without ever making a mistake. They have already taken over many dull and repetitive jobs in offices and factories. Computers are also helping us to increase our knowledge in all kinds of fields. When steam engines and factory machines were

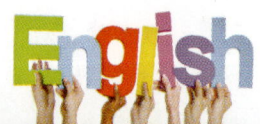

first invented, they gave people much greater physical power to do things. They made possible the industrial revolution, as a result of which people's lives were greatly changed.

The development of computers in the late 20th century has given us greater mental power. Computers can do a lot of extra thinking and remembering for us, just as engines push and pull for us. Computers have already changed our way of life and work. This change is often given the name of 'Computer Revolution.' Like the Industrial Revolution in the 1700s and 1800s, it is changing our lives in the 2000s. And this change is so fast that a device developed during one year begins to look obsolete the next year provided it is fitted with the right kind of input and output units.

A computer can be programmed to carry out almost any task. As computers become more advanced, more uses for them are being found. Here are just a few examples showing the uses of computers. In factories, computers have been used for maintaining the quality of goods. Robots controlled by computers are being increasingly used to do routine jobs day after day, without making mistakes or getting bored. Computer can help design new machines. These machines can also be tested by computer before they are actually built.

Another important field in which computers are proving very useful is the running of business. Large business houses make use of computers in calculating their payrolls, sending bills. checking payments and keeping track of the way the business is being run.

Computers can also hold stores of information called databases. Any part of the information can be obtained very quickly by anyone using the computer.

Computers are playing an important role in teaching also. They can be very helpful in teaching school pupils and testing their knowledge. Many schools have classes for computer studies where children are taught how to handle computers correctly.

One of the most important uses of computers is in medicine. They are used in scanners which can look inside the body to find if anything is wrong. They are also helpful in deciding the causes of illnesses. They can ask patients about their symptoms and work out the most likely cause of them. They can help doctors in making new drugs to fight an illness. Computerised machines can help disabled people to work and live fuller lives. A special computer, for example, is able to read books to blind people.

Role of Advertisements

Advertisements play a very important role in the promotion of one's business. But a business advertisement should be drafted, designed and laid out in an artistic manner that will tempt the reader to go through it even if he has no desire to buy the advertised product.

In fact, it is not possible to think of the modern world without advertising. In its wider sense, advertising is as much applicable to the world of politics and religion as to that of business and trade. But when we speak of advertisements we generally refer to business and commerce. They have become the backbone of the world of trade. Extensive markets depend on large-scale advertising. It is through colorful advertisements that trading companies create demand and secure sales for their products.

In the past, there was not much need to advertise goods. Markets were limited. The traders or manufacturers had only local customers. At best, they took the services of town criers or they used hand-bills or posters. But now advertising itself has become a specialized form

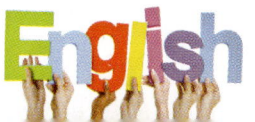

of business. Many advertising agencies have come up. These agencies help businessmen to promote their sales.

Small traders still use hand-bills and posters. They also use wall-paintings for the purpose. But, big traders and industrialists use sophisticated devices for this purpose. They advertise their products through the silver screen of the cinema. They telecast sponsored programmes. They give catchy advertisements on the radio. Colorful and life-size hoardings are displayed on the roadsides. Many gift schemes are started to push the sale of products.

In fact, trade advertisements are everywhere around us. They are seen at every street corner, at the bus stands, at the railway stations. Businessmen know that they can't do without advertisements. It is not enough to produce goods. Much more important is the creation of markets. A businessman or manufacturer, who thinks that he can do without advertisement, will soon be wiped out of the market.

Advertisements give a boost to the country's economy. They encourage production. Increase in business brings about more employment opportunities. With greater sales. Manufacturers can improve the quality of products. They can also make researches in fresh areas.

Now, there is nothing wrong in advertising. But trouble arises when false claims are made by the manufacturers' for their products. Such traders and manufacturers earn profits by deception. It is really sad that harmful and sub-standard products should be sold to innocent customers by the sheer force of advertisements.

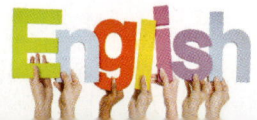

Practice Exercises

I. Write essays on the following topics:

1. Pollution
2. A healthy mind in a healthy body
3. Harmful consequences of deforestation
4. Corruption
5. Hazards of television watching
6. Discipline
7. Rising prices
8. Nursing as a profession
9. Advantages of co-education
10. Child labour
11. Honour killing or horror killing
12. Evils of smoking
13. Fair treatment to girl child
14. A television programme you enjoyed most
15. Stress caused by faulty examination system
16. Importance of training in education
17. An hour before the examination in front of the examination hall
18. Games and sports
19. Value education should be a part of the curriculum
20. Women's rights

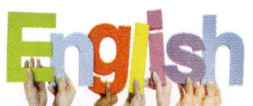

NOTES

Chapter 31

Resume and Cover Letter

INTRODUCTION

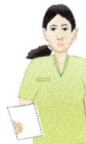

The word 'resume' has two different connotations. 'Resume' as a noun is pronounced differently which stands for "curriculum vitae" whereas 'resume' as a verb is pronounced in a different way, which means "restart". It is not about your past jobs, but how you performed them. It tells about your accomplishments that are most relevant to the work you want to do in the near future. It predicts that how well you can perform in the desired future job. It's an inkling of your personality. Moreover, we should not forget a highly celebrated dictum "its not the cup of tea that matters, but with whom you are taking that matters". So your presentation is of paramount importance. Your resume should be attention-seeking. Few years back the number of vacancies was more than the aspirants, but now the trends have been changed. At present there are hundreds of applicants for a job. Few get appointment and for the rest there is only disappointment. The first barrier is a call for an interview. Employers generally skip resumes. They don't spend more than a minute on your resume. Hence you must tell everything in the fewest possible words. Your resume is a key to enter an interview chamber. So, it turns to be rather more important.

Resume ....

- ❑ Is results-driven document that is relevant and essential to prove that you have the requisite credentials to perform the job.
- ❑ Is educational tool that exemplifies the essence of you and enlightens readers about the who, what, when, where, why, how and how much about you.
- ❑ Shares information while selling and supporting your values, benefits and worth to the organisation.
- ❑ Tells uniqueness of you, the inimitable individual and captured imprint.
- ❑ Is meaningful marketing tool designed to fulfill your goal of getting an interview with your target audience.
- ❑ Is evokes a positive response from the prospective employer ... 'we'd like to interview you.'

TYPES OF RESUMES

Chronological Resume

A chronological résumé enumerates a candidate's job experiences in reverse chronological order.

The chronological résumé format is by far the most common résumé layout in use. In using this format, the main body of the document becomes the **professional experience** section, starting from the most recent experience and going chronologically backwards through a succession of previous experience. The chronological résumé works to build credibility through experience gained, while illustrating career growth over time.

Functional Resume

A functional résumé lists work experience and skills sorted by skill area or job function.

The functional résumé is used to assert a focus on skills that are specific to the type of position being sought. This format directly emphasizes specific professional capabilities and utilizes experience summaried as its primary means of communicating professional competency. In contrast, the chronological résumé format will briefly highlight these competencies prior to presenting a comprehensive timeline of career growth via reverse-chronological listing with most recent experience listed first.

Combination Résumé

The combination résumé balances the functional and chronological approaches. A résumé organized this way typically leads with a functional list of job skills, followed by a chronological list of employers.

Curriculum Vitae

In the United States, a CV is expected to include a comprehensive listing of professional history including every term of employment, academic credentials, publications, contribution or significant achievements. In certain professions, it may even include samples of the person's work and may run to many pages.

Within the European Union, a standardised CV model known as Europass has been developed (in 2004 by the European Parliament) and promoted by the EU to ease skilled migration between member countries.

CONTENTS OF RESUME

A resume is the most important document you will ever create. Just like a gardener you will have to choose every blossom with proper attention. **Garbage in, garbage out.** If the choice of contents is erroneous, the impact is bound to be off beam. So you have to set every flower in such a way that it becomes a beautiful bouquet. Before writing, take time to do a self-assessment on a paper. Pen down your skills, abilities, work experience if any, co-curricular activities and whatever you feel relevant for the employer. For every single post there should be a different resume. So the contents vary from resume to resume. The resume must contain the following:

❑ *Name:* Mention the name that has been written on your certificates. Avoid nicknames.

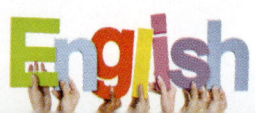

❏ ***Address:*** Use a permanent address. If there is any alternative address you may add that also. Mention if there is any landmark nearby.

❏ ***Telephone:*** Use a permanent telephone number including area code. If you keep an answering machine then record a neutral greeting. If you have a mobile phone, don't hesitate to mention the number.

❏ ***E-mail address:*** Always add your e-mail address because it shows that you are well versed with the modern technology as many employers will find it highly useful. You should mention an e-mail only if you check it frequently. You can add your website address also, if you keep one.

❏ ***Objective:*** Keep it as short as possible. Conclude it in one or two sentences. It tells a potential employer the sort of work you are interested to do. Your objectives should throw adequate light on your interests and abilities. Tailor your objective to each employer you target and every job you plan to seek. Mind that a single cap can't be fitted on every head.

❏ ***Work experience:*** Briefly give the employer an overview of the work that you have done. The choice of diction plays an important role in it. Use action words to state your job duties. Mention your work experience in reverse chronological order, i.e., put your last job first and work backward to the first one. You should add the designation, name of the organization, location, tenure and work responsibilities.

❏ ***Education:*** If you have some work experience to your credit then you can place your academic qualifications after the work experience. Add most recent educational information first. Don't abbreviate your degrees. Mention the percentage and the year of passing.

❏ ***Co-curricular activities:*** You need to add the co-curricular activities in which you have participated. You can mention the achievements in sports as well as positions in cultural programmes.

❏ ***Accomplishments:*** Here you can add all the honors and awards that you have got. You should tell about every possible feather that comprises your cap. Never underestimate your achievements.

❏ ***Strengths:*** Muse about your positive points and enlist them.

❏ ***Hobbies and interests:*** This is optional. Don't include hobbies in a resume unless the activity is somehow relevant to your job objective. For example, the hobby of skydiving might seem relevant for the job of a 'security guard' but not for a teacher.

❏ ***Languages known:*** Mark your fluency in speaking, writing and reading different languages.

❏ ***References:*** Make sure to have the consent of the people who you are going to use as references. It's not mandatory to mention references. Moreover 'References furnished on request' may be added at the bottom.

GUIDELINES FOR MAKING A RESULT-ORIENTED RESUME/HELPFUL HINTS

A high-quality resume can create a gigantic difference. These days resume writing has become very important because of an extreme division of labour and areas of specialization. Employers are always on the look for the selection of specialists for specific jobs. It's more of an art and less

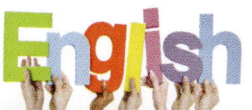

of a mechanical format. In order to get a job, one has to pass various obstacles and resume is not only the first but also the most significant one. There are a number of tips that we should consider while creating a resume.

Do's

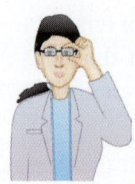

- ❑ Try to restrict your resume in one page. You can go for another page only if it is inevitable.
- ❑ Precise it because employers typically skim resumes, spending average time of just 15–45 seconds on each. So make it a 30 second personal commercial.
- ❑ Sentences should begin with action verbs. Deeds speak louder than words.
- ❑ It should appeal to the needs of a potential employer.
- ❑ Make a raw list of all your experiences, activities, achievements, courses (including summer jobs), internships, volunteer works, etc. This will eventually help you in drawing a result-oriented resume.
- ❑ If overestimation is wrong, so is underestimation. Don't sell yourself short.
- ❑ List your technical knowledge in an organized manner. Your technical strengths must stand out vividly at the beginning of your resume.
- ❑ Stick to the past tense, even for descriptions of currently held positions.
- ❑ Use white or off- white paper.
- ❑ Use a standard size paper i.e., 8½ × 11 inches.
- ❑ Print only at one side of the page.
- ❑ Have a laser or a high quality print.
- ❑ Stick to the font size from 10 to 14.
- ❑ Choose one typeface and stick to that.
- ❑ Run a spell check on your computer before anyone glances at it.
- ❑ Proofread, proofread and proofread it plenty of times to catch a hidden error.
- ❑ Send your resume in a large envelope.
- ❑ If you are to fax it, set the fax on 'fine' or 'super fine'. Always send original, not a photostat one.
- ❑ Make sure that you send your resume to the right person.

Don'ts

- ❑ Avoid decorative type faces
- ❑ Avoid glittering and colorful pages
- ❑ Avoid excessive italics, scripts and underlining
- ❑ Avoid horizontal or vertical lines
- ❑ Avoid graphics and shading
- ❑ Avoid folding and stapling
- ❑ Avoid too light or dark printing
- ❑ Avoid mentioning your age, marital status, health, irrelevant awards, etc. purposelessly

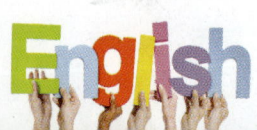

COVER LETTER

A cover letter is equally important. Whenever you send your resume it should be accompanied with a cover letter. It will tell the employer the exact purpose of your resume and the benefit that they can have by reading it. As your resume is supposed to be in a formal style so you can add certain more details about yourself in the cover letter. It gives you a chance to show your communication skills and different facets of your personality. Always send your resume and cover letter together because each has a unique function to do. If the purpose of a resume is to inspire an employer to call you for an interview, then the purpose of a cover letter is to instigate him to go through your resume. Both go hand in hand. Be specific in your cover letter.

SAMPLE COVER LETTER, CURRICULUM VITAE AND RESUME

COVER LETTER

Cover Letter for the post of a lecturer in a college.

279, Sector 37A
Chandigarh
July 15, 2021
Director-cum-Principal
IHM
Banur

Sub: Application for the Post of a Lecturer in Communication Skills.

Dear Sir/Madam

With reference to your advertisement dated: July 13, 2021 published in **The tribunal** present my candidature for the post of a lecturer in Communication Skills. Finding my candidature eligible, I am intended to offer my services for the same. I have done M.A. in English and qualified the UGC (NET). My PhD in linguistics is in progress. I have had the teaching experience of 5 years to my credit. I have participated and conducted numerous co-curricular activities.

If given the chance to serve your esteemed institution under your kind control, I assure you that I would leave no stone unturned for your kind satisfaction. Please give a generous consideration to my application. I would very much appreciate on giving me a chance to be interviewed. I would then be able to give you further details about my work. I muse that it is going to help you in judging my suitability for the above-said post. Consider favorably and oblige.

Yours sincerely

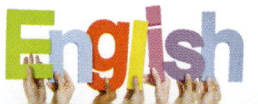

Manisha

RESUME

Write a resume (by a nurse) applying for a job of senior ward nurse at a hospital.

#279, Sector-15,
Chandigarh.
May 25, 2021
Mehak Sood
Human Resource Manager
Gian Sagar Hospital
Ram Nagar, Banur

Sub: Applying for the post of a Senior Ward Nurse.

Dear Madam

With reference to your advertisement in the Daily Tribune on 20th May, I wish to apply for the post of senior ward nurse in your hospital. I am currently a ward nurse in Mukat Hospital in Chandigarh. In addition to my normal ward nurse duties, I am responsible for triage assessment. My resume is attached for your perusal.

I am committed to pursuing a career in nursing and am particularly interested in the above-mentioned post as it would help me gain the experience of working in a larger hospital. It would also give me opportunities to give quality care to a large number of patients.

I look forward to hearing from you.

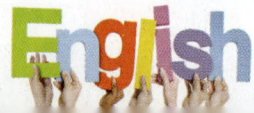

Yours sincerely
Deepika Sharma
Enc. CV

CURRICULUM VITAE

Name	:	**Deepika Sharma**
D.O.B	:	August 15, 1990
Address	:	279, Sector 15, Chandigarh
Phone	:	0172-2690279, Mobile – 9876543201
Email	:	*deepika@gmail.com*
Profile	:	A registered nurse with 3 years work experience in ward nursing.
Marital Status	:	Unmarried

Educational Qualification

❑ June 2012 – BSc Nursing Gian Sagar College of Nursing, Banur.
❑ June 2008 – Senior Secondary from DAV School, Chandigarh.
❑ June 2006 – Secondary Examination, MRA Sr. Sec. School, Chandigarh.

Work Experience

June 2016 till present ward nurse at Mukat Hospital, Chandigarh.

Responsibilities

Mukat Hospital is a 50 bed Hospital with ICU, operation theatre and labour room facilities. As a nurse, I am responsible for the welfare and care of patient in the ward. I have experience of working in the causality, emergency and post-operation wards.

Skills	:	Languages-fluent in English, Hindi and Punjabi
Interests	:	Regular volunteer at local health awareness camps
References	:	Dr Rao. HOD Medicine, Gian Sagar Hospital, Banur, 9285432548
		Dr Preeti HOD Skin, Mukat Hospital, Chandigarh, 9779585878

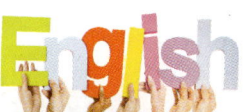

India Assurance Company, New Delhi has given an advertisement in "The Hindustan Times" for recruitment of management trainees to be groomed as managers of their company. Apply for the same, giving your detailed bio-data (curriculum vitae). Invent all necessary details. You are Aman/Aditi, 54-A, Gulab Road, Lucknow.

54-A, Gulab Road
Lucknow
March 10, 2021
The Personnel Manager
India Assurance Company
New Delhi

Sir,

Sub: Recruitment of Management Trainee.

With reference to your advertisement in The Hindustan Times dated March 5, 2021 for management trainees to be groomed as managers for your company, I would like to be considered for the said post.

My bio-data is enclosed for your perusal and consideration. If I am found suitable, I can appear for the interview at your convenience. In case of selection, I assure you of my unstinted cooperation and devotion in the discharge of my duties.

Yours faithfully
Aditi

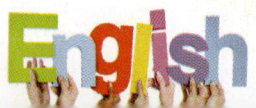

RESUME

Name	:	**Aditi Kukreja**
Father's Name	:	Prof. SN Kukreja
Address	:	54-A, Gulab Road, Lucknow
Date of Birth	:	August 7, 1975

Educational Qualification

(i) BCom, Delhi University
(ii) MBA from Symbiosis University
(iii) Diploma in Computer Application from NIIT Lucknow

Experience	:	1 year
Present Employment	:	Working with Global Telesystems, Lucknow
Marital Status	:	Married
Personal Details	:	Height 5'-3"
		Weight 60 kg
		Mother Tongue—Hindi
Language known	:	English, Punjabi, French
Hobbies	:	Reading, listening to music, painting
References	:	1. Professor Suresh Mohan, IT College, Lucknow, 09459384566
		2. Professor Kapil Ranjan, Symbiosis, Pune, 09417307668
Contact No	:	9216684689
Email. ID	:	*Aditi75@gmail.com*

 Practice Exercises

I. A post of Computer Operator is lying vacant in Gian Sagar College of Physiotherapy. Send a resume with application for the same.

II. A post of Principal is lying vacant in a Nursing College in Jalandhar. Send a Resume applying for the post.

III. A post of Professor is lying vacant in Sukhmani College of Nursing in Derabassi. Send a Resume along with application.

IV. A post of Clinical Instructor is lying vacant in Gian Sagar College of Nursing. Send your resume for the same.

V. You are Anita, send an application with resume for the post of Nursing Tutor in Swift College of Nursing.

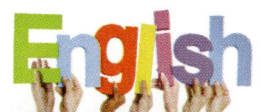

NOTES

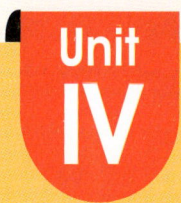

Unit
IV

Spoken English

Unit Outline

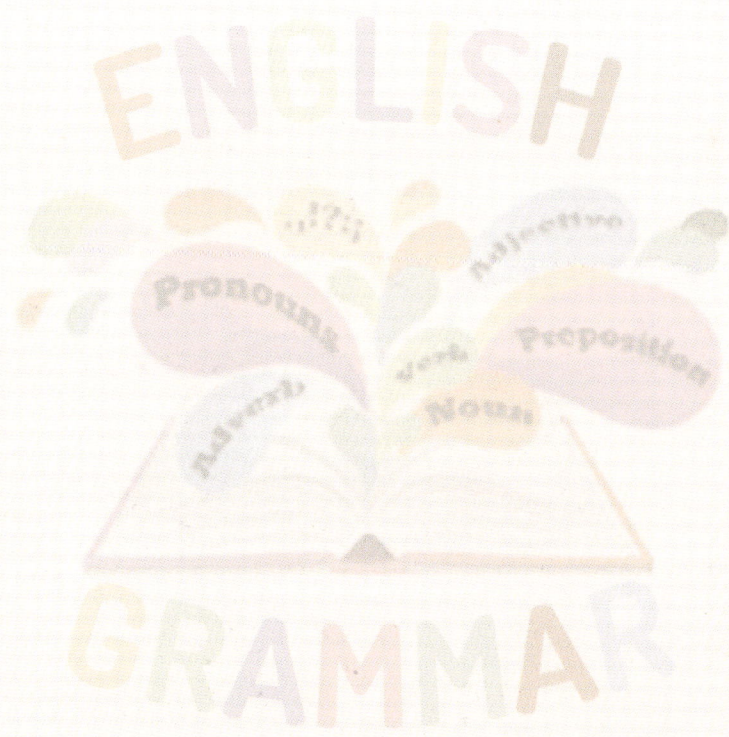

Chapter 32

Telephonic Conversation

In telephonic conversation we rely on two things: (a) listening and concentrating on what we hear and (b) the tone and words of the voice of the caller. The element of concentration in telephonic talk is of crucial importance. How much we remain alert in talking to a person, we soon forget the details of what we have just listened. Therefore, have a telephone pad and pen next to the telephone at all times and fix them in some way to the desk so that they do not get lost. There is nothing more frustrating than scribbling around for something to write on or with after the call has started. Taking notes right from the beginning of conversation saves repeating small but vital facts later on and minimizes the effect of distractions going on around us.

We also need to make sure that the caller knows that we are listening to. When speaking face to face we use many non-verbal signs to indicate this, such as nodding. On the telephone, "Verbal nods" like "I see", "yes", "Okay", "right", etc. are uttered to indicate that the listener is listening attentively.

It is not just what we say but the way we say it. The tone is important in creating the right image. So do the following:

- Identify yourself and your organization:
    "Anjali Singh speaking".
    "I am Lovepreet from Computer Section".
- Be tactful:
    "May I know Sir/Madam, your name please".
    "Do you wish him to call you when the meeting is over?"
- Be helpful:
    "Could I leave my message for him?"
    "Mr Nikhil is out just now. Can I give your message to Mr Salman?"
- Give a greeting: This should consist of:
    "Good morning/afternoon; our department; our name".
    "Good morning, Mukat Hospital, Abishek speaking".

When we answer like this, callers respond immediately by telling us their names. This is useful to acquire early on because we can use that person's name throughout the call as well as for future reference. *i.e.,*

    "I'll make sure you receive the information by tomorrow."

This way of ending telephone conversation is tremendously friendly and helpful.

❏ Use appropriate questions to maintain control. There are basically two types of questions: open and closed. Open questions are those which require more than a straight 'yes' or 'No'. Closed questions require a 'Yes/No' answer. They generally start... did you, was it, have you, etc. we need to use appropriate questioning techniques to elicit the relevant information from the caller. *i.e.,*

"Do you want more information on that?" may just get "yes".

"What more information would you like?" will elicit specifics.

❏ Keep people informed. If, for any reason we have to leave our caller holding on, we should tell him how long it will be and offer to call him back with information he needs.

The following 'Don'ts need to be observed in telephonic conversation:

• Never hold two conversations. It does not matter what else is happening in the office, talk to person on the line, ignore other problems around you. Don't shout or mumble.

• Don't get too close to the receiver.

• Don't say "Hello." This can start a chain reaction of hellos.

• Don't forget to say "Thank you", If it is called for.

• In the case, the telephone gets cut off and conversation again started, don't show irritation nor discuss whose fault it was that we got cut off.

Never say:	Say:
"Hello"	The name of the firm, department or office.
"Who?"	"Who is speaking, please?"
"Who are you?"	"What is your name, please?"
"Who do you want?"	"Who do you wish to speak to?"
"He is out."	"I am sorry Mr ... is not available. Can I help you?"
"He is not here".	"I am sorry Mr ... is not available. Can I help you?"
"Hold on"	"Would you hold the line, please?"

Tone of the voice conveys the way we are feeling about the conversation, the caller or the way we feel on that particular day. One good way of making sure that we sound right is to smile while we are talking. Smiling relaxes the vocal chords and has a dramatic effect on the voice, instantly making us sound more friendly and relaxed.

Difficult Callers

The "difficult caller" is misnomer of the term. When the dealing between the customer and firm/organization comes to a dead end, either of the party may be rude and aggressive in his/her behavior. Difficult call arises in the face of the failure of transaction or owing to the misunderstanding in the process of transactions. For example, a customer wants refund for booking of the car he had done six months back. He had been promised that he would get the car three weeks after booking, but the car is nowhere in sight after six months. The receptionist has to bear the burnt of the ire of the customer.

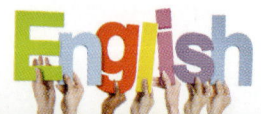

One should remain professional in a difficult situation like this. Accept responsibility for whatever is being complained about. You are part and parcel of the organization to the caller. Don't shrink the onus of failure to meet the contract. Don't say: "I agree with you that our finance section is rather not helpful in solving such problems. "Nor get irritated and scold the caller: "You are the tenth person this week who has complained about that". Apologize. It takes out half the heat of the complaint. Avoid taking any insult personally. After all, the caller does not have any personal grudge with you as you have not tried to insult or unnecessarily argue with him.

Finish the call positively by telling the caller what will happen next. Take follow-up action immediately and make sure you ring back if you said you would. Offer alternatives to the caller, if you can. For example, if you don't have the information, the caller wants saying, "would you like to hold on, or shall I call you back?" may help.

Always use the name of the so-called difficult caller in your conversation. He may feel treated efficiently and politely.

Do Ring Back

The major complaint in telephonic conversation is that the party has not called back the customer as he had been promised. Not calling back the person that he has been promised for is the greatest bane of Indian bureaucracy as well as business class in the eyes of professionals and foreign business concerns. In order to remedy this perception, the following tips are suggested:

- ❑ It should be a normal habit in telephonic conversation that you offer to take a message for the concerned person, offering to take a message is the lowest form of help. In answering someone else's phone, some people simply say: "I am sorry he is out, can I take a message?" This is impolite way of offering help. It could be: "I am sorry, he is out. Can I help at all?" and very often one can, and the call is dealt with there and then.

- ❑ For taking special message, there must on the table be a special pad or form, otherwise special messages get lost in the pad of general messages. It is preferable to have them printed on colored paper, so that they could stand out.

- ❑ When we take down any information like telephone numbers, names, purpose, etc. We should repeat them to the caller to make sure that we have noted down correctly and in legible handwriting.

Then belonging to an organization, the receptionist/taker of the message must do something to reach the message to the right person and that something happens to it. This requires a high level of good business ethics and sound work culture ... unfortunately both are deficient in our country. For example, the Chief Executive should not feel offended, if the receptionist enquires about the message he/she passed on to him. The notion of infra dig does not exist in the modern/global business culture.

The American executive like their secretaries to answer the telephone on their behalf. In such cases the secretary announces the name of the office, e.g., "Mr Prescott's office. Good morning."

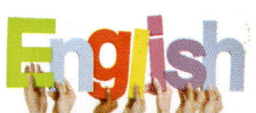

Telephone Etiquettes

The call centres and Multi-National Companies normally expect the following telephone etiquette skills:

❑ **Telephone Talking Tips**

- Speak slowly and clearly into the mouthpiece. Do not chew gum, eat, or drink while talking.
- Let your voice communicate that you are interested in the caller. Be friendly, but do not waste time.
- Get to the point of the cell. Be a good listener and pay attention to the person on the other end of the line.
- Turn off background noise, if any. Remain calm during the conversation, even if the person on the other end is not.
- End the conversation with a courteous comment such as "Thank you or Good-bye". Then replace the receiver softly.

❑ **When Placing a Call**

- Identify yourself. ("Hello, this is Amit Goyal from Transoft Office.")
- If you have several items to discuss, make a list beforehand, so that you do not forget anything. Have all necessary information near you.
- If the person you are calling sounds busy, ask if you can call back at a more convenient time.
- If you want your call returned, give your name, your telephone number and a time when you can be reached.

❑ **When Answering a Call**

- Try to answer the telephone by the second or third ring.
- Identify yourself and the organisation that you represent.
- If the call needs to be transferred, politely ask who is calling and do not leave the caller on hold for long.
- Keep note-taking material near your telephone. If you need to take a message, be complete and accurate.

❑ **Writing Telephone Messages:** Telephone messages in the workplace must be taken carefully and delivered promptly. Double-check the numbers and spellings with the caller and use the five words as a checklist:

- What is the message and when was it taken?
- Who is in the message from and for?
- When is the meeting or appointment mentioned in the message?
- Where is the receiver of the message to go or call back?
- Why is the message important—what is the purpose?

After you have taken the message, deliver it promptly. You may fill out a standard message from by hand or use e-mail, depending on the situation.

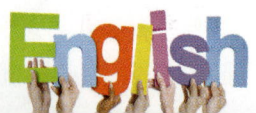

Chapter 33

Seminar

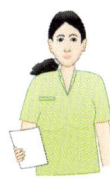

A seminar is a lecture or presentation delivered to an audience on a particular topic or set of topics that are educational in nature. A lecture is delivered by one person, usually a professor talking and the students making notes. There may be discussion sessions related to the class. A seminar involves equal participation of students, instead of the professor overseeing or guiding the class or leading it. To do well at seminar usually means that you not only have to read but also should be able to discuss it.

- ❏ The seminar uses problem-solving approach. It gives students an opportunity to participate in methods of scientific analysis and research procedures.
- ❏ Students are expected to do considerable library research, if feasible obtain primary source data. Data is analyzed critically, evaluated and conclusions are reached under the direction of the teacher guide.
- ❏ The teacher should help the student to select, formulate and organize the most significant student problems and to suggest available sources of information.
- ❏ As the seminar progresses, the students will assume increased responsibilities for preparing problems and for conducting the discussion.
- ❏ Group should be composed of 10–15 students and duration is 1–2 hours.

Meaning and Definition

- ❏ The word seminar is derived from the Latin word *seminarian*, meaning 'seed plot'
- ❏ Formal presentation by one or more experts in which the attendees are encouraged to discuss the subject matter.
- ❏ Seminar is generally a form of academic instruction either at an academic institution or offered by a commercial or professional organization.
- ❏ The seminar maybe defined as an assemblage' of teacher with a number of selected advanced students where methods of original research are expounded and where the creative faculty is trained where the spirit of scientific independence is inculcated.
- ❏ A small group of advanced students in a college or graduate school engaged in original research or intensive study under the guidance of a professor who meet regularly with them to discuss their reports and findings.

Requirements of Seminar

- ❏ A teacher is a leader (student can also function as a leader)
- ❏ Ten to fifteen members are participants
- ❏ The topic is presented by the students taking 15–20 minutes time each
- ❏ Duration is 1–2 hours
- ❏ Leader should keep the discussion within the limits of the problem discussed
- ❏ Students present their data in an informal way under the leadership of the teacher
- ❏ Care should be taken to avoid stereotype
- ❏ All members take part in discussion in an informal way in an orderly manner
- ❏ The chairman should be skilled in encouraging the timid participants
- ❏ A student secretary should record the problems which arise and the solution is given.

Approaches Used for Conducting Seminar

Class Discussion

Seminar can take a number of forms and are generally run on somewhat less restricted lines than class discussion, with the group members themselves having much more control over the course and content of the discussion. One common method of running a seminar is to base it on an essay, paper or prepared talk presented by one of the students in the group and then discussing the presentation in-depth.

Fishbowl Technique

Another variation of the seminar approach is the fishbowl technique. Hence half the members of the class who are involved in seminar, sit in an inner circle and conduct a discussion while the remainder sit in an outer circle and act as non participating observers. Both sections of the group then combine for a general discussion.

Brain Storming

Yet another approach of organistaion of a seminar is brainstorming. This involves group member spontaneously noting down or suggesting a range of possible solutions to a problem or question posed by the teacher.

Advantages

- ❏ **Learning experience:** A wealth of knowledge is usually presented by many speakers at one time in one place. A lot of 'learning' at one clip, with most material compressed into two or three days is real worth of time.
- ❏ **Sense of companionship:** Individuals meet together and create sense of companionship.
- ❏ **Morale booster:** Being with others that 'understand' individual's problems or concerns, is usually a great morale booster!
- ❏ **Alternative to other learning experiences:** A great way for those who don't like to read or attend classes to improve their knowledge of a specific subject.

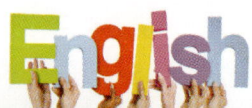

Disadvantages

- ❑ **Costly** in terms of time and money.
- ❑ **Rely on resource person's knowledge:** The chance that the speakers may be sharing incorrect knowledge or not at all knowledgeable themselves (it pays to make your own assessments of presented topics, not just blindly 'follow the pack'). Tips, tricks and strategies need to be weighed as to 'worth' and 'accuracy' therefore before using carefully weight these.

Essentials for Seminar

A situation seems to have to arise mainly from the presumptions that technique demands maturity in terms of language, social and emotional make up and the facility to deal with abstractions. The value of seminar should be seen in terms of the basic mechanism of the involvement of learners. Here the learners are expected to present others, their ideas or experiences who would react to them in the light of their own experiences.

Types of Seminar

The said mechanism is employed in conducting a seminar but seminars are organized at different levels. On the basis of levels or organization, the seminars are of four types:

1. Mini seminar
2. Main seminar
3. National seminar
4. International seminar

Mini Seminar

A seminar organized to discuss a topic in class is known as mini-seminar. The purpose of the mini seminar is to train the students for organizing the seminar and play different roles. It is simulated situation for the students. In institution, such seminars should be organized before the main seminar.

Main Seminar

Such seminars are organized at departmental level or institutional level on a major theme. All the students and staff members take part in such seminars. These seminars are organized weekly or monthly in departments. Generally specific themes are selected for main seminar.

National Seminar

A national seminar is organized by an association or organizations at national level. The experts are invited on the theme of the seminar.

International Seminar

Generally, such seminars are organized by UNESCO and other international organizations. The topic or the theme of seminar is very broad, e.g., students unrest or activisms, innovations in teacher-education and examination reforms. A nation can also organize such seminars on international theme.

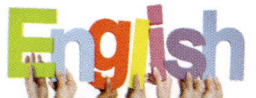

NOTES

Chapter 34

Panel Discussion

INTRODUCTION

The panel is another approach to discussion teaching. Different from general discussion, question and answer, and buzz groups, the panel is almost always used with a large group, and generally utilizes panel members who have either different points of view on the subject or special training and experience which equip them to speak authoritatively about the matter. The panel method became popular on such radio programs as The University of Chicago Round Table, and in the education field it became a regular classroom method Mc Burney wrote that while a lecture may be more orderly and compact, "the panel discussion insures breadth and variety spontaneity and freedom." This is also known as **Socratic method of teaching.**

THE PANEL

This method was originated by Prof. Hasy A Overstreet.

- ❏ Panel is a discussion in which a few persons carry on a conversation in front of an audience, when the group is too large to work effectively through the usual round-table procedure.
- ❏ Purpose to reproduce the features for the benefit of a larger group.
- ❏ It is a socialized group conversation in which different points of view are presented.
- ❏ When handled intelligently and creatively, the panel stimulates thought and discussion and clarifies thinking. Because several people engage in a free exchange of opinions, the panel influences the audience to an open-minded attitude and respect for the opinion of others. The quick exchange of facts, opinions and plans tends to develop more critical attitude and better judgment. It can be helpful to stimulate discussion, encouraging thinking and developing group opinion.

Techniques of Panel Method

- ❏ The members of the panel
- ❏ The chairman
- ❏ The audience

The panel consists of 4–8 members seated in a semicircle facing the audience.

The members of the panel should be quick thinkers and facile talkers, representing different points of view.

The members should prepare by knowing the limits of the topic to be discussed and the regulations which are to guide the discussion.

The chairman should be selected carefully, as much of the success of the panel will depend on her leadership. She should be a person with wide mental flexibility who has a sense and is able to determine the relevance of remarks as they are made.

Chairman must keep the discussion to the subject and see that all members of the panel have an equal opportunity to express their views. She should act as a neutral referee.

The chairman begins the panel discussion by exploring the whole proceeding. First, the members of the panel are introduced by name and background of the experience. The topic is announced, and the limits of the discussion are stated. The chairman may start the procedure rolling by making a comment or two or by directing a question to a particular person. After that she keeps the conversation to the topic encouraging expression of the difference of opinion and organizes the discussion with occasional summaries. A general summary before discussion is opened to the audience.

The panel discussion should provide a natural setting in which the audience will have an opportunity to ask questions, evaluate replies and make constructive contributions.

Questions from the audience may be directed to certain speakers.

Objectives of Panel Discussion

- ❑ To provide information and new facts.
- ❑ To analyze the current problems from different angles.
- ❑ To identify the values.
- ❑ To organize for mental recreation.

It is used to find out the solution of current problem of important nature and provide the full understanding of significant topic. It is an effective instructional technique which creates situation to facilitate higher cognitive learning.

TYPES OF PANEL DISCUSSION

The group discussion is organized in different forms; for different levels, for different purposes and on different themes. It may be of two types:
1. Public panel discussion
2. Educational panel discussion

Public Panel Discussion

This type of panel discussion is organized for common men problems. Three types of objectives are achieved by these kinds of discussions.
a. To provide factual information regarding current problems
b. To determine the social values
c. To recreate the common man

The public panel discussions are organized in television programs. The current problems like educated unemployment, annual budget, increase in prices of things, jobs delinking with degrees, emerging issues, etc.

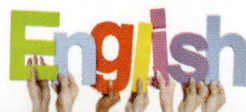

Educational Panel Discussion

It is used in educational institutions to provide factual and conceptual knowledge and clarification of certain theories and principles. Sometimes these are organized to find out the solution of certain problems. The following two objectives are achieved by the educational technique:

- ❏ To provide factual information and conceptual knowledge.
- ❏ To give awareness of theories and principles.

PROCEDURE OF PANEL DISCUSSION

A panel discussion consists of four types of participants. It means four roles are played in organizing panel discussion.

i.   Instructor
ii. Moderator
iii. Panelist
iv. Audience

Instructor: In the panel discussion, most important role is of an instructor. It is the responsibility of an instructor to decide how, where and when panel discussion will be organized. The schedule of panel discussion is prepared by him. Sometimes he has to plan the rehearsal of discussion.

Moderator: In the panel discussion, moderator has to do significant job. He has to keep discussion or theme and encourage the interaction among the members. He has to summarize and highlight the discussion more often. The moderator must have the mastery on theme or problem of the discussion.

Panelists: There are four to ten panelists in the panel discussion. The members of the panel sit in semicircle before the audience. The moderator sits in the middle of the panelists. The panelists must have the mastery of theme of the discussion.

Audience: After the panel discussion, audience are allowed to put question to seek clarification. They can present their point of view and their experiences regarding the theme or problem. The panelists attempt to answer the question of the audience.

In some questions, moderator also tries to answer the questions.

At the end of the discussion, moderator summarizes the discussion and presents his point of view. He expresses thanks to the panelists and audience.

USE OF PANEL DISCUSSION TECHNIQUE

- ❏ This instructional technique encourages social learning.
- ❏ The higher cognitive and effective objectives are achieved.
- ❏ It is used to develop the ability of problem solving and logical thinking.
- ❏ It develops the interests and light type of attitude towards the problem.
- ❏ It develops the capacity to respect other's ideas and feelings and ability of tolerance.
- ❏ It provides the opportunity of the theme and content.

The following topics may be used for this purpose:

- ❏ Education as an instrument of social change
- ❏ 'Student teaching' in teaching education program

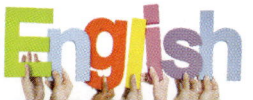

- Population education
- Scope of educational technology in our country
- Adult education
- Delinking jobs to degrees
- Examination reform
- National health policy
- National population policy

LIMITATIONS OF PANEL DISCUSSION TECHNIQUE

The following are the limitations of this technique:
- There are chances to deviate from theme at time of discussion, hence the purpose of the panel discussion is not achieved.
- Some members dominate the discussion and do not provide the opportunities to others to participate in discussion.
- There is possibility to split the group into two sub groups, i.e., for and against the theme. It does not maintain the conductivity situation of learning.

SUGGESTIONS FOR ORGANISING PANEL DISCUSSION

The following suggestions should be taken into consideration to organize effective panel discussion:
- There should be rehearsal before the actual discussion.
- The moderator should be matured person with full understanding of theme or problems. He should have control over the situation.
- The seating arrangement for panelists and audience should be such that everyone should be at equal distance so that they can observe each other.
- The moderator should encourage the discussion on the points which may lead to contractive aspect of the problem. He should encourage the constructive discussion among panelists and audience.

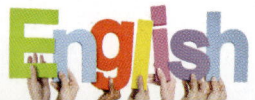

Chapter 35

Symposium

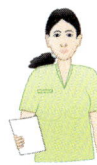

Symposium originally referred to a drinking party (the Greek verb sympotein means 'to drink together') but has since come to refer to any academic conference, whether or not drinking takes place.

Symposiums are conferences or meetings that feature various experts who speak on a particular topic for a specified period of time. Afterwards, the speaker answers questions from the audience. A moderator or session chair oversees the symposium and ensures that the speakers and audience stay on track. It is:

❑ A formal meeting at which several specialists deliver short addresses on a topic or on related topics.

❑ A meeting or conference for the discussion of some subject, especially a meeting at which several speakers talk on or discuss a topic before an audience.

❑ A collection of opinion expressed or articles contributed by several persons on a given subject or topic.

Purpose

The main purpose of the symposium is to provide the understanding to the students or listeners on theme or problem specifically to develop certain values and feelings.

Uses of Symposium

❑ **Information:** Symposiums are the ideal environment for information gathering and sharing.

❑ **Presentation:** Panel discussions allow attendees to hear various experts defend their position or offer their opinions.

❑ **Exposition:** The expositions provide an opportunity for attendees to view product demonstrations and the vendors detailed questions.

❑ **Networking:** Symposiums offer an opportunity for attendees to network and socialize with their peers and these relationships can form the basis for collaboration on future projects.

Objectives of Symposium

The following are main objectives of the symposium technique:
- ❑ To identify and understand two various aspects of theme and problems
- ❑ To develop the ability of decision and judgment regarding a problem
- ❑ To develop the values and feelings regarding a problem
- ❑ To enable the listeners to form policies regarding a theme or problem

Technique

Characteristics of Symposium Technique

The symposium technique has the following main characteristics:
- ❑ It provides the broad understanding of a topic or a problem.
- ❑ The opportunity is provided to the listeners to take decision about the problem.
- ❑ It is used for higher classes to specify themes and problems.
- ❑ It develops the feeling of cooperation and adjustment.
- ❑ The objectives as synthesis and evaluation (creativity) are achieved by employing the symposium technique.
- ❑ It provides the different views on the topic of the symposium.

Mechanism of Symposium Technique

The symposium is a type of discussion, in which two or more speakers, talk for 10–20 minutes, develop individual approaches or solutions to a problem or present aspects of a policy, process or program. The speeches are followed by questions or comments from the audience, as in the panel forum. The speeches may be persuasive, argumentative, informative or evocative.

Technique of Symposium

- ❑ Teacher should plan the program ahead of time.
- ❑ Each member of the class, as well as the student speakers should know the objectives of the symposium and breadth of the topic.
- ❑ Each student should prepare on the given accepted topic.
- ❑ The teacher should have a conference with each of the student speakers.
- ❑ The teacher or a student may function as a chairman.
- ❑ The symposium starts with the chairman introducing the topic.
- ❑ Next, chairman introduces the speakers.
- ❑ Then the topic is presented by the students taking 15–20 minutes time each.
- ❑ As a conclusion (at the end), the chairman gives brief summary of all the speeches and opens the discussion to the students.
- ❑ A question or contribution may be addressed by the chairman.

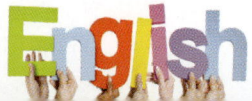

Precautions for Symposium

We suggest three conditions in the use of the symposium technique:

Firstly, the moderator should be sure to prepare the speakers or see that they are prepared. They should know the rules of procedure, sequence of speaking and way in which the forum will be conducted and they should be aware of the ideas, and background of the other performers.

Secondly, the chairman or both (moderator and chairman) are responsible for preparing the agendas. He should not attempt to stack the cards by omitting or ignoring vital phases of the problem as he selects or delegates his speakers.

Thirdly, the chairman in all the forum situations must plan very carefully for the questioning period that follows the prepared speeches, unless he wishes to risk boredom/bedlam.

Scope for the Use of Symposium

The symposium technique is used to realize the higher cognitive and affective objectives. The nature of the topic should be such that the audience should be interested in the theme.

Advantages

- It is suited to a large group or classes.
- This method can be frequently used to present broad topics for discussions at conventions and organization meetings.
- Organization of symposium is good if the set speeches are prepared beforehand.
- Gives deeper insight into the topic.
- Directs the students to continuous independent study.
- Lends itself to the teaching of clinical subjects.
- This method can be used in political meetings.

Disadvantages

- Inadequate opportunity for all the students to participate actively.
- The speech is limited to 15 or 20 minutes.
- Limited audience participation
- Question and answer are limited to 3 or 4 minutes.
- Possibility of overlapping of subjects.

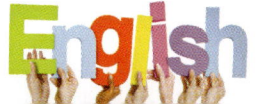

NOTES

Chapter 36

Workshop

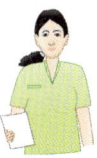

A group of individuals who work together towards the solution of problems in a given field during a specific period of time. Workshop is defined as assembled group of 10–25 persons who share a common interest or problem. They meet together to improve their individual skill on a subject through intensive study, research, practice and discussion.

Workshop Technique

Educational process has two aspects: theoretical and practical. The instructional techniques are used to develop the theoretical aspects of the students. The conference and seminars are organized for achieving higher cognitive and affective objectives. The psychomotor aspect is developed through training. Teaching is a continuum from conditioning to indoctrination and training is also inclusive in it. The new innovations and practices of education are introduced by organizing workshop in which persons are trained to use new practices in their teaching-learning process. The workshops are organized to develop the psychomotor aspects of the learner regarding practices of new innovations in area of education. Under this technique participants have to do some practical work to produce instructional teaching and testing material.

Source of Workshop Technique

The word, 'Workshop' has been borrowed from engineering. There are usually workshops in the engineering. In these workshops persons have to do some task with their hands to produce something, e.g., railway workshop. Under railway workshop, these workshops railway engines are *repaired* and *manufactured*. Similarly workshops are organized in education to prepare questions on the subjects in Question Bank Workshops. The participants of the Workshop prepare questions on their subjects. The participants are given knowledge and training for preparing questions in the workshop.

VALUES OF GROUP DISCUSSION

- ❏ It creates analytical and critical abilities, creativity and encourages the students to think for themselves.
- ❏ It develops critical habits of study.
- ❏ It interprets problems of the past, throws light on the problems of the present to gain insight into ways for shaping the future.
- ❏ It keeps students advanced in creative thoughts by their own efforts and helps in making progress as a result of the responses.
- ❏ It enables the students to enrich their own participation.
- ❏ It gives the students an opportunity to learn how to adjust to social situations.
- ❏ The students acquire new knowledge from discussion and develop the ability to reexamine and analyze their own reasons and contributions in the light of ideas presented by others.
- ❏ It helps in increasing self-activity as students are participating.
- ❏ Group benefits as there is a pooling of ideas and harmonizing of attitudes in the solution of a common problem.
- ❏ Cooperation in highest sense is developed, since open-mindedness, respect for the other person's opinions and concern for the effective group discussion is there.

Essentials of Good Group Discussion

- ❏ A clear formulation of realistic goals.
- ❏ A permissive atmosphere conductive to full participation. Planning in terms of time and resources is available.
- ❏ Work on specific problems rather than broad general problem area.
- ❏ Participation by each group member.
- ❏ Physical conditions facilities, so that each member is seen and heard.
- ❏ Opportunity for members to get acquainted.

Scoring Maximum Results from Group Discussion

- ❏ Prepare for discussion
- ❏ Come to the discussion with questions in mind
- ❏ Speak your mind freely
- ❏ Listen thoughtfully to others
- ❏ Be brief, do not monopolize the discussion
- ❏ Strike while the idea is hot, don't wait for the leader to reorganize before speaking
- ❏ Don't let the discussion get away from you
- ❏ Indulge in friendly disagreement
- ❏ Give credit to others by acknowledging their contributions
- ❏ Interaction is important
- ❏ Group discussion depends upon sharing ideas and experiences

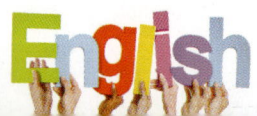

Good Group Discussion Depends Upon

- Good leadership
- Clear identification of the problem to be discussed or the goal to be reached
- Preparation by the leaders and the participants
- Active participation by all members of the group
- Accurate information

Values: Increased knowledge, intellectual abilities, skills, interests, changes in attitudes and values, better personal and social adjustment, increased cooperation.

Characteristics of Workshop

- Activity based
- Active engagement of participants during the workshop
- High production values
- Information-sharing meeting
- Limited number of participants
- Less formal, include more discussion
- Emphasizing practical applications
- Requiring some preparation in advance of the workshop
- Thorough minute-by-minute planning of workshop sessions

Advantages

- Focuses on the real-world needs of the participants
- Involves collaborative problem-solving
- Makes the participants feel they are part of a learning community
- Helps in group building
- Useful for small groups where there is a common interest or concern
- Makes the participants understand that they are valued for their learning efforts
- Involves shared learning where the participants can talk directly and meaningfully to one another
- Encourages communication and acceptance of other viewpoints
- It is useful when the solutions to problems are not clear.

Disadvantages

- Dominance by members
- It can be difficult to remain focused and clear about the purpose and desired outcome.

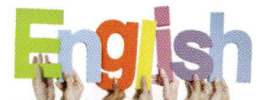

NOTES

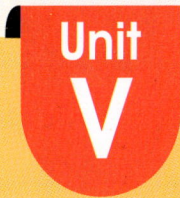

Unit V

Listening Comprehension Skills

Unit Outline

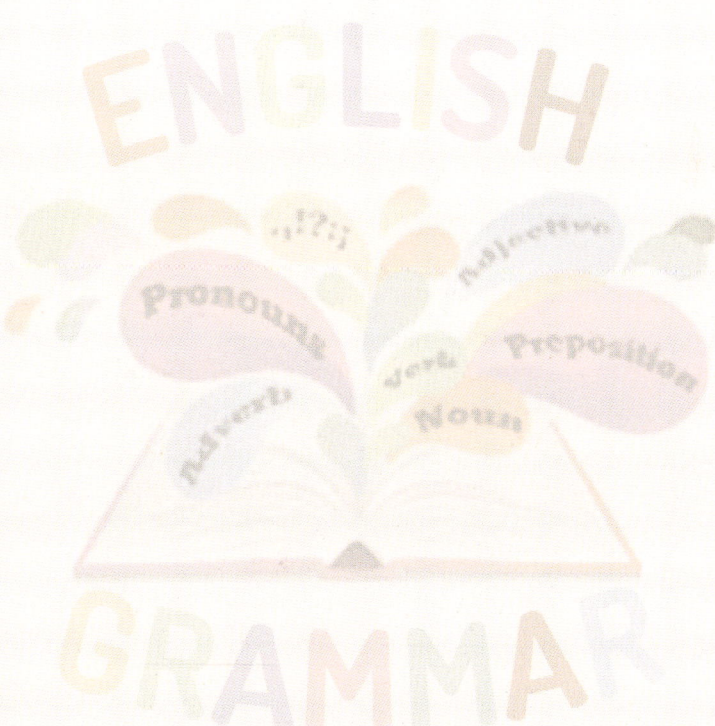

Chapter 37

Listening Comprehension Skills

Listening is a significant part of the communication process. Communication cannot take place until and unless a message is heard and retained thoroughly and positively by the receivers/ listeners. Listening is a dynamic process. Listening means attentiveness and interest perceptible in the posture as well as expressions. Listening implies decoding (i.e., translating the symbols into meaning) and interpreting the message correctly in the communication process.

Listening differs from hearing in sense that:

- Hearing implies just perceiving the sounds while listening means listening with understanding whatever you are listening. Both the body as well as mind is involved in the listening process.
- Listening is an active process while hearing is a passive activity.
- Hearing is an effortless activity while listening is an act requiring conscious efforts, concentration and interest. Listening involves both physical and psychological efforts.

Effective listening requires both deliberate efforts and a keen mind. Effective listeners appreciate flow of new ideas and information. Organizations that follow the principles of effective listening are always informed timely, updated with the changes and implementations and are always out of crisis situation. Effective listening promotes organizational relationships, encourages product delivery and innovation, as well as helps organization to deal with the diversity in employees and customers it serves.

To improve your communication skills, you must learn to listen effectively. Effective listening gives you an advantage and makes you more impressive when you speak. It also boosts your performance.

Type of Listening

There are three main types of listening.

1. **Active listening:** The listener gives verbal or non-verbal feedback by asking questions and by paraphrasing what the speaker said. In this situation, the listener uses his other senses to go beyond the words spoken. Hearing alone does not provide enough information. It is about understanding the speaker's point of view without necessarily agreeing with it. Active listening is the most civil type of listening because you must acknowledge emotions and feelings.

Active listening is used to ensure a mutual understanding. In fact, in a conversation, the interlocutor is rarely fully committed. It is very common for the listener to be distracted by preoccupations, noise and other distractions. Overall, the interlocutor is only providing his full attention 50% of the time.

This type of listening is the most valuable during a conflict. When a conflict occurs, we concentrate on our arguments and how we will respond instead of listening to the speaker. This means that we are unable to effectively comprehend the speaker's message. Active listening doesn't mean we have to agree with the speaker, simply understand what they are trying to convey.

A good way to see if you have understood the speaker's words is to paraphrase. This way, misunderstanding can be detected and solved quickly.

2. **Critical listening:** Critical listening is also known as evaluative, judgmental or interpretive listening.

The main goal of this type of listening is to evaluate the message with logic while analyzing the different arguments provided by the speaker. It requires some analysis, judgment and critical thinking. It is necessary in order to be able to criticize the strength of the evidence and to determine that motive of the speaker. However, critical listening is not an easy task to accomplish because it is needed to absorb and evaluate the information together.

When applying critical listening, the key point is to first of all understand the speaker before evaluating. Questioning oneself about the credibility, the validity and the strength of the evidence is vital. Some other questions such as: "Is this speaker biased? Is he a trusted expert in his domain of expertise?" can help separate the facts from the personal opinions of the speaker.

In this situation, it is important to be open-minded because it is important to stay objective.

3. **Content listening:** This type of listening involves understanding and retaining the information provided by the speaker. It also requires to identify the key points of the message and to find cues by doing a summary of it. Moreover, it is important to understand different sounds and tones provided by the speaker. However, some other factors need to be taken under consideration such as phonology, vocabulary, grammar, general discourse, and informational discourse.

To effectively apply content, it is needed once again to identify the main idea or the key points of the message. Then, the next thing to do is to ask questions for clarifications if the message was misunderstood. This will increase the level of understanding of the message transmitted.

Characteristics of Good and Effective Listener

A good and effective listener tries to give maximum amount of thought to the speaker's ideas being communicated, leaving a minimum amount of time for mental exercise to go off track.

❑ **Be attentive:** A good listener must pay attention to the key points. He should be alert. He should avoid any kind of distraction.

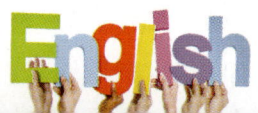

- **Do not assume:** A good listener does not ignore the information he considers is unnecessary. He should always summarize the speaker's ideas so that there is no misunderstanding of the thoughts of the speaker. He avoids premature judgements about the speaker's message.
- **Listen for feelings and facts:** A good listener deliberately listens for the feelings of the speaker. He concentrates totally on the facts. He evaluates the facts objectively. His listening is sympathetic, active and alert. He keenly observes the gestures, facial expressions and body language of the speaker. In short, a good listener should be projective (i.e., one who tries to understand the views of the speaker) and empathic (i.e., one who concentrates not only on the surface meaning of the message but tries to probe the feelings and emotions of the speaker).
- **Be kind and generous:** A good listener makes deliberate efforts to give a chance to other speakers also to express their thoughts and views. He tries to learn from every speaker. He evaluates the speaker's ideas in spare time. He focuses on the content of the speaker's message and not on the speaker's personality and looks.
- **Grab the opportunities:** A good listener tries to take benefit from the opportunities arising. He asks, "what is it for me?"

    To conclude, effective listening enhances the communication quality. It makes all attentive.

    It encourages optimistic attitude, healthy relations and more participation. It leads to better decision making in an organization. Effective listening is directly related to our ability to do team work. It must be noted that we listen at about an efficiency rate of 25 percent maximum, and we remember only about 50 percent of what is delivered during a ten minutes speech/lecture communication.

Effective Listening Skills

- Discover your field of interest.
- Grasp and understand the matter/content.
- Remain calm. Do not lose your temper. Anger hampers and inhibits communication. Angry people jam their minds to the words of others.
- Be open to accept new ideas and information.
- Jot down and take a note of important points.
- Work upon listening. Analyze and evaluate the speech of others in spare time.
- Rephrase and summarize the speaker's ideas.
- Keep on asking questions. This demonstrates how well you understand the speaker's ideas and also that you are listening.
- Avoid distractions.
- "Step into the shoes of others", i.e., put yourself in the position of the speaker and observe things from his view point. This will help creating an atmosphere of mutual understanding and improve the exchange of ideas in communication process.

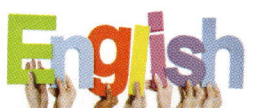

Barriers to Effective Listening

While there are many subtitles to communication between people, some basic skills can help us to be a more effective communicator. Let us explore the barriers to listening.

◻ **Focus on a personal agenda:** When we spend our listening time formulating our next response, we cannot be fully attentive to what the speaker is saying.

◻ **Experiencing information overload:** Too much stimulation or information can make it very difficult to listen with full attention. Try to focus on the relevant information, and the central points that are being conveyed.

◻ **Criticizing the speaker:** Do not be distracted by critical evaluations of the speaker. Focus on what they are saying—the message—rather than the messenger.

◻ **Getting distracted by emotional noise:** We react emotionally to certain words, concepts and ideas, and to a myriad of other cues from speakers (appearance, non-verbal cues).

◻ **Getting distracted by external "noise":** Audible noise may be extremely distracting. Some things can be minimized—e.g., turn down the ringer on your phone, and the e-mail beep on the computer while meeting someone. Other noises maybe unavoidable—e.g., construction, other people. Also, there may be figurative "noise" from the external environment, such as distracting or inappropriate decor in a room, or environmental conditions such as the room being too hot or cold.

◻ **Experiencing physical difficulty:** Feeling physically unwell or experiencing pain can make it very difficult to listen effectively. You can wish to communicate that this is not a good time and reschedule the discussion. Otherwise, you may just need to concentrate even more on the task of listening.

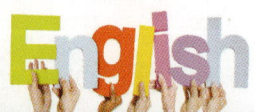